Register Now for Online Access to Your Book!

SPRINGER PUBLISHING
CONNECT™

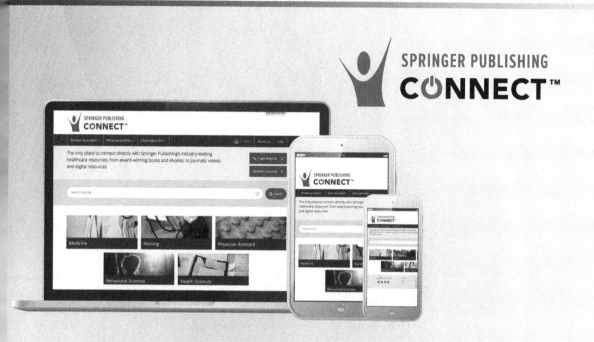

Your print purchase of *Evaluation of Quality in Health Care for DNPs, Third Edition,* **includes online access to the contents of your book**—increasing accessibility, portability, and searchability!

Access today at:
http://connect.springerpub.com/content/book/978-0-8261-7523-6
or scan the QR code at the right with your smartphone. Log in or register, then click "Redeem a voucher" and use the code below.

6ETDJ8LA

Scan here for quick access.

Having trouble redeeming a voucher code?
Go to https://connect.springerpub.com/redeeming-voucher-code

If you are experiencing problems accessing the digital component of this product, please contact our customer service department at cs@springerpub.com

The online access with your print purchase is available at the publisher's discretion and may be removed at any time without notice.

Publisher's Note: New and used products purchased from third-party sellers are not guaranteed for quality, authenticity, or access to any included digital components.

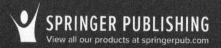

SPRINGER PUBLISHING
View all our products at springerpub.com

Evaluation of Quality in Health Care for DNPs

Joanne V. Hickey, PhD, RN, FAAN, FCCM, is professor emerita, after recently retiring from the University of Texas Health Science Center at Houston, Cizik School of Nursing. In addition to teaching at the master, clinical practice and clinical research at the master, Doctor of Nursing Practice (DNP), and PhD levels, she has held a number of administrative positions including track director for the Acute Care Nurse Practitioner and Critical Clinical Nurse Specialist programs, department chairperson and assistant dean for Acute and Continuing Care, and program director for the DNP Program, the first DNP program in Texas. She held the Patricia L. Starck/PARTNERS Professorship in Nursing. Dr. Hickey received a diploma in nursing from Roger Williams General Hospital School of Nursing, a baccalaureate degree in nursing from Boston College, in MSN from the University of Rhode Island, an MA in counseling from Rhode Island College, a PhD from the University of Texas at Austin, and a post-master's certificate, acute care nurse practitioner from Duke University. She is a Fellow of the American Academy of Nursing and a Fellow of the American College of Critical Care Medicine. She is a member of numerous professional organizations including the American Nurses Association, Sigma Theta Tau International, Society of Critical Care Medicine, and American Association of Neuroscience Nursing.

Eileen R. Giardino, PhD, MSN, APRN, RN, ANP-C, FNP, is associate professor at Rush University and retired from the University of Texas Health Science Center at Houston, Cizik School of Nursing. In addition to teaching at the bachelor, master, and Doctor of Nursing Practice (DNP) levels, she has held a number of administrative positions including director of Undergraduate Programs and track director for the Clinical Nurse Specialist and Family Nurse Practitioner programs. Dr. Giardino received a baccalaureate degree in nursing from the University of Pennsylvania, an MSN from Widener University, a PhD from the University of Pennsylvania, and post-master's certificates as an adult nurse practitioner and family nurse practitioner from LaSalle University. She is a member of numerous professional organizations including the American Nurses Association and Sigma Theta Tau International.

Evaluation of Quality in Health Care for DNPs

Third Edition

Joanne V. Hickey, PhD, RN, FAAN, FCCM
Eileen R. Giardino, PhD, MSN, APRN, RN, ANP-C, FNP

EDITORS

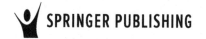 SPRINGER PUBLISHING

First Springer Publishing edition 2012; subsequent edition 2016.

No part of this publication may be reproduced, stored in a retrieval system, or transmitted in any form or by any means, electronic, mechanical, photocopying, recording, or otherwise, without the prior permission of Springer Publishing Company, LLC, or authorization through payment of the appropriate fees to the Copyright Clearance Center, Inc., 222 Rosewood Drive, Danvers, MA 01923, 978-750-8400, fax 978-646-8600, info@copyright.com or on the Web at www.copyright.com.

Springer Publishing Company, LLC
11 West 42nd Street, New York, NY 10036
www.springerpub.com
connect.springerpub.com/

Acquisitions Editor: Joseph Morita
Compositor: S4Carlisle Publishing Services

ISBN: 978-0-8261-7522-9
ebook ISBN: 978-0-8261-7523-6

DOI: 10.1891/9780826175236

SUPPLEMENTS:
Instructor Materials:

Qualified instructors may request supplements by emailing textbook@springerpub.com

Instructor's PowerPoints ISBN: 978-0-8261-7525-0

21 22 23 24 25 / 5 4 3 2 1

The author and the publisher of this Work have made every effort to use sources believed to be reliable to provide information that is accurate and compatible with the standards generally accepted at the time of publication. Because medical science is continually advancing, our knowledge base continues to expand. Therefore, as new information becomes available, changes in procedures become necessary. We recommend that the reader always consult current research and specific institutional policies before performing any clinical procedure or delivering any medication. The author and publisher shall not be liable for any special, consequential, or exemplary damages resulting, in whole or in part, from the readers' use of, or reliance on, the information contained in this book. The publisher has no responsibility for the persistence or accuracy of URLs for external or third-party Internet websites referred to in this publication and does not guarantee that any content on such websites is, or will remain, accurate or appropriate.

Library of Congress Cataloging-in-Publication Data

Names: Hickey, Joanne V., editor | Giardino, Eileen R., editor.
Title: Evaluation of quality in health care for DNPs / [edited by] Joanne
    V. Hickey, Eileen R. Giardino.
Other titles: Evaluation of health care quality in advanced practice nursing.
Identifiers: LCCN 2021016458 (print) | LCCN 2021016459 (ebook) | ISBN
    9780826175229 (cloth) | ISBN 9780826175236 (ebook)
Subjects: MESH: Nursing Audit | Advanced Practice Nursing | Evaluation
    Studies as Topic | Program Evaluation | Quality of Health Care
Classification: LCC RT85.5 (print) | LCC RT85.5 (ebook) | NLM WY 100.5 |
    DDC 610.73068–dc23
LC record available at https://lccn.loc.gov/2021016458
LC ebook record available at https://lccn.loc.gov/2021016459

Publisher's Note: New and used products purchased from third-party sellers are not guaranteed for quality, authenticity, or access to any included digital components.

Printed in the United States of America.

We dedicate this book to:

- *Students and colleagues (current and future) . . . and particularly advanced practice nurses, who have an unprecedented opportunity to impact new models of health care that will influence health care organizations, clinical practice, and health policy for an ultimate transformation of the health care system.*

- *Our contributing authors . . . recognized experts in their disciplines; these leaders are much sought after for their expertise in practice, education, research, and consultation. Our request to share their knowledge through writing was met with gracious acceptance and production of excellent manuscripts. Their passion for the quality of health care and especially the role of evaluation in achieving health care quality is the heart and soul of this book.*

- *Our husbands supported our passion and commitment for working on this book. Jim Hickey and Angelo Giardino served as wise listeners and counsels as we grappled with the best ways to organize ideas and find the right words to illuminate the work of evaluation.*

CONTENTS

CONTRIBUTORS

Joyce L. Batcheller, DNP, RN, NEA-BC, FANOL, FAAN Adjunct Professor, School of Nursing, Texas Tech University Health Sciences Center, Lubbock, Texas; Executive Nurse Advisor, AMN Healthcare; President, CNO Space
Dr. Batcheller has years of high-level experience in nursing administration as a chief nursing officer and leader in health policy.

Juliana J. Brixey, PhD, MPH, RN Associate Professor of Biomedical Informatics and Nursing, Department of Graduate Studies, Cizik School of Nursing and School of Biomedical Informatics, University of Texas Health Science Center at Houston, Houston, Texas
Dr. Brixey is director of the informatics track in the Doctor of Nursing Practice program at the School of Nursing and also teaches in the School of Informatics.

Nancy Manning Crider, DrPH, MS, RN, NEA-BC Assistant Professor, Department of Graduate Studies, Cizik School of Nursing, University of Texas Health Science Center at Houston, Houston, Texas
Dr. Crider has a long career in nursing administration, nursing education, and research. She teaches in the nurse executive track in the Doctor of Nursing Practice program.

M. Roseann Diehl, PhD, DNP, CRNA Professor of Professional Practice, Harris College of Nursing & Health Sciences, Texas Christian University, Nurse Anesthesia Program, Fort Worth, Texas
Dr. Diehl teaches in the nurse anesthesia program, practices as a CRNA, and is an expert in simulation education.

Angelo P. Giardino, MD, PhD, MPH Wilma T. Gibson Presidential Professor and Chair of the Department of Pediatrics at the University of Utah School of Medicine, Salt Lake City, Utah
Dr. Giardino is chief medical officer at Intermountain Primary Children's Hospital in Salt Lake City, Utah.

Eileen R. Giardino, PhD, RN, APRN, NP-C, ANP-BC   Associate Professor, Adult Health & Gerontological Nursing, Rush University College of Nursing, Chicago, Illinois; Retired Associate Professor, Department of Family Health, Cizik School of Nursing, University of Texas Health Science Center at Houston, Houston, Texas
Dr. Giardino has years of experience in the development of advanced practice, master, and DNP programs. She is the editor in chief of the Journal of Nursing and Interprofessional Leadership in Quality and Safety.

Joanne V. Hickey, PhD, RN, FAAN, FCCM   Professor Emerita, recently retired from the Cizik School of Nursing, University of Texas Health Science Center at Houston, Houston, Texas. Dr. Hickey was professor of nursing in the Department of Research.
Dr. Hickey has many years of experience in the development of advanced practice, master, and DNP programs and has taught at both levels as well as the PhD program. She is also recognized as an expert in neuroscience nursing and is the author of The Clinical Practice of Neurological and Neurosurgical Nursing *now in its eighth edition.*

Ronda G. Hughes, PhD, MHS, RN, FAAN   Associate Professor, Director Center for Nursing Leadership and Director for the Executive Doctorate of Nursing Practice Program, College of Nursing, University of South Carolina, Columbia, South Carolina
Dr. Hughes's career has included a blend of roles in academia, administration, and research. She served in the U.S. Department of Health and Human Services for almost two decades, primarily at the Agency for Healthcare Research and Quality and the Health Resources and Services Administration.

Peggy L. Landrum, PhD, RN, CS   Clinical Professor, College of Nursing, Texas Woman's University, Denton, Texas
Dr. Landrum's clinical focus areas are mental health, behavioral change, and the impact of policy engagement by nurses on practice. Research interests include motivation and behavior change in primary care settings. She maintains a clinical private practice and conducts workshops and trainings in the use of motivational interviewing throughout the United States and Europe. She also practices in Landrum and Associates, Clinical Psychotherapy Practice.

Kristen Starnes-Ott, PhD, CRNA, FNAP   Vice Dean for Academic Affairs and Professor, Betty P. Akins Endowed Chair in Nursing, University of Texas Medical Branch (UTMB) School of Nursing, Galveston, Texas
Dr. Starnes-Ott has received numerous grants to support her scholarly focus on patient safety using simulation methodology, telehealth applications in nursing education, communication and situational awareness among health care providers, patient-centered communication and team leadership. She has taught a variety of graduate level courses including nurse anesthesia, quality and patient safety, translational science, and evidence-based practice.

V. Gail Roberson Turner, DNP, MBA, RN-BC   Lead Project Manager, Memorial Hermann Health System, Houston, Texas
Dr. Turner has years of experience in informatics within health care organizations and is an expert in informatics and health care technology.

Beth Ulrich, EdD, RN, FACHE, FAONL, FAAN Professor, Department of Graduate Studies, Cizik School of Nursing, University of Texas Health Science Center at Houston, Houston, Texas
Dr. Ulrich has a long career in nursing administration, leadership, nursing education, and research. She teaches in the nurse executive track in the Doctor of Nursing Practice program and is editor in chief, Nephrology Nursing Journal.

Patricia S. Yoder-Wise, EdD, RN, NEA-BC, ANEF, FANOL, FAAN Professor and Dean Emerita, School of Nursing, Texas Tech University Health Sciences Center, Lubbock, Texas
Dr. Yoder-Wise has taught health policy at the doctoral level at two schools of nursing to both PhD and DNP learners. She is a past president of the Texas Nurses Association and convenor of a coalition of nursing organizations interested in public policy. She has influenced policy at the organizational, state, national, and international level. Dr. Yoder-Wise is also president of The Wise Group, editor in chief of The Journal of Continuing Education in Nursing *and* Nursing Forum, *and president of the National League for Nursing.*

PREFACE

The preface for the third edition builds on the intent described in the preface for the second edition, which is to provide a high-quality resource on evaluation for nurses. The intent of this book is to address the special needs of DNP nurses to understand the principles of conducting large-scale evaluations and translating those principles into developing smaller projects, such as unit-based projects or projects required in DNP degree programs. Five years after the preparation of the second edition of this book, some things (principles/concepts/content) have stayed the same, while significant changes in other areas of content and knowledge are noteworthy. First, what has stayed the same is the expectation of competency in evaluation of patient outcomes of all professional nurses. However, the competency bar is raised for Doctor of Nursing Practice (DNP) nurses for evaluating health care and health care systems from a systematic and comprehensive science-based, data-driven perspective. Evaluation occurs in all areas of health care including populations, organizations, systems, programs/projects, health informatics, practice guidelines/protocols, health policy, and other health-related entities. Along with the higher expectations for DNP nurses come greater opportunities to lead evaluation teams and influence high-level decision-making in all areas of health care.

We recognize that the reader does not necessarily read a book from the first chapter through the last. Therefore, the chapters in this book are self-contained in that all the information needed to address the topic are included in the chapter. Some content in one chapter may be included in another chapter and presented as it applied to the particular chapter content. We trust that there is a balance between content that clarifies the focus of the chapter and what some may call redundancy. Our experience with students and graduates suggests that the more inclusive approach to chapter content is helpful for the reader.

The intended audiences for this book are students enrolled in master and doctoral level programs, including APRN and DNP programs; DNP graduates and practicing APRNs; nurse administrators; directors of quality improvement; faculty teaching evaluation; and others interested in evaluation of health care from a practice and clinical perspective. In selecting content for the topics of each chapter, our intent is to provide an overview of the state of the science and knowledge of evaluation and its application to common practice issues in which DNP, APRN, and master's-prepared nurses lead and participate. Students, graduates, and colleagues provided information about their particular needs, which was greatly appreciated.

The intent of this book is to lay a foundation in evaluation for DNPs/APRNs to assume their important role in the process. Evaluation principles (concepts) as applied to health care continue to be underdeveloped and evolving. Evaluation is a nonlinear and messy process. While there is no one right way to conduct an evaluation, it is driven by the intended purpose and use of the evaluation findings. In this current and complex health care environment, there is now more than ever the urgent need to systematically evaluate all aspects of health care entities. The purpose of the evaluation is to determine effectiveness and value based on established criteria, in order to guide and inform decision-making. DNPs/APRNs can make significant contributions to developing the science, methods, and uses of evaluation in health care.

Before submitting what is new in the third edition, a few comments on a major update from the American Association of Colleges of Nursing (AACN). On April 7, 2021, AACN approved *The Essentials: Core Competencies for Professional Nursing Education*. The press release noted that bold action was taken to transform nursing education and strengthen the nation's health care workforce. This eagerly anticipated updated *Essentials* reflects bold new thinking and direction for professional nursing education. *The Essentials of Doctoral Education for Advanced Nursing Practice* was published in 2006 by the AACN and has served the nursing profession well in establishing and developing DNP programs nationally. However, the concurrent changes in health care delivery, practice, and nursing education have driven the need to update the *Essentials*. The structure of these new *Essentials* includes both prelicensure and advanced practice into one document. The new 2021 *Essentials*, as they apply to advanced practice, will briefly be discussed in Chapter 1.

Another much anticipated publication is *The Future of Nursing 2020–2030* from the National Academy of Medicine. Previously expected for release in 2020, it has been postponed until 2021 to allow for incorporation of emerging information of the nursing role in pandemics such as COVID-19. The report is designed to make recommendations to extend the vision for the nursing professions into 2030. According to the website, the report will chart a path for the nursing profession "to help our nation create a culture of health, reduce health disparities, and improve the health and well-being of the U.S. population in the 21st century." The previous *Future of Nursing* report in 2010 has had a profound influence on the nursing profession and health care. The new report is anticipated to guide the development of nursing for the decade.

Now to what is new in the third edition. In general, every existing chapter has been extensively revised to reflect the development of evaluation science as evidenced by the updated and new content and references to the need of nurses to evaluate smaller projects such as unit-based projects, or for DNP students to evaluate their DNP projects.

Section I addresses the foundations of evaluation. Chapter 1 elaborates on the role of the DNP mandate in evaluation. Through a brief history, overview of evaluation, mandate, and competencies for high-level, science-based evaluation, the DNP is brought to the table of evaluation. Chapter 2 addresses the nature of evidence, the basic building block of data for evaluation, and provides a critical review of characteristics, sources, and quality of evidence as they apply to rigorous evaluation. The conceptual foundations and models for evaluation are discussed in Chapter 3. A number of frameworks are described to provide the reader with new models for addressing evaluation including those for evaluation of smaller projects. Chapter 4 addresses evaluation and outcomes and the current challenges to identifying meaningful outcomes. The national imperative for cost-effectiveness and value is addressed in Chapter 5 through a comprehensive and practical discussion of financial evaluation specific to evaluating quality in health care.

The focus of Section II is on evaluation of organizational imperatives in health care. Chapter 6 examines the evaluation of organizations and systems, while Chapter 7 addresses health care informatics and patient care technology. With the redesign of health care delivery, organizations and systems are being restructured and redesigned to be more responsive to patient–family-centered care models. An integral part of health care is health informatics, as well as patient care technology integration and evaluation. The current national trends for electronic medical records and telehealth are having a huge impact on how health care is delivered and how health professionals practice. Chapter 8 details planning of a program evaluation along with planning a smaller scope evaluation, a common focus for DNP professional work.

Chapter 9 focuses on quality improvement as a developing science and an important focus in all health care delivery. Quality improvement projects must be evaluated, and often that responsibility falls to the DNP nurse. Chapter 10 discusses the important area of patient care standards, guidelines, and protocols from the perspective of how they are developed, implemented, and evaluated as well as how they are used as standards/criteria to judge performance for evaluation. Chapter 11 examines the critical role of interprofessional teams as instrumental in the delivery of high-quality and safe care. The practice of traditional teams is changing and cutting across organizations and systems to create new models of teamwork. Chapter 12 is new to address competency assessment and the burgeoning use of simulation as an educational method for health care professionals. The historical development of simulation, methods, and evaluation models is discussed.

Section III, evaluation of populations and health policies, discusses evaluation at the macro level and the impact of policy changes. Chapter 13 addresses characteristics, risk factors, determinants of health, and evaluation methods from the lens of populations and population health. Chapter 14 elucidates the steps of translating a problem to policy changes to practice as a way of evaluating health policy. DNPs are encouraged to seek opportunities for advocacy and leadership in influencing health policy development, implementation, and evaluation. Chapter 15 examines drivers of change, impact, and challenges to evaluation now and for the future, including the increased demand for comprehensive high-level evaluation by DNPs and the related competencies required to be successful.

Some of the unique features of the book are definitions of key terms, examples to illustrate a point, and case studies to provide exemplars of comprehensive evaluations, including clinical applications and recommended resources for further perusal. Most importantly, this book is focused on the needs of DNPs and their responsibility for evaluation in health care. Our esteemed contributors are well-recognized and respected as content experts and scholars in their respective fields. Contributing authors were gracious in accepting our requests to share their knowledge by contributing to this third edition. As members of the nursing profession, we assume our responsibility to educate current and future nurses in the best evidence-based knowledge available that will be utilized to improve high-quality health care for the nation.

Our sincere hope is that this edition will meet our primary aim of providing a relevant, evidence-based resource to assist DNPs in assuming their responsibility and accountability for competency in the conduct of high-level evaluation that will inform decision-making for those engaged in health care delivery and practice.

Joanne V. Hickey
Eileen R. Giardino

Qualified instructors may obtain access to supplemental PowerPoints by emailing textbook@springerpub.com

ACKNOWLEDGMENTS

We are indebted to many wonderful people who shared their expert knowledge and helped make this book possible through their contributions to the first and/or second edition. We express our thanks and gratitude to the following:

Christine A. Brosnan, DrPH, RN Associate Professor, Retired, Cizik School of Nursing, University of Texas Health Science Center at Houston, Houston, Texas, who was the coeditor of this book for the first two editions.

Patrick G. Brosnan, MD Professor of Pediatrics, Retired, Department of Pediatrics, School of Medicine, University of Texas Health Science Center at Houston, Houston, Texas

Deanna E. Grimes, DrPH, RN, FAAN Professor Emerita, Cizik School of Nursing, University of Texas Health Science Center at Houston, Houston, Texas

Richard M. Grimes, PhD, MBA Adjunct Professor, McGovern Medical School, University of Texas Health Science Center at Houston, Houston, Texas

Sharon McLane, PhD, MBA, RN-BC Retired Informatician and Nursing Services Administrator, Lakeland, Florida

J. Michael Swint, PhD Professor of Health Economics, George McMillan Fleming Professor, Director, Division of Management, Policy, and Community Health, School of Public Health, University of Texas Health Science Center at Houston, Houston, Texas

Nancy F. Weller, DrPH, MPH, MS, RN Assistant Professor, Retired, Department of Nursing Systems, Cizik School of Nursing, University of Texas Health Science Center at Houston, Houston, Texas

We also wish to thank Ann Scanlon-McGinity, PhD, RN, FAAN, for her thoughtful counsel on administrative nurse leaders, innovation, and leadership for Chapter 15.

FOUNDATIONS OF EVALUATION

ONE

EVALUATION AND ADVANCED NURSING PRACTICE: THE MANDATE FOR EVALUATION

Joanne V. Hickey

> *What we call the beginning is often the end.*
> *And to make an end is to make a beginning.*
> *The end is where we start from.*
> —*T. S. Eliot*

INTRODUCTION

The mandate for evaluation is a critical component of any project to determine the achievement of desired outcomes. However, evaluation is often a neglected component in the design and execution of many endeavors. The word "evaluation" has various connotations for different audiences and the nature of the type and process for the conduct of an evaluation that adds to the lack of clarity about the evaluation. Doctor of Nursing Practice (DNP) graduates are expected to understand evaluation processes and assume responsibility and accountability for multiple facets of evaluation in health care organizations. Therefore, competency in evaluation is critical to the value that DNP graduates bring to health care. This chapter provides an overview of evaluation and discusses major health care issues driving the mandate for enhanced evaluation.

The terms *project* and *program* are used interchangeably in this book although they have a slightly different focus. A *project* is defined as a group of activities intended to achieve a specific goal, typically over a shorter duration, that is more specific and narrower in scope than a program (McGuire, 2016, p. 6). By comparison, the term *program* is defined as a group of clear, related, complementary activities that are intended to achieve a desired outcome among the target group(s) (McGuire, 2016, p. 5). The scale of a program can vary. A program may deliver a specific service (e.g., a new model for professional competency assessment for operating room nurses) in an organization or a broader collection of related services (e.g., a new model for professional competency assessment throughout an organization). The reader can determine the most appropriate term to be used for their purposes.

THE MANDATE FOR EVALUATION AND PROFESSIONAL NURSING PRACTICE

All professional registered nurses evaluate care provided to individual patients as part of the nursing process. The American Nurses Association (ANA, 2015, p. 87) defines *evaluation* as the process of determining the progress toward attainment of expected outcomes, including the effectiveness of care. The ANA's definition of evaluation is a *discipline-focused* description of the patient's responses to interventions and specific outcomes, as well as the care provided by the professional nurse. However, this definition is focused primarily on the patient–nurse relationship. The emergence of the DNP degree in the last decade has expanded the scope of evaluation for the graduates of these programs. The following briefly describes the background and expected competencies of DNP graduates in evaluation.

Health Care Issues Influencing Doctor of Nursing Practice Education

Graduate nursing education occurs within the context of societal demands and needs as well as the interprofessional work environment (American Association of Colleges of Nursing [AACN], 2011, p. 5). The seminal report, *To Err Is Human,* published by the Institute of Medicine (IOM, 1999), focused national attention on the state of patient safety, noting that between 44,000 and 98,000 people die each year from medical errors. A 2013 report suggests that these numbers were grossly underestimated. In a review of four studies published between 2006 and 2012 using the Global Trigger Tool, between 210,000 and 400,000 preventable deaths per year were reported (James, 2013). In 2001, *Crossing the Quality Chasm: A New Health System for the 21st Century* (IOM, 2001) addressed the problematic state of the health care system and leadership for nursing practice. These seminal reports highlight the medical errors and financial burden caused by fragmented care and system failures in health care. Among the recommendations resulting from these reports were that health care organizations, providers, and groups should promote health care that is safe, effective, patient-centered, timely, efficient, and equitable. These six elements have become the six domains of health care quality and a framework for judging quality in health care (IOM, 2001).

The *Health Professions Education: A Bridge to Quality* report from the IOM (2003) and the National Research Council of the National Academies (2005, p. 74) identified competencies that all health professionals must have for practice in the 21st century. Included are competencies to provide patient-centered care, work in interdisciplinary teams, employ evidence-based practice, utilize quality improvement methodologies, and integrate informatics in providing care. The IOM called for dramatic restructuring of all health professionals' education and noted that the best prepared senior-level nurses should be in key leadership positions and participate in executive decisions.

The *Future of Nursing: Leading Change, Advancing Health* (2010), published by the IOM, was the first report from the IOM focused solely on the profession of nursing. This report set a vision for nursing through 2020. Major recommendations included the following: advanced practice registered nurses should be able to practice to the full extent of their education and training; expand opportunities for nurses to lead and diffuse collaborative improvement efforts; double the number of nurses with a doctorate by 2020; nurses should be full partners with physicians and other health care professionals in redesigning health care in the United States; and prepare and enable nurses to lead change to advance health. Along with the IOM's recommendations were actions that needed to be taken to achieve these goals. The impact of this report was remarkable in that it was widely read and taken seriously by the profession of nursing, other health providers and leaders, legislators, and high-level decision makers. The recommendations for the nursing profession in the *Future of Nursing* report (2010) provided a window of opportunity for nursing to step up and meet the needs of society through practice at the highest level of nursing practice.

Many of the actions recommended in the report have been carried out, but there are still others awaiting action. A new committee convened by the National Academy of Medicine extends the vision for the nursing profession into 2030 through the Future of Nursing 2020-2030: Charting a Path to Achieve Health Equality consensus committee. The goals of the consensus committee are similar, as experts convene to continue to define a course for the nursing profession while working with others to create a culture of health, reduce health disparities, and improve the health and well-being of the U.S. population in the 21st century (https://nam.edu/publications/the-future-of-nursing-2020-2030/).

Influencers of Nursing and Nursing Education for the 21st Century

Several contemporary factors have been identified as influencers of the desired characteristics of the nursing workforce for the 21st century and thus must be integrated into the educational preparation of future nurses. They include diversity, equity, and inclusion; four spheres of care; systems-based practice; informatics and technology; engagement and experience; academic practice partnerships; and career-long learning (AACN, 2021, pp. 6–10). These are well described in *The Essentials: Core Competencies for Professional Nursing Education* (2021) and further in this chapter and book.

American Association of Colleges of Nursing's Leadership in Nursing Education

The American Association of Colleges of Nursing (AACN) has published the Essentials series that provides the educational framework for the preparation of nurses for undergraduate, graduate, and doctoral programs. In the past, three versions of the Essentials were published: *The Essentials of Baccalaureate Education for Professional Nursing Practice;* last published in 2008; *The Essentials of Master's Education in Nursing,* last published in 2011; and *The Essentials of Doctoral Education for Advanced Nursing Practice,* last published in 2006. Each Essentials document has provided specific guidance for the development and revision of nursing curricula at each degree level. Given changes in higher education, learner expectations, and the rapidly evolving health care system outlined in the *AACN's Vision for Academic Nursing* (2019), bold new thinking and new approaches to nursing education are needed to prepare the nursing workforce of the future (AACN, 2019, 2021).

The Essentials of Doctoral Education for Advanced Nursing Practice (AACN, 2006) outlines expectations for DNP graduates, including evaluation and expected competencies. The document is organized around eight specific areas of practice called "Essentials." Each essential includes a description of the area of practice and related expected competencies. These Essentials have served the nursing profession well since 2006 as the blueprint for DNP education and its expected outcome competencies. However, times change, and periodic rethinking and revisions are required to keep the Essentials current and useful for nursing.

Realignment With Professional Practice Changes: Updated Essentials 2021

Late in November of 2020, AACN released a draft of *The Essentials: Core Competencies for Professional Nursing Education*. This draft document reflected new thinking about the profession of nursing and contemporary practice with a focus on competencies. In the introduction to the document, several points are made. First, the new Essentials document is a singular document that addresses professional nursing preparation across the continuum from prelicensure education through advanced practice education. In this document, there are 10 domains that all professional nurses are expected to develop, although the expected competencies are presented at two levels, prelicensure and advanced practice. Second, each domain includes a descriptor of the competency, key concepts, the competencies, and subcompetencies. See definitions and further description at AACN (2021; https://www.aacnnursing.org/Portals/42/AcademicNursing/pdf/Essentials-2021.pdf). The draft was posted for discussion and comment.

As of early 2021, nursing faculties, employers, practicing nurses, and others thoughtfully reviewed and commented on this document. The final version of the new Essentials was approved and released in April 2021 and is available on the AACN website (https://www.aacnnursing.org/Portals/42/AcademicNursing/pdf/Essentials-2021.pdf). The new structure of domains, concepts, and competencies is part of the final document. Therefore, this content has been included in this chapter. The basic tenets included in the 2006 DNP Essentials have not been deleted. Rather, they have been expanded, and new thinking of contemporary nursing practice has been infused. Change is inevitable and will continue as the profession stays abreast with societal needs for professional nursing practice.

Impact of Doctor of Nursing Practice Graduates

The DNP degree has been in existence since 2006 and is now 15 years old. The DNP is recognized as the terminal practice degree in nursing, which has caused nursing leaders to rethink the education of nurses and the optimal utilization of the growing number of DNP graduates. Graduates of DNP programs represent the traditional advanced practice nursing roles of nurse practitioner, clinical nurse specialist, nurse anesthetist, and nurse midwife, and also nurse executive and nurse informaticist roles. Although the early DNP programs were designed as post-master programs, the emergence of the BSN to DNP curriculum has rapidly developed. Students in a post-master program often come to the DNP program with years of clinical experience in advanced practice roles. However, the student enrolling in the BSN to DNP program does not bring experience in an advanced practice role and may enter a DNP program directly from the BSN program or with little clinical experience. BSN to DNP students have different professional experience backgrounds, and educational programs must recognize the differences in designing the curriculum so that both groups of students can achieve the required competencies to be awarded the DNP degree.

The DNP graduate has an expanded scope for evaluation as the graduate moves beyond the single patient/client and discipline-specific focus to also address evaluation at a population, organizational, and systems level. From this lens, DNP graduates expand the depth and scope of evaluation to include the theoretical and scientific approaches utilized by behavioral, social, and organizational scientists to evaluate more complex multidisciplinary questions. The theoretical foundation of evaluation is grounded in science and the rigorous methodologies used to conduct systematic evaluations of phenomena of interest to those engaged in the delivery and utilization of health care services. In order for any evaluation to have credibility, it must be based on the best practices of evaluation of science and methodologies considered to be valid and reliable by industry standards.

The DNP graduate must engage in evaluation at this level of expertise to be viewed as a credible health professional by health and other professionals, administrators, legislators, insurers, and leaders to demonstrate expertise in evaluation science and methodology. The results of evaluations provide information to decision makers whose decisions affect the health care system.

The focus of an evaluation can be broad and comprehensive and may include quality indicators, clinical outcomes, and the risks–benefits of health care for a population, organization, or system. Table 1.1 provides examples of the scope of evaluation possibilities in which DNPs might engage. DNPs must develop the competencies to engage in high-level evaluation processes both independently and as members of an interprofessional team because their contributions are integral to

TABLE 1.1 Examples of Evaluations by DNPs

Focus	Description	Evaluation Example
Patient/client or groups/populations		
Groups of patients/ clients	• A group may be defined as a set of patients who have in common a provider(s), disease, or are receiving care in a particular setting. • The focus of patient-centered evaluation is usually directed at response to care and health outcomes.	• In a diabetic group within a practice, how do the patients'/ clients' outcomes compare with national, evidence-based guidelines such as targeted HbA1c, weight, and blood pressure levels?
Populations	• A set of persons having common, personal, economic, or environmental characteristics. • The common characteristic may be anything that influences health, such as age, diagnosis, level of disability, or socioeconomic status.	• The outcomes of patients with ischemic stroke in a multifacility health care system as compared with national guidelines. • Patient satisfaction with care and with their encounter with the health care system.
Organization		
Models of care	• A conceptual model or diagram that broadly defines the way health services are delivered.	• The effectiveness of models of practice such as interprofessional teams or solo practice in decreasing length of stay.

(continued)

TABLE 1.1 Examples of Evaluations by DNPs (continued)

Focus	Description	Evaluation Example
Evidence-based practice	• The integration of best research evidence, expert opinion, and patient values in making decisions about the care of individual patients (IOM, 2003).	• The adherence to evidence-based guidelines for myocardial infarction as patients move from one unit to another along the continuum of care.
Quality improvement	• A formal approach to the analysis of performance and systematic efforts for improvement through a planned program within an organization.	• Integration of health care technology and information systems into point of service care for a particular diagnosis or condition.
Systems		
Cost-effectiveness analysis (CEA)	• A comparative evaluation of two or more interventions in which costs are calculated in dollars (or the local currency) and end points are calculated in health-related units (Drummond et al., 2005).	• Assists health professionals in making decisions about equipment purchases or establishing new programs or services.
Responsiveness to community needs	• The ability of a person, unit, or organization to address the expressed needs of a community. • The community is usually described as external to the health care organization or system and may be people living in the same area as the facility, a facility such as a housing project, or an ethnic group with ties to the health care facility.	• Develops programs based on expressed needs of the community of interest through a partnership with that community so that the community partners are stakeholders in the program. • Examples of such programs are starting a Saturday clinic for immunization at the local school, a prenatal clinic for high-risk mothers in a community with a high incidence of premature deliveries, or a hypertension clinic at a local industrial plant for workers.

achieving a high-quality health care system for the nation. Only then will the full potential of DNP graduates to achieve high-quality and safe outcomes be realized.

It is the primary purpose of this book to assist DNP students and graduates to understand evaluation as an integral component of their practice and to master the theoretical and scientific underpinnings of evaluation in health care. In *The Future of Nursing: Leading Change, Advancing Health* report (IOM, 2010), Dr. Harvey Fineberg, then president of the IOM, said, "achieving a successful healthcare system in the future rests upon the future of nursing." If nurses are going to lead the transformation of health care, as *The Future of Nursing* report suggests, then that transformation must be based on credible evaluation data. DNP graduates have the knowledge and competencies to assume a leadership role in evaluation of the current and future health care delivery system and its components.

PRINCIPLES OF EVALUATION

This chapter now turns to the discussion of evaluation, including its scope, conceptual and theoretical bases, types, processes, methods, and practices to provide the DNP student and graduate with the necessary knowledge to conduct evaluations.

Evaluation and Related Terms and Concepts

Evaluation is the systematic determination of the quality or value of something (Scriven, 1993). Among the many definitions of evaluation, some are reflective of a specific type of evaluation, whereas others are more generic. Generic definitions of evaluation include a process that requires judgments to be made about the extent to which something satisfies a criterion or criteria; the systematic application of scientific and statistical procedures for measuring program conceptualization, design, implementation, and utility; making comparisons based on these measurements; and the use of the resulting information to optimize program outcomes (Centers for Disease Control and Prevention [CDC], 2010). Other terms and concepts often used in evaluation have some commonalities as well as differences with the scope of evaluation. They include program evaluation, quality assurance, quality improvement, and outcomes research. Table 1.2 includes terms commonly referred to in evaluation.

TABLE 1.2 Definitions of Frequently Used Terms in Evaluation of Health Care

Term	Definitions
Assessment	A systematic process of collecting information about an entity from diverse sources; it is an appraisal.
Accountability	The obligation to demonstrate and take responsibility for performance in light of agreed expectations.
Analysis	An investigation of the component parts of a whole and their relationships in making up the whole; the process of breaking a complex topic or substance into smaller parts to gain a better understanding of it.
Assessment	The appraisal or estimation of the nature, quality, or ability of someone or something.
Benchmarking	The process of comparing one's processes and performance metrics with industry bests and/or best practices from other industries.
Best practices	The most up-to-date patient care interventions that result in the best patient outcomes and minimal patient risk of complications or death (Robert Wood Johnson Foundation [RWJF], 2013).

(continued)

TABLE 1.2 Definitions of Frequently Used Terms in Evaluation of Health Care (*continued*)

Term	Definitions
Context	The background, environment, conditions, setting, framework, or surroundings in which events or occurrences take place. The circumstances that form the setting for an event, statement, knowledge, idea, or project so that it can be fully understood and assessed. In evaluation, it is the characteristics of the local setting in which the evaluation takes place that influence the planning, implementing, and evaluating processes.
Criterion	"… an attribute of structure, process, or outcome that is used to draw an inference about quality" (Donabedian, 2003, p. 60).
Critique	A critical review of an object, process, literature, or performance; a critical examination or estimate of a thing or situation in order to determine its nature and limitations or its conformity to standards or criteria.
Culture	A pattern of learned, group-related perception—including both verbal and nonverbal language—that is added to values, the belief system, and the disbelief system (Ogrinc et al., 2018, p. 62).
Dose	The amount of an intervention and the frequency of delivering that dose. For example, if the intervention used in a project includes an educational program for staff, what is the intervention (what does it include), and how often is it administered in order to achieve the expected outcome?
Effectiveness	The extent to which planned outcomes, goals, or objectives are achieved as a result of an activity, strategy, intervention, or initiative intended to achieve the desired effect, under ordinary circumstances (not controlled circumstances such as in a laboratory). • A measure of the accuracy or success of a diagnostic or therapeutic technique that occurs in an average clinical environment. • The extent to which a treatment achieves its intended purpose.
Efficacy	The extent to which a specific intervention, procedure, or service produces the desired effect, under ideal conditions (controlled environment, lab circumstances).
Efficiency	• The ratio of the output to the inputs of any system. • An efficient system or person is one who achieves higher levels of performance (outcome, output) relative to the inputs (resources, time, money) consumed.
Evaluation	• The process of determining progress toward attainment of expected outcomes, including the effectiveness of care (ANA, 2010, p. 63). • "The systematic application of scientific and statistical procedures for measuring program conceptualization, design, implementation, and utility; making comparisons based on these measurements; and the use of the resulting information to optimize program outcome" (CDC, 2010).
Fidelity	The degree to which a measurement system consistently indicates changes in the measured item without any error.
Indicators	A quantitative or qualitative variable that provides a simple and reliable means to measure achievement, monitor performance, or reflect changes.
Monitor	The process of observing and checking the progress in quality of specific characteristics over a period of time.

(*continued*)

TABLE 1.2 Definitions of Frequently Used Terms in Evaluation of Health Care (*continued*)

Term	Definitions
PDSA cycle	A Plan–Do–Study–Act (PDSA) cycle is designed for small-scale testing of a change or intervention to see if works toward desired outcome achievement. P phase: Design the item to be tested; it might be testing the data collection plan by asking a few individuals to try to follow the plan and give you feedback about the clarity of the instructions. D phase: Carry out your plan. S phase: What does the collected data tell you about the acceptance and ease of the intervention? A phase: What changes do you want to make based on what you have learned from this PDSA cycle? (Ogrinc et al., 2018)
Quality	Medical quality is the degree to which health care systems, services, and supplies for individuals and populations increase the likelihood for positive health outcomes and are consistent with current professional knowledge (IOM, 1990).
Quality assurance	Quality assurance is an older term that is still used in the literature, although quality improvement is the term seen more frequently. A program for the systematic monitoring and evaluation of the various aspects of a project, service, or facility to ensure that standards of quality are being met. "All actions taken to establish, protect, promote, and improve the quality of health care" (Donabedian, 2003, p. xxiv).
Quality of care	A measure of the ability of the provider, health care facility, or health plan to provide services for individuals and populations that increase the likelihood of desired health outcomes and that are consistent with current professional knowledge (RWJF, 2013).
Quality improvement	An assessment process examining a patient's care or an organizational or systems problem for the purpose of improving processes or outcomes. Initiatives with a goal to improve the processes or outcomes of the care being delivered. *Clinical quality improvement* is an interdisciplinary process designed to raise the standards for the delivery of preventive, diagnostic, therapeutic, and rehabilitative measures in order to maintain, restore, or improve health outcomes of individuals and populations (IOM, 1990).
Stakeholders	Individuals, groups, or organizations with a significant interest in how well the project or program functions.
Standard	Authoritative statement defined and promoted by the profession or other credible entity by which the quality of practice, service, or education can be evaluated (ANA, 2015, p. 89).
Synthesis	The composition or combination of parts or elements so as to form a whole; the combining of often diverse conceptions into a coherent whole.
Transparency	"The process of collecting and reporting health care cost, performance, and quality data in a format that can be accessed by the public and is intended to improve the delivery of service and ultimately improve the health care system" (RWJF, 2013). Ensuring openness in the delivery of services and practices with particular emphasis on valid, reliable, accessible, timely, and meaningful data that are readily available to stakeholders, including the public.

Comparison of Assessment and Evaluation

In the English language, some words are misused or used interchangeably because two words may be close in meaning in some respect but yet quite different from each other. This is true of the words *assessment* and *evaluation*. *Assessment is* a systematic process of collecting information about an entity from diverse sources; it is an appraisal. By comparison, *evaluation is* concerned with making a judgment about quality, skills, or importance of some entity. When you assess, you assess the level of performance of a particular entity, but when you evaluate, you determine the level of achievement according to a standard or criterion.

Evaluation Defined

Evaluation is a systematic determination of a subject's merit, worth, and significance, using criteria governed by a set of standards. Simply put, an evaluation is the systematic determination of the quality or value of something (Scriven, 1991, pp. 1, 4–5). In evaluation, you judge something based on a standard or criterion to determine compliance or shortcomings with the standard or criterion. The evaluation process assists an organization, program, project, or other initiative to examine an aim, objectives, proposal, or expected outcomes to help in decision-making regarding the merit of a planned project. Evaluation can also be used to ascertain the degree of achievement or results or outcomes of a completed work. The process of evaluation is systematic in that it is organized around a group of steps logically sequenced to accomplish its purpose. It requires quality data collection, methodology consistent with the aims, and a defensible choice of indicators of quality to support the credibility of the findings (D'Errico et al., 2020).

Standards/Criteria for Evaluation

Any evaluation must be based on some established standards or criteria that reflect the merit of a work. The overall purpose of any evaluation is to support data-driven decision-making by providing the practitioner and other stakeholders with the information needed to make informed decisions about future actions. In addition, it provides an understanding of the structural components and processes of the work to support the need for changes to accomplish stated goals (Wikipedia, 2020a, 2020b). The application of evaluation is universal in that it can be used for a variety of entities, such as science, the arts, and business as well as health care organizations, health policy, foundations, human services, and healthcare quality. Although evaluation is often thought of something conducted at the end of a project, a plan for evaluation must be considered in the planning phase of a project. There are various forms of evaluation, which will be discussed later in the chapter, include formative evaluation that may be conducted at various time points in the project. Although evaluation is inherently a theoretically informed process (whether explicitly or not), the definition and parameters of evaluation are tailored to its context; that is, the theory, needs, purpose, methodology, and quality indicators of the evaluation process itself (Wikipedia, 2020a). A discussion of evaluation in professional nursing practice is an example of an evaluation definition tailored to a specific context.

Ethics of Evaluation

The integrity of the evaluation is critical to the credibility, trust, and confidence one has of the findings. The American Evaluation Association (AEA) has published guiding principles for evaluators to follow (AEA, 2018). They point out that guiding principles and evaluation standards are different. *Guiding principles* refer to the ethical conduct of the evaluator, whereas *evaluation standards* refer to the quality of the evaluation. The AEA describes five principles for evaluators that are interdependent and interconnected to guide evaluation in all stages of the evaluation from initial discussion of focus and purpose through design, implementation, reporting, and, ultimately, the use of the evaluation (AEA, 2018). Each principle includes substatements to amplify the meaning of the principle and to guide application. The following are the five guiding principles for evaluators; the reader is encouraged to visit the AEA website (see resources) for further illumination of each principle:

- *Systematic Inquiry*: Evaluators conduct data-based inquiries that are thorough, methodical, and contextually relevant.
- *Competence*: Evaluators provide skilled professional services to stakeholders.
- *Integrity*: Evaluators behave with honesty and transparency in order to ensure the integrity of the evaluation.
- *Respect for People*: Evaluators honor the dignity, well-being, and self-worth of individuals and acknowledge the influence of culture within and across groups.
- *Common Good and Equity*: Evaluators strive to contribute to the common good and advancement of an equitable and just society.

Bias

Integrity involves honesty and moral and ethical principles. This means that the principle of freedom from bias in evaluation is integral to the overall evaluation. Freedom from bias includes three dimensions that address impartiality, independence, and transparency. *Impartiality* refers to equitable treatment, which in evaluation means an open-mindedness to follow the evaluation process fairly without prejudice or preconceived ideas. *Independence* refers to freedom from outside control that could influence or pressure someone to make decisions contrary to the evidence. Examining for presence of conflict of interest must be addressed to determine any threat to impartiality. *Transparency* is the free, uninhibited flow of information that is open to the scrutiny of others (National Patient Safety Foundation, 2015, p. xii) and implies clarity and openness of processes, clear ongoing communications, and accountability so that something can be easily replicated by others. As applied to evaluation, transparency means stakeholder awareness of the reason for the evaluation, an openness and clarity of the processes employed, and the accountability for criteria by which the findings will be judged. Elimination of bias cannot be exercised equally in all projects (LoBiondo-Wood & Haber, 2014, p. 171). For example, one may be charged with developing practice guidelines for the spread of coronavirus with a special focus on how long the organism lives on surfaces such as tabletops. There may be limited high-quality literature about a topic of interest, so one may need to look for direction at qualitative studies, gray literature, and social media. Since the sources of the information are subject to opinions and bias, the guidelines need to be reflective of reliable current knowledge to minimize the possibility of bias. In such a situation, the potential for bias must be clearly identified along with an openness to revising the practice guidelines based on more credible information, as it appears. In summary, the key elements of evaluation, regardless of type of evaluation, include the following:

- Characterized by a systematic, rigorous, and meticulous application of scientific methods to assess the aim, design, methodology, implementation, data collection, and outcomes of a project.
- Requires time, focus, expertise, and resources to conduct an evaluation.
- Based on some clearly identified criteria or standards.
- Conducted in an objective ethical manner, free of bias to the extent possible, regarding the degree to which the components of the project fulfill the stated goals (Rossi et al., 2019).

TYPES OF EVALUATIONS

There are many different types of evaluation, so it is important to choose the right evaluation process to address the needs of the project and the stage of the project's development over the life cycle of the project. The most common types of evaluation include formative, process, outcome, economic, impact, and summative evaluations, whereas the stages or phases of a project include the conceptualization phase, implementation phase, or project closure phase. Evaluation methods need to be customized according to the purpose of the evaluation and what needs to be evaluated. Each type of evaluation can assist in providing the right kind of data at the right time so that evaluators and stakeholders can make the best informed data-driven decisions. An assumption for any evaluation is that the aim, objective, structure, methods, and audience of the project are clearly defined and reflect the overall purpose of the project.

In listing and describing the following common types of evaluation, there are some description variations noted among authors, although, generally, there is agreement on the main characteristics of a type of evaluation.

Formative Evaluation

A formative evaluation is conducted when the project is still in the developmental stage or early stages of implementation. It helps to determine whether the project is feasible and appropriate before it is fully implemented. It is usually conducted when a new project or activity is in the developmental stage or when an existing project is being adapted or modified (CDC, n.d.). A formative evaluation provides data about the need for the project and develops the baseline for subsequent monitoring. By conducting small trials of the project and discussions with stakeholder or focused groups, formative evaluations may identify areas for revision to improve the likelihood of success before implementation (Nanda, 2017). These small trials or Plan–Do–Study–Act (PDSA) cycles are cycles for learning and can be very informative for making changes to strengthen the evaluation.

Process Evaluation

Process evaluation is conducted to "measure the activities of a project, project quality, and who it is reaching" (Hawe et al., 1990). It occurs once the project is being implemented and helps determine whether project activities have been implemented as intended and whether the target population has been reached. The data generated can be used to identify gaps and to improve the future implementation by correcting ineffective activities and processes as well as providing information about how well the project is working to external stakeholders. Data can be gathered for a process evaluation from a review of internal reports, from discussions with project team members, and by conducting small samples of the implementation from project participants. For example, as part of a hospital program to prevent nosocomial infections, a practitioner conducts a process evaluation to determine whether the correct protocol for handwashing is being used by the staff. Hawe et al. (1990) recommends that a process evaluation of a system be conducted prior to any other type of evaluation.

Outcome Evaluation

Outcome evaluation measures project effects and benefits in the target population by assessing the progress in achieving outcomes during the implementation of the program. It generates data about the project outcomes and the degree to which those outcomes are attributable to the project interventions as compared with set benchmarks. Insights from outcome-focused feedback can help increase project effectiveness. Data collected include both qualitative and quantitative data. These data answer the question about what are the short-term and long-term results of the project. They also examine the presence of any unintended consequences resulting from the project so that action can be taken to address them.

Economic Evaluation

Also called cost analysis, cost-benefit analysis, cost-utility analysis, and cost-effectiveness evaluation, an economic evaluation is used during the project's implementation and measures the benefits of the project against the costs. Economic evaluation generates useful quantitative data that measure the efficiency of the project and identify inefficiencies. The many forms of economic evaluation include cost analysis, cost-benefit analysis, cost-utility analysis, and cost-effectiveness evaluation. Each type has a different focus and methodology to achieve its objectives. These data can be compared to an audit and provide useful information to stakeholders to identify inefficiencies and information about how the costs translate into desired outcomes (Nanda, 2017).

Impact Evaluation

An impact evaluation assesses the extent to which the outcomes were caused by the intervention in question rather than other factors present in the environment such as socioeconomic trends, environmental or political conditions, or other interventions (Clarke et al., 2019). It is a systematic and empirical process that assesses how effective a project was in achieving its ultimate outcomes (CDC, n.d.). Impact evaluation is useful for measuring sustained beneficial changes brought about by the project, including its impact on policy, and is conducted at the end of a project. These data can be collected from surveys of participants and comparison of the project aims with outcomes.

Summative Evaluation

The term *summative evaluation* is used less often than in the past, whereas the terms *outcome evaluation* and *impact evaluation* are used more often in the health care literature. By definition, summative evaluation is conducted after the project has been completed or at the end of a project cycle. It provides data about how well the project delivered benefits to the target population. It is useful for project leaders to justify the project, show what has been achieved, and garner support for project continuation or expansion (Nanda, 2017).

THE DYNAMIC NATURE OF EVALUATION: A COMPREHENSIVE VIEW OF THE PROCESS

Specific types of evaluation are designed to be conducted at different stages in the life cycle of a project to make judgments about the progress of the project in achieving desired outcomes. Sidani and Braden (2011) emphasize the dynamic nature of projects by noting that the process for designing, evaluating, and translating interventions is systematic and rigorous yet flexible. Although the phases are logically sequenced, the results of each phase drive the work forward toward the next phase or backward toward an earlier stage. For example, conducting a small PDSA cycle in a quality improvement initiative can determine whether an intervention was acceptable to a group of nurses to provide meaningful data. When evaluation determines that the interventions are acceptable to this target audience, then efficacy has been established. Moving forward to the next step of implementation is appropriate. However, if the nurses indicated that the intervention did not work or was not acceptable to them, then it is back to a previous stage of the project to rethink and revise previous steps in the process. The previous stage that may require reexamination could be problem identification or needs assessment. In either case, the evaluator must go back to rectify ineffectiveness or inefficiencies and test again, before moving forward.

OVERALL PROJECT WITH STAGES OF DEVELOPMENT

In order to examine the overall plan and implementation of a project, the following steps in a project will be reviewed: problem identification; needs assessment; project aim or purpose; design, including methodology; implementation; and evaluation. A useful resource for evaluation is W. K. Kellogg Foundation's *The Step-by-Step Guide to Evaluation: How to Become Savvy Evaluations Consumers—November 2017* (Kellogg Foundation, 2017).

Problem Identification

A *problem* is a perceived deficiency or conditions that negatively influence the achievement of the desired outcome. The particular problem may not be evident to all stakeholders. It suggests that the conditions constitute a problem that requires deliberate attention, deliberation, and an organized intervention (Rossi et al., 2019, p. 34). A problem may be ignored, accepted as part of reality, or addressed with work-arounds. All potential problems are based on some assumptions about what is good, what is quality, and what can be changed. A *problem statement* is a short, clear explanation of the issue to be addressed. It sets up the context, relevance, and aims of the project (Wikipedia, 2020b). Unless the nature and scope of a problem is clearly and accurately identified, any subsequent phases of a project may be ineffective. Assumptions and intended target population must be clearly identified.

Needs Assessment

A *needs assessment* is a planned, systematic process of examination that answers questions about the condition a project intends to address, the appropriate target population, and the nature of the need for the project. It identifies the gaps between current and desired conditions. According to Altschuld and Kumar (2010), a needs assessment has three distinct phases: preassessment, assessment, and postassessment. The preassessment phase is designed to get organized and establish what is known. It focuses on the following areas: exploration of the scope of the problem, identification of key stakeholders to serve as members of a work group, defining the gap between the desired outcomes and existing conditions, synthesis and communication of the evidence, and decisions about the next steps.

The purpose of a needs assessment is to develop a deeper understanding of the needs of the target population, service deliverers, and organization's responsibilities and then identify likely causes of the needs. A needs assessment determines the gaps between what is and what should be and identifies who is responsible and what is affected. It answers the question of what additional information is needed, what criteria should be used for choosing solutions, and what resources are needed. The assessment phase also includes the plan needed to collect data, actual data collection, data analysis, and synthesis of data leading to decisions and next steps. The purpose of the postassessment phase is to take action to resolve the problem that needs to be rectified. It includes review of the needs of stakeholders to determine whether their concerns have been addressed; analysis of potential causes of the needs and remedies for removal of the gaps; and selection of the solution to be implemented (Rossi et al., 2019, pp. 265–267).

Aim or Purpose

A clearly stated SMART (i.e., specific, measurable, achievable, realistic, and timely) aim statement provides direction for the project. *Specific* refers to the precise statement about what you hope to accomplish. *Measurable* poses the question to determine whether the objectives are measurable so that it is clear that the changes or interventions implemented produced the desired results. *Achievable* answers the question, is the project doable given the time you have available to you? *Realistic* refers to the reality check of determining whether you have the time, resources (human, financial, and other), and support needed for the project. *Timely* refers to the timeline for the scope of the project and answers the question of when each portion of the project will be completed. A SMART aim statement directs the project, clarifies what the project will and will not accomplish, and states expected outcomes (Institute of Healthcare Improvement [IHI], 2020a, 2020b).

In the *planning* phase, the *purpose* of the evaluation must be clear. The purpose may be to examine only one approach (e.g., the outcome of care) or to examine all three approaches to quality assurance (the structure, process, and outcome of care). An outcome evaluation may focus on the *effectiveness* of an intervention, program, or policy. *Effectiveness* refers to a change in health status resulting from an intervention provided under usual conditions, whereas effectiveness describes a change in health status resulting from an intervention provided under controlled conditions (Brook & Lohr, 1985; Donabedian, 2003).

The team may choose to conduct a formative evaluation, a summative evaluation, or both. *Formative evaluation* refers to an appraisal occurring during the implementation of a program in which the results are used to revise and improve the rest of the program. *Summative evaluation* refers to an appraisal that occurs at the end of a program in which the results are used to determine the benefit and future use of the program. The term *formative* is often used interchangeably with "process evaluation," and "summative evaluation" is used interchangeably with "outcome." The interchangeable terms do not always mean the same thing (Fitzpatrick et al., 2004).

Design

Design is simply the plan or blueprint for the conduct of a project. It includes the target audience, contextual environment, conceptual or theoretical basis, plan for the intervention, operational definitions, what data need to be collected and by whom, instruments for data collection, data storage, and analysis plan. A prerequisite is a clear and thorough understanding of the problem that is in need of remediation. The problem may be an ineffective policy guideline, practice, or procedure, to name a few. The design is your plan, as you view the project prospectively, and reflects how you think the project will unfold.

The *target audience* of a program (or an evaluation) must be clearly identified for the intervention and could be nurses, patients, interdisciplinary team members, or others. The target audience always involves stakeholders; that is, people who are directly or indirectly affected by the project. Clear and effective communications with stakeholders in a project (e.g., sender, message, recipient, method, and timing) is paramount to the success of the project.

Context refers to the environment or setting in which the project will take place. The *contextual environment* is not only the physical characteristics, but also the psychological elements in which the project is conducted. The *physical characteristics* include the setting, such as a clinic, a care unit within an acute care facility, rehabilitation or long-term care facility, or community agency. It may be a for-profit or not-for-profit organization, and funding sources may be private payers, Medicare, or Medicaid. The project site may be in an urban or rural environment, and the setting may be resource rich or resource poor to support the project. The mix of types and levels of health care providers also are contextual characteristics. The *psychological environment* refers to the culture of an organization. You want to know how open the culture is to change, the working relationship, transparency, and core values. Both the physical and the psychological characteristics will influence the openness to the acceptance of new approaches and changes.

The *conceptual/theoretical basis* refers to what credible information is known about the problem and related solutions to remediating it. Middle-range theories, data-based consensus guidelines, research reports, and other sources help the designer in framing the problem in relation to what is known about the problem and exploring possible solutions. In the collection of data, expert opinion and local opinion are also useful.

The *plan* or *blueprint* for the intervention includes the logically organized steps and timeline for the progression and completion of the project. The discrete steps of the project can be organized on a Gantt chart, which includes a timeline for completion. This helps to keep people informed and on target.

Operational definition refers to the specifications of the characteristics of a concept and how the concept will be measured. The operational definition defines what instruments will be used to assess the presence of the concept and to what degree the concept exists (LoBiondo-Wood & Haber, 2014, p. 78). An example of an operational definition of the weight of an object is the number in pounds that appears on a home step-on scale when a person steps on a weighing scale.

Data collection includes what data will be collected, by whom, when, and how. In the conduct of a project, a large amount of data can be collected that is not useful and wastes time and resources. Therefore, the selection of data elements to be collected along with why they are necessary must be established. Another important consideration is who will collect the data. This implies that data collectors will be trained to ensure interrater reliability, and if data are collected over time, period checking of interrater reliability is conducted. As timing is a critical factor in capturing change, it is important to specify when, or at what point in time, data are collected. One can collect data too soon after an intervention is implemented for a change to be evident. Finally, the question of how the data will be collected must be addressed to specify whether the data will be captured at the data collection site to be downloaded into a database or entered on forms to be entered later into a database. The fewer the steps from data collection to entry into the database, the lesser the chance of error.

The *instruments for data collection* may be standardized tools, such as the Hamilton Depression Rating Scale to diagnose depression, or an evaluator developed tool, such as a checklist of key characteristics of a problem. The instrument must be a match for the data of interest. Examining operational definitions can help in determining the right tool for the right data source. *Data storage* must be planned so that it meets the requirements for ethical management of data and security measures for protection of human subjects, especially regarding any proprietary, sensitive, or personal information. Data stored on a computer should have password protection and provide limited access to only those directly involved with the project.

A plan for *data analysis* is needed. *Analysis* refers to the procedures and calculations used to describe or make inferences about the data collected. The selection of statistical analysis methods depends on the type of data collected (e.g., qualitative or quantitative data), the amount of data, and the purposes of the project. The data analysis may use descriptive or inferential statistics with quantitative data, whereas if one is looking for major themes, qualitative analysis methods are appropriate for data analysis. It is helpful to consult with a statistician in the planning phase of a project to ensure that the data you plan to collect and the type of statistical analysis meets the objectives of the project and statistical analysis requirements. Depending on the perspective and scope of the analysis, the analysis may be as simple as comparing the results of the evaluation against a national standard or benchmark such as *The Healthcare Effectiveness Data and Information Set* (HEDIS). For example, in a medical health care practice, data obtained from a retrospective review of medical records might be analyzed to determine the mean value for a variable of interest such as HbA1c from the diabetic patients in that practice. The percentage of patients who maintained an HbA1c <7% would then be determined and the results compared with a standard set for the practice. In contrast, data analysis of studies with complex designs may require application of sophisticated statistical techniques.

Implementation

The plan for the project is mobilized during the implementation phase. Sidani and Braden (2011, p. 11) conceptualized project implementation in three phases. In phase one, it is necessary to determine a clear and thorough understanding of the project's presenting problem, a point that has been underscored several times. Constant attention to gain the depth of understanding of a problem keeps the focus on the nature of the problem, the specific indicators of the problem, the range of severity with which it can be represented or be experienced, the determinants or factors that contribute to the problem, and potential consequences of the problem (Sidani & Braden, 2011, p. 11). An understanding of the problem is acquired through both deductive and inductive methods. Deduction is used to identify relevant middle-range theories, whereas induction explores a problem as it is experienced by the target population or the problem's local effects. In systematically exploring the problem, knowledge is gained about aspects of the problem that may be amenable to change and those that are not amenable to change. Understanding what is and what is not amenable to change in the problem helps to identify the interventions that may be useful in the remediation within that environment.

In phase two, the process of designing the interventions is related to elaborating the specifics of the intervention to the setting and culture in which it will be implemented. Relevant middle-range and practice theories can be very helpful in elucidating the critical details of the intervention and the best way to deliver those interventions. It also includes an understanding of the components of the intervention needed to promote the desired change.

In phase three, the project director and team develop an intervention theory specific to their project that describes the specific interventions and mechanisms to achieve the changes that will be implemented within the particular environment and local culture to achieve the desired outcomes. This is the project team's best estimate of how the intervention should work.

Sidani and Braden's (2011) three phases of project development are built on theoretical and empirical knowledge to design the intervention; project planners must not undervalue the input from the target population and other stakeholders involved in the project. Their valuable input, in all phases of the implementation, helps to clarify the presenting problem and the activities and mode for delivering the interventions that are acceptable to the involved stakeholders within the local setting (Sidani & Braden, 2011, p. 12).

Evaluation

Although positioned at the end of a project, evaluation is an integral part of the ongoing project from the beginning to the end. The types of evaluations previously discussed suggest that evaluations are conducted throughout every phase of the project. In addition, summative evaluation processes should be part of the planning of the project so that the elements of interest are clearly integrated into the project. A *criterion* refers to characteristics used to appraise the quality of care. A *standard* refers to a measurable reference point that is used for comparison. Generally, criteria are expressed in relation to standards (Donabedian, 2003; Fitzpatrick et al., 2004). For example, if an evaluation is focused on diabetes mellitus management, an appropriate criterion could be the level of HbA1c, whereas the standard might be that 95% of clinic patients will maintain an HbA1c <7%.

Dissemination

During the *dissemination* stage, the team submits a report that clearly are describes the results, including the strengths and weaknesses of the evaluation, conclusions, recommendations, and implications. The report may be submitted to the administrator or sponsor who requested the evaluation, presented at a professional meeting, or prepared for publication.

DOMAINS OF EVALUATION: QUESTIONS AND METHODS

In conducting an evaluation, a series of thoughtful questions are developed to give structure to the evaluation leads to appropriate planning. They become the basis for discussion about questions of interest to particular stakeholders, and the answers to those questions are used to elucidate and strengthen the planning and implementation of the project (Rossi et al., 2019, pp. 16, 17). The questions fall into five domains designed to elucidate the critical elements of each domain. These five domains include the following:

1. *Need for the project/program:* Questions that focus on determining the need for the project and conditions a project is intended to ameliorate.

- What are the nature and magnitude of the problem?
- Who thinks there is a problem in the system? What are the characteristics of the population being affected?
- How is the problem impacting the population? What are the population's unmet needs?
- What needs to change to eliminate the problem? What are the desired outcomes?
- What help is needed to ameliorate the problem?

2. *Program theory and design:* Questions about the project's conceptualization and design.

- What outcomes does the project intend to affect, and how do they relate to the nature of the problem or conditions the program aims to change?
- What theory supports the expectation that the project can have on the intended effects on the target outcomes?
- Is the project directed at the appropriate population? Will that population be willing to participate through the life of the project?
- What interventions does the project intend to implement? What is the probability that the interventions will be effective and why?
- How will the intervention be delivered, and will these modes be acceptable to the intended population?
- How will the project be resourced, organized, and staffed? Are these adequate to reach and serve the intended population?

3. *Program process:* Questions about project operations, implementation, service delivery, and recipient experience to the project services.

- Is the intended intervention or service being provided to the intended persons?
- Are we missing any individuals or groups who should be receiving the intervention? If so, why?
- Do you expect the participants to complete the intervention aspect of the project, or do you expect attrition before the project is completed? If attrition, why do participants drop out?
- Are the participants satisfied with the intervention? Are they finding it useful or helpful?
- Is the project well organized and well managed? If not, what action needs to be taken to rectify the deficiencies?

4. *Program impact:* Questions about the project change in the targeted outcomes and the project's impact on those changes as it relates to effectiveness.

- Are the expected outcomes and goals of the project being achieved?
- Are the refinements made to the project (e.g., PDSA cycles) demonstrating gradual progress toward achievement of the desired outcomes?
- Are positive gains from the project for the target population not identified in the goals or outcomes statements?
- Are there unexpected consequences of the project? If so, what are they?
- Are problems being addressed by the project leader in a timely fashion?

5. *Program efficiency:* Questions about the project's cost and cost-effectiveness.

- What are the total costs (e.g., staff time, equipment, transportation) of implementing the project, and who pays for it?
- Were resources used efficiently without waste or excess?
- Is the cost reasonable in relation to the size of the project and the value added gained from the project?
- Could this project be conducted for a lower cost yet still reap the benefits?

The questions for each of the five domains are examples of what questions the evaluator or team conducting the evaluation might ask to determine the effectiveness, outcomes, and value added from a project, and the number of questions asked are dependent on the purpose and scope of the project. However, these five domains provide a generic framework for posing critical questions for the evaluation.

TRENDS AND HEALTH CARE PRIORITIES INFLUENCING EVALUATION

The current transformation of the U.S. health care system has led to a realignment of the key priorities that are shaping the transformation of health care. Some of the drivers include the determinants of health, prevention, population health, patient/community engagement, quality and safety, a value-based health care system, and system performance (Artiga & Hinton, 2018; Salmond & Echevarria, 2017) These drivers of health care are noted because evaluations are often centered on aspects of the drivers to determine their impact on health care. These drivers are described in the following section.

Determinants of Health

Although the current understanding is that dimensions of health and illness are multifactorial, that holistic alternative to a biomedical model was a new and innovative approach almost 50 years ago (Borrell-Carrió et al., 2004). In 1977, Engel published an article in *Science* suggesting that health and illness were actually the products of a complex interaction among biological, psychological, and social factors (Engel, 1977). This idea was a major shift in thinking and reflected a gradual move in science away from a reductionist worldview of a simple cause-and-effect relationship toward a systems orientation. Engel (1977) proposed the *biopsychosocial model* as a way to understand how illness, disease, and suffering are affected by multiple levels of organization and to develop a holistic approach to understanding and treating patients (Borrell-Carrió et al., 2004). The biopsychosocial model was transformational in its conceptualization of health and illness and was a paradigm shift in thinking about the interaction of health and illness. Current concepts around "patient centeredness" evolved from this model (Burke, 2013, p. 137).

Patient-centered care means "providing care that is respectful of and responsive to individual patient preferences, needs, and values and ensuring that patient values guide all clinical decisions" (IOM, 2001). It is an approach to care that relies on a partnership between the provider and the patient based on a comprehensive view of the patient and their values and goals. It is based on effective communication, respect, and empathy, with the goals of improving patient care outcomes and reducing unnecessary costs (Bau et al., 2019; Rickert, 2012). The term *person-centered care* is now being used because it is more inclusive of a comprehensive view of an individual in health and illness. Person-centered care is about developing a plan of care with people that fits with what that person is ready, willing, and able to do. Person-centered care means the person is an equal partner in planning their care (Royal College of Nursing, 2020). It also implies equity.

Equitable care means "providing care that does not vary in quality because of personal characteristics such as gender, ethnicity, geographic location, and socioeconomic status" (IOM, 2002).

Medical care is estimated to account for only 10% to 20% of the modifiable contributors to health outcomes for a population (Hood et al., 2016). The other 80% to 90% is due to the social determinants of health (SDOH) that include health-related behaviors, socioeconomic factors, and environmental factors. The World Health Organization (WHO) defines SDOH as "conditions in which people are born, grow, live, work, and age. The[ir] circumstances are shaped by the distribution of money, power, and resources at global, national and local levels" (WHO, 2012).

Magnan (2017) lists five concepts that are influencing the integration of SDOH into health care. What is known about the SDOH is that medical care in itself is insufficient for achieving better health outcomes and that SDOH are influenced by policies and programs and associated with better health outcomes. New payment models are prompting interest in SDOH. Innovative models are connecting health care, social services, and some SDOH to improve health outcomes while new frameworks for integrating SDOH in health care are emerging.

Several national and international organizations have embraced a determinant of health framework to address current and future population health initiatives. For example, the *Healthy People 2030* initiative is designed to guide national health promotion and disease prevention efforts to improve the health of the nation. Released by the U.S. Department of Health and Human Services (HHS) every decade since 1980, *Healthy People 2030* identifies science-based objectives with targets to monitor progress and motivate and focus action. *Healthy People 2030* is the current iteration of the *Healthy People* initiative and is available from the HHS at https://health.gov/healthypeople and from the National Center for Health Statistics (2020).

Healthy People 2030 builds on *Healthy People 2020* and is a set of science-based, 10-year national objectives for improving health and well-being in the United States. It provides a framework that includes its vision, mission, foundational principles, and overarching goals; core objectives with targets; and research and developmental objectives. The foundational principles explain the thinking that guides decisions about *Healthy People 2030* and include the following:

● Attain healthy, thriving lives and well-being, free of preventable disease, disability, injury, and premature death.
● Eliminate health disparities, achieve health equity, and attain health literacy to improve the health and well-being of all.
● Create social, physical, and economic environments that promote the attainment of full potential for health and well-being for all.
● Promote healthy development, healthy behaviors, and well-being across all life stages.
● Engage leadership, key constituents, and the public across multiple sectors to take action and design policies that improve the health and well-being of all.

For a more detailed discussion of *Healthy People 2030*, see Chapter 13.

WHO also addressed determinants of health. According to WHO, the determinants of health include the social and economic environment, the physical environment, and the person's individual characteristics and behavior (WHO, 2012). The determinants underscore that many factors interact to affect the health of individuals and communities. Whether people are healthy or not is determined by their circumstances and environment. Income and social status, education, physical environment, social support networks, genetics, and health services are all components of the determinants of health. Recognition of the complexity of health and illness is important for anyone wishing to evaluate health-related attributes of populations, communities, organizations, or systems (WHO, 2012).

Prevention

To prevent literally means to keep something from happening. In clinical practice, the term *prevention* is used for those interventions that occur before the initial onset of disorder. A common classification of prevention includes the following:

● *Primary prevention*—To promote health prior to the development of disease or injuries through institution of interventions designed to avoid occurrence of disease either through eliminating disease agents or increasing resistance to disease.
● *Secondary prevention*—To detect disease in the early stages prior to the development of symptoms.
● *Tertiary prevention*—To reverse, arrest, or delay progression of disease through rehabilitation or treatment.

Interestingly, the scope of prevention has changed from what was once the domain of public health to a current major focus on prevention in clinical practice. The health care system is also reconceptualizing itself from an illness-based health care system to focus on wellness and health maintenance.

Population Health

Clinical care is increasingly moving toward population-based care. As clinical practices become larger, with defined populations, these large practices are dealing with the realities of a transition from individual-based care to population-based care

(Starfield et al., 2008). The redefining of public health and population health has been stimulated by the development of patient-centered medical homes. To understand the concept of population health, we begin with the basic concept of health. WHO (2019a, 2019b) published the most commonly cited definition of health: "Health is a state of complete physical, mental and social well-being and not merely the absence of disease or infirmity." This definition asserts that physical and mental well-being are a human right, enabling a life without limitation or restriction (WHO, 2019a, 2019b).

Population health is defined as "the health outcomes of a group of individuals, including the distribution of such outcomes within the group" (Kindig & Stoddart, 2003). The groups may be based on geographic populations such as countries or communities but can also refer to patients, patients with particular health problems, organizations, or any other defined group (Kindig & Stoddart, 2003). The health outcomes of such groups or institutions are of relevance to policy makers in both the public and the private sectors as well as to evaluators for purposes of decision-making.

Confusion often exists between the concepts of population health and public health. The traditional view of public health has been that it provides the critical functions of local and state health departments such as prevention of epidemics, control of environmental hazards, and the encouragement of healthy behaviors. The new and broader definition of the public health system offered by *The Future of the Public's Health in the 21st Century* (IOM, 2002) calls for "building a new generation of intersectoral partnerships that draw on the perspectives and resources of diverse communities and actively engage them in health action" (IOM, 2002) for the population.

Patient/Community Engagement

The IOM (2001) defines *patient-centered care* as "providing care that is respectful of and responsive to individual patient preferences, needs, and values, and ensuring that patient values guide all clinical decisions." This definition implies a goal of advocacy for the patient. Patient-centered care is one of six interrelated elements constituting high-quality health care that the IOM (2001) report identified. The term *patient-centered* means considering patients' cultural traditions, personal preferences, values, family situations, social circumstances, and lifestyles. It supports active involvement of patients and their families in the design of new care models and in decision-making about individual options for treatment (IOM, 2001).

The CDC defines *community engagement* as "the process of working collaboratively with groups of people who are affiliated by geographic proximity, special interests or similar situations with respect to issues affecting their well-being" (CDC, 2011). Community engagement is a fundamental value of public health based on the belief that the public has a right to participate. The public health community believes that by using "collective intelligence" and working together, problems will be more accurately identified and more effective solutions developed. Through this process, people have an opportunity to understand and to engage collaboratively in the processes of change.

Both patient-centeredness and community engagement are critical elements in the design of a health care system for the 21st century. The question is how to measure and evaluate these lofty concepts. Work is underway to develop effective tools for these purposes.

Quality and Safety

Within the current national imperatives for health care quality and safety, the mandate for evaluation of care has never been more vital to meeting societal needs (Izumi, 2012). Quality care is safe care, and safe care is a hallmark of quality. Evaluating the quality of care delivered to clients/patients is a necessity that emerges from the social contract between health professionals and society. Implicit in this social contract is the accountability of all health professionals to their clients/patients for the quality and safety of the services they render and for the expectation of care with predictable outcomes (Sidani & Braden, 2011).

Although there is a clear mandate for providing high-quality health care, the ambiguity associated with defining quality is surprising. How the word *quality* is defined depends on the context and perspective of the stakeholder such as the patient, family member, provider, program, insurer, accreditor, evaluator, institution, or system. For example, quality can be *outcomes* in which quality is defined as meeting the overall clinical results reasonably expected by a patient. Quality can be viewed from the lens of *interpersonal engagement* of the patient and the provider. Another major definition of quality may be *satisfaction* by the consumer with providers and payers. *Efficiency* of health care delivery is another dimension of quality, while *utilization*, which refers to underuse, overuse, or misuse of medical services, may be a focus of interest. Finally, *safety* is often considered synonymous with quality and may be defined as avoidance of medical error. The IOM (2001) defines *quality in health care* as "the degree to which health services for individuals and populations increase the likelihood of desired health outcomes and are consistent with current professional knowledge." This definition is from a national population perspective for the goal of health care in the United States. A clear operational definition of quality, reflective of focus, along with the metrics for measurement is important for evaluation. Quality is often viewed as a surrogate for value, another word with multiple meanings. It will be discussed from the perspective of system-level changes in the U.S. health care system.

Value-Based Health Care System

The U.S. health care system is moving from a volume and fee-for-service model to one using value-based payment (quality/outcomes and cost/price). A core issue in health care is the value of health care delivered. *Value* is defined as patient health outcomes per dollar spent or the cost of delivering desired outcomes (Porter, 2010). Porter (2010) described *outcomes* as the health results that matter for a patient's condition over the care cycle and *costs* as the total expense of care for a patient's condition over the care cycle. A full care cycle includes outpatient, inpatient, rehabilitative care, and support services such as social work and nutrition.

According to Porter (2010), the transition to a value-based health care system will require fundamental changes that include organizing care into integrated practice units around patients' medical conditions (e.g., organizing primary and preventive care to serve distinct patient groups); measurement of outcomes and related cost for every patient; bundled price reimbursement for a care cycle; integration of care delivery across separate facilities; and building and enabling an information technology platform to support access to and integration of information.

At a time when it is clear that the high cost of U.S. health care is unsustainable, especially in light of poor outcomes, a new way of financing health care concurrent with better outcomes is needed. Noted experts (Berwick et al., 2008; Porter, 2010) say it is possible to have better outcomes and lower cost simultaneously. Cost is the actual expense of patient care and must be measured around the patient and the full cycle of care. That means the cost of all resources used in providing care, including out-of-pocket expenses incurred by the patient, must be taken into account. Tools such as detailed process maps help to graphically display the steps in the process of care provided and offer a team the opportunity to analyze and recommend revisions to the process that improves value and decreases costs (http://www.ihi.org/resources/Pages/Tools/Flowchart.aspx). This may be done by addressing fragmentation of care, inefficiencies in delivery, and underuse and overuse of services that do not contribute to improved outcomes and value for the patient.

Bundled reimbursement rather than fee-for-service can be based on a *single payment* for a full cycle of care for an acute medical problem, or on *time-based reimbursement* for the overall care of a chronic condition or for primary/preventive care for a defined patient population (Porter, 2010). This approach discourages unnecessary use of resources and encourages efficient and effective use of resources and processes of care that result in good outcomes at reasonable costs.

From this brief overview of a few key points of value-based health care, it is clear that health informatics will play a major role in the future. Health informatics is much more than the electronic medical record. It is technology that integrates various forms of data that will support data-based decision-making and the integration of services across settings and cycles of care (Saba & McCormick, 2015). It is evident that systems-level evaluation by knowledgeable health professionals such as DNPs is needed to guide the transformation of health care.

Performance of Health Care Systems

Significant effort has been directed at optimizing the performance of health care systems to achieve improved organizational and patient outcomes. One framework used to guide organization and systems performance is the Triple Aim initiative (Berwick et al., 2008; IHI, 2012). The IHI Triple Aim is a framework developed by the Institute of Healthcare Improvement (IHI) that describes an approach to optimizing health system performance. The underlying premise is that new designs must be developed to simultaneously augment the three dimensions that are referred to as the "Triple Aim": improving the patient experience of care (including quality and satisfaction); improving the health of populations; and reducing the per capita cost of health care (Berwick et al., 2008; IHI, 2012).

According to the Commonwealth Fund and other reputable sources, the U.S. health care system is the most expensive in the world, with over 17% of the gross domestic product currently devoted to health care. However, the United States ranks low on many health indicators compared with other countries that spend far less on health care (Commonwealth Fund, 2015). The idea that spending alone will equal better health care performance and outcomes is just not true. The Triple Aim is not only focused on better experiences for patients and a healthier population, but is also based on the assumption that these goals can be accomplished at a lower cost than our current financial investment in health care. The Triple Aim provides a broad and comprehensive framework for evaluation of health care. Both the IHI and Commonwealth Fund have indicators that demonstrate achievement of objectives that are helpful for evaluation purposes.

In summary, this section has addressed major trends and priorities in health care at the level of the current health care delivery system. All of these trends will need ongoing evaluation to determine whether they are impacting health care delivery. The next section examines systems through a three-level approach at the micro-, meso-, and macrolevels.

A SYSTEMS PERSPECTIVE FOR EVALUATION: MICROSYSTEMS, MESOSYSTEMS, AND MACROSYSTEMS

A *system* is a set of interdependent and interrelated elements (e.g., both human and nonhuman) working together to achieve a common goal. Nelson et al. (2007) proposed a six-nestled-level model of health care systems diagrammed by a concentric circle fanning out from the epicenter, the patient. Ogrinc et al. (2018) note that this model helps to address the question of what system is the unit of practice, intervention, and measurement that we are studying, improving, or evaluating? The model is described in what follows.

The center of the concentric circles views the patient as a *self-care unit* (level 1), which includes the patient, the information, and the information technology needed to act to maintain health or increase the level of wellness. For example, a person who has diabetes mellitus will take insulin daily and monitor blood glucose levels that are used to determine the need for adjustment in additional insulin to keep the patient stabilized and optimally functional. Moving from the center to the next level is the *individual care provider and patient system* (level 2). This is the system level of the clinician's relationship with the patient and family and includes the goal of their interaction. In the example of diabetes mellitus, the goal is control of disease to prevent complications such as diabetic retinopathy or ketoacidosis.

The next level (level 3) is the *health care clinical microsystem*, which refers to the small, functional frontline units that provide most health care to most people. A health care clinical microsystem is a "small group of people including health professionals and patients and their families who work together in a defined setting on a regular basis to create care for discrete subpopulations of patients" (Nelson et al., 2011, p. 2). The health professionals include clinical and administrative support and information technology personnel who work with a defined group of patients who come together for a specific health care purpose (Ogrinc et al., 2018).

Moving outward to the next higher level is the *mesosystem* (level 4), which is the layer between the microsystem and the macrosystem and is often the interface between the two. A *mesosystem* is a larger system composed of linked clinical and supporting microsystems and is part of an embedded mesosystem within larger organizations (Nelson et al., 2011, p. 7). A mesosystem is often identified as a service line such as the neuroscience care center. Midlevel leaders are responsible for large clinical programs, clinical support services, informatics, and administrative services. Mesosystems may overlap in their clinical programs and support services, thus adding to the complexity of the systems and organization for responsibility and accountability.

The next larger system is the *macrosystem level* (level 5). A *macrosystem* refers to broader, overarching sectors such as a single hospital, a large corporate, state, national organization, or systems. Its leaders are responsible for organization-wide performance (Nelson et al., 2011).

The final level (level 6) is the *society, community, market, and social policy system*. Ogrinc et al. (2018, p. 63) describe this level as "the geographic, political, and/or economic group of macro-organizations (e.g., hospitals, payers, government) that have the aim of providing health care and fostering health in a community." The functionality and aims of these macroorganizations are governed by health policies and laws that influence the care provided to patients. In addition, insurers, clinical facilities, microsystems, and individual providers all have policies that directly influence individual patient care.

Importance of Recognizing the System Level

The differentiation of system levels greatly influences evaluation by providing a lens for understanding systems from a contextual and cultural perspective that will influence evaluation. When planning an evaluation, the DNP must consider its purpose and focus. The evaluation can focus on a single level (e.g., patient, care provider and patient, microsystem, mesosystem, macrosystem, or societal level), or it can include multiple levels, adding to the complexity. For example, at the micro level, the emphasis is on evaluating the quality of a particular intervention for a group of similar patients and often involves examining its effectiveness in achieving expected outcomes (Sidani & Braden, 2011). An evaluation addressing a problem at the mesosystem level may focus on a division, such as surgical services, in which multiple units that provide clinical care to surgical patients are included. An example of a possible evaluation focus might be policies and procedures for fall prevention on one particular clinical service. At the macro level, the emphasis shifts to a broad and comprehensive focus in which evaluation of the quality of programs or initiatives at the organization or systems level is addressed. For example, an evaluation might investigate the organizational policies on drug reconciliation as patients transition from one unit to another.

A BRIEF HISTORY OF HEALTH CARE EVALUATION

Individuals change history, and the modern history of health care evaluation was particularly influenced by three visionaries: Florence Nightingale, Ernest Codman, and Avedis Donabedian. Each brought to health care the idea that interventions should be more than worthy efforts and should deliver real benefit to patients. It is said that Florence Nightingale not only took care of patients, but also counted them. Born in 1820, she was drawn to mathematics, nursing, and public health, none of which was considered a desirable career for a wealthy woman living in 19th-century England (Spiegelhalter, 1999). As a professional nurse, she had the vision to integrate her keen observational skills with her knowledge of statistics and public health to improve patient care. Nightingale is a recognized pioneer in the evaluation of health care outcomes because she clearly understood the goal of care.

She said, "In dwelling upon the vital importance of *sound* observation, it must never be lost sight of what observation is for. It is not for the sake of piling up miscellaneous information or curious facts, but for the sake of saving life and increasing health and comfort" (Nightingale, 1859).

Born in 1869 into a prominent family, Ernest Codman was a Harvard-educated physician who accepted a position at Massachusetts General Hospital soon after completing his medical education. He seemed to be following the path of a successful physician of his day (American College of Surgeons, 2010; Donabedian, 1989). However, he began to wonder if the prevailing medical interventions actually improved patient health and soon focused on the idea of measuring end results, an idea that was not well received by colleagues or hospital administrators. Without the necessary support to proceed, he left Massachusetts General Hospital and founded his own hospital in which he put his theories about evaluation into practice. In 1924, he described his concept of "end result": "It is that every hospital should track each patient with the object of ascertaining whether the maximum benefit has been obtained and to find out if not, why not" (Codman, 2009, pp. 2766–2770).

Dr. Codman kept cards on each of his patients in his newly established hospital. On each card he wrote how he had treated the patient and whether his treatment helped or hurt. Patients with similar conditions were placed on the same wards, and he suggested that they be placed under the care of a physician with specialized knowledge about the condition. Codman collected patient information during a hospital stay and analyzed it to determine the success or failure of medical care. He encouraged his colleagues to do as he did, but very few shared his enthusiasm or curiosity. The more he exhorted members of the medical community to examine the results of their interventions, the more they distanced themselves from him. The preoccupation with using patient outcomes to learn about improving care changed the course of his life and resulted in some success. Codman integrated his ideas into projects and published works, which received acclaim during his lifetime. However, he was never able to convince his colleagues that evaluating medical care would lead to improved patient health (Donabedian, 1989).

A more recent physician leader in quality improvement was Avedis Donabedian, who developed a model for health care evaluation that is still widely used. Born in 1919, Dr. Donabedian spent a major portion of his professional career teaching and writing at the University of Michigan (Suñol, 2000). He discerned that health care outcomes could not be measured in isolation (Mulley, 1989); rather, they must be viewed within the context of the quality of care (Donabedian, 1980). He understood that methodologies must differ on the basis of the perspective of the evaluation. That is, the methods used to evaluate the quality of care provided to an individual patient are different from the methods used to evaluate system or population outcomes (Donabedian, 1980).

Donabedian (1980) defined *quality* as "a judgment concerning the process of care, based on the extent to which care contributes to valued outcomes." He outlined indicators of *structure, process*, and *outcome* as pathways to evaluating quality of care. He described *structure* as "the relatively stable characteristics of the providers of care, of the tools and resources they have at their disposal and of the physical and organizational settings in which they work" (Donabedian, 1980). He described *process* as "a set of activities that go on within and between practitioners and patients" and *outcomes* as "a change in a patient's current and future health status that can be attributed to antecedent health care" (Donabedian, 1980).

Each of these leaders had an unswerving dedication to improving patient health outcomes. They all had the clarity of vision to see the link between practitioner–patient-system interactions and health status and the perseverance to continue their work regardless of the obstacles. Their influence continues to impact health care evaluation and quality improvement science today.

NEGLECT OF EVALUATION

There are many reasons for the considerable amount of resources being spent on developing new interventions and programs whereas comparatively little is being spent on evaluating them. First, the concept of evaluation itself is threatening. Most practitioners follow care protocols they believe will produce good outcomes if applied competently. Evaluating care can be seen as questioning the practitioners' personal dedication, knowledge, and skills.

Second, the available evidence may be insufficient to determine whether a treatment or project is really effective. Practitioners may follow protocols and still have poor outcomes because they are doing the wrong thing right. The standard of care is only as good as the evidence supporting it.

Third, evaluation is difficult, complex, and dynamic (Mulley, 1989). For example, in the intensive care unit, practitioners must adjust to patient demographic characteristics and prior health status before measuring patient outcomes. Age, gender, socioeconomic status, and severity of illness all factor into developing a case mix. Feasibility must also be considered. Tracking indicators of care over a long period of time may be essential to determine whether a program benefits a population, but this may be seen as too costly and impractical.

Fourth, technology keeps changing at a rapid pace. Practitioners may find themselves in the middle of evaluating a program when new information or a new technique makes the current program obsolete. Finally, innovation is exciting and often brings funding and acclaim to a system or institution. Evaluation can seem to be a necessary but tedious process that diverts resources and time away from patient care (Bloom et al., 1999).

The case of hormone replacement therapy (HRT) is a good example of the complexities inherent in evaluating interventions. Practitioners had long recognized that HRT provided relief to menopausal women from the effects of vasomotor symptoms such as hot flashes and night sweats. During the 1990s, reviews of mainly observational studies suggested that HRT had additional benefits, including a decrease in both cardiovascular disease and hip fractures (Barrett-Connor et al., 2005; Shook, 2011). HRT treatment for all menopausal women became the standard of care, and prescriptions soared, climbing to 91 million in 2001 (Hersch et al., 2004). Practitioners followed protocols and diligently recommended HRT to their patients because they thought it was the right thing to do. Patients learned about the importance of hormone therapy from newspaper articles, the Internet, and TV and were glad to take a pill that might prevent serious and debilitating disorders. A few practitioners may have observed adverse events among their patients but probably not enough to be alarming. An individual practitioner lacked the sample size to detect a significant increase in morbidity or mortality.

Findings from the Women's Health Initiative Estrogen Plus Progestin Trial (WHI-EPT) and the Heart and Estrogen/Progestin Replacement Study (HERS) were released (Hulley et al., 1998; Rossouw et al., 2002). These studies were randomized controlled trials and involved thousands of women. Depending on the kind of hormone medication prescribed, the results indicated that women on HRT had an increased risk for certain cardiovascular diseases and cancers. The number of prescriptions plummeted as the standard of care changed, and practitioners became more cautious in their treatment. This case illustrates that an individual practitioner frequently lacks the resources and expertise to evaluate a new and widely accepted intervention that becomes the standard of care. It is also an example of practitioners unwittingly doing the wrong thing right.

SUMMARY

This chapter acquainted DNP students and graduates with the basic definitions, conceptual/theoretical dimensions, and processes related to evaluation, and highlighted the expectation to evaluate within the Essentials (AACN, 2006) documents for DNP education. The message is clear: DNPs are responsible and accountable to conduct evaluations. The fundamental purpose of evaluation is to provide information for decision-making. Within the backdrop of a developing body of knowledge about evaluation, the DNP must understand what is possible methodologically and what outcomes one can expect. The 2021 Essentials further underscore the role of advanced practice nurses in evaluation.

There are many ways to conduct evaluations, and professional evaluators tend to agree that there is no "one best way" to do any evaluation. Instead, good evaluation requires carefully thinking through the questions that need to be answered, what is being evaluated, and the way in which the information generated will be used. Subsequent chapters will lead the DNP down a path to an increased understanding of evaluations in specific areas of interest in health care.

RESOURCES

American Evaluation Association. (2018). American Evaluation Association guiding principles for evaluators 2018 updated guiding principles. https://www.eval .org/p/cm/ld/fid=51

- Links to Assessment and Evaluation Resources—List of links to resources on several topics
- Glossaries

REFERENCES

Altschuld, J. H. W, & Kumar, D. D. (2010). *Needs assessment: An overview.* Sage.
American Association of Colleges of Nursing. (2006). *The essentials of doctoral education for advanced nursing practice.* Author.
American Association of Colleges of Nursing. (2011). *The essentials of master's education in nursing.* Author.
American Association of Colleges of Nursing. (2019). *AACN's vision for academic nursing.* Author.

American Association of Colleges of Nursing. (2021). *The essentials: Core competencies for professional nursing education*. Author. https://www.aacnnursing.org/Portals/42/AcademicNursing/pdf/Essentials-2021.pdf

American College of Surgeons. (2010). *History and archives of the American College of Surgeons: Ernest A. Codman*. https://www.facs.org/about%20acs/archives/pasthighlights/codmanhighlight

American Evaluation Association. (2018). *Principle of evaluation*. Retrieved March 15, 2020, from https://www.eval.org/p/cm/ld/fid=51

American Nurses Association. (2015). *Nursing: Scope and standards of practice* (3rd ed.). Author.

Artiga, S., & Hinton, E. (2018). Beyond health care: *The role of social determinants in promoting health and health equity*. Henry J Kaiser Family Foundation. Retrieved April 24, 2020, from http://files.kff.org/attachment/issue-brief-beyond-health-care

Barrett-Connor, E., Grady, D., & Stefanick, M. L. (2005). The rise and fall of menopausal hormone therapy. *Annual Review of Public Health*, 26, 115–140. https://doi.org/101146/annurev.publhealth.26.021304.144637

Bau, I., Logan, R. A., Dizil, C., Rosof, B., Fernandez, A., Paasche-Orlow, M. K., & Wong, W. F. (2019). Patient-centered integrated health care quality measures could improve health literacy, language access, and cultural competence. NAM Perspectives. Discussion Paper, National Academy of Medicine. https://researcherprofiles.org/profile/79296679

Berwick, D. M., Nolan, T. W., & Whittington, J. (2008). The triple aim: Care, health, and cost. *Health Affairs*, 27(3), 759–769. https://doi.org/10.1377/hlthaff.27.3.759

Bloom, M., Fischer, J., & Orme, J. G. (1999). *Evaluating practice-guidelines for the accountable professional*. Allyn & Bacon.

Borrell-Carrió, F., Suchman, A. L., & Epstein, R. M. (2004). The biopsychosocial model 25 years later: Principles, practice, and scientific inquiry. *The Annals of Family Medicine*, 2(6), 576–582. https://doi.org/10.1370/afm.245

Brook, R. H., & Lohr, K. N. (1985). Efficacy, effectiveness, variations, and quality. Boundary crossing research. *Medical Care*, 23(5), 710–722. https://doi.org/10.1097/00005650-198505000-00030

Burke, J. (2013). *Health analytics: Gaining the insights to transform health care*. John Wiley and Sons.

Centers for Disease Control and Prevention. (n.d.). *Types of research*. Retrieved March 12, 2020, from https://www.cdc.gov/std/Program/pupestd/Types%20of%20Evaluation.pdf

Centers for Disease Control and Prevention. (2010). *Defining public health research and public health non-research*. https://www.cdc.gov/od/science/integrity/docs/cdc-policy-distinguishing-public-health-research-nonresearch.pdf

Centers for Disease Control and Prevention. (2011). *Principles of community engagement* (2nd ed.). http://www.atsdr.cdc.gov/communityengagement/pdf/PCE_Report_508_FINAL.pdf

Clarke, G. M., Conti, S., Wolters, A. T., & Steventon, A. (2019). Evaluating the impact of healthcare interventions using routine data. *BMJ (Clinical Research ed.)*, 365, l2239. https://doi.org/10.1136/bmj.l2239

Codman, E. A. (2009). The registry of bone sarcomas as an example of the end-result idea in hospital organization. *Clinical Orthopaedics and Related Research*, 467, 2766–2770. https://doi.org/10.1007/s11999-009-1048-7

Commonwealth Fund. (2015). *Mirror, mirror on the wall: 2014 update: How the U.S. health care system compares internationally*. http://www.commonwealthfund.org/publications/fund-reports/2014/jun/mirror-mirror

D'Errico, S, Geoghegan, T., & Piergallini, I. (2020). Evaluation to connect national priorities with the SDGs: *A guide for evaluation commissioners and managers*. IIED. https://evalsdgs.org/wp-content/uploads/2020/02/Evaluation-to-connect-national-priorities-with-the-SDGs.pdf

Donabedian, A. (1980). *Explorations in quality assessment and monitoring. Vol. 1. The definition of quality and approaches to its assessment*. Health Administration Press.

Donabedian, A. (1989). The end results of health care: Ernest Codman's contribution to quality assessment and beyond. *Milbank Quarterly*, 67(2), 233–261. PMID: 2698445.

Donabedian, A. (2003). *An introduction to quality assurance in health care*. Oxford University Press.

Drummond, M. F., Sculpher, M. J., Torrance. G. W., O'Briend, B. J., & Stoddart, G. L. (2005). *Methods for the economic evaluation of health care programmes*. Oxford University Press.

Engel, G. (1977). The need for a new medical model: A challenge for biomedicine. *Science*, 196, 129–136. https://doi.org/10.1126/science.847460

Fitzpatrick, J. L., Sanders, J. R., & Worthen, B. R. (2004). *Program evaluation: Alternative approaches and practical guidelines*. Pearson Education.

Hawe, P., Degeling, D., & Hall, J. (1990). *Evaluating health promotion: A health worker's guide.* MacLennan & Petty.

Hersch, A. L., Stefanick, M. L., & Stafford, R. S. (2004). National use of postmenopausal hormone therapy. *JAMA, 291*(1), 47–53. https://doi.org/10.1001/jama.291.1.47

Hulley, S., Grady, D., Bush, E., Furberg, C., Herrington, D., Riggs, B., & Vittinghoff, E. (1998). Randomized trial of estrogen plus progestin for secondary prevention of coronary heart disease in postmenopausal women. Heart and Estrogen/Progestin Replacement Study (HERS) Research Group. *JAMA, 280*(7), 605–613. https://doi.org/10.1001/jama.280.7.605

Hood, C. M., Gennuso, K. P., Swain, G. R., & Catlin, B. B. (2016). County health rankings: Relationships between determinant factors and health outcomes. *American Journal of Preventive Medicine, 50*(2), 129–135. https://doi.org/10.1016/j.amepre.2015.08.024

Institute of Healthcare Improvement. (2012). IHI triple aim initiative. http://www.ihi.org/Engage/Initiatives/TripleAim/pages/default.aspx

Institute of Healthcare Improvement. (2020a). Flowchart. Retrieved April 22, 2020, from http://www.ihi.org/resources/Pages/Tools/Flowchart.aspx

Institute of Healthcare Improvement. (2020b). IHI model for improvement. Retrieved March 31, 2020, from http://www.ihi.org/resources/Pages/HowtoImprove/default.aspx

Institute of Medicine. (1990). *Medicare: A strategy for quality assurance* (Vol. 1). National Academies Press.

Institute of Medicine. (1999). *To err is human: Building a safer health system.* National Academies Press.

Institute of Medicine. (2001). *Crossing the quality chasm: A new health system for the 21st century.* National Academies Press.

Institute of Medicine. (2002). *The future of the public's health in the 21st century.* National Academies Press.

Institute of Medicine. (2003). *Health professions education: A bridge to quality.* National Academies Press.

Institute of Medicine. (2010). *The future of nursing: Leading change, advancing health.* National Academies Press.

Izumi, S. (2012). Quality improvement in nursing: Administrative mandate or professional responsibility? *Nursing Forum, 47*(4), 260–267. https://doi.org/10.1111/j.1744-6198.2012.00283.x

James, J. T. (2013). A new, evidence-based estimate of patient harms associated with hospital care. *Journal of Patient Safety, 9*(3), 122–128. https://doi.org/10.1097/PTS.0b013e3182948a69

Kellogg Foundation. (2017). *The step-by-step guide to evaluation: How to become savvy evaluations consumers—November 2017.* https://www.wkkf.org/resource-directory/resources/2017/11/the-step-by-step-guide-to-evaluation--how-to-become-savvy-evaluation-consumers

Kindig, D., & Stoddart, G. (2003). What is population health? *American Journal of Public Health, 93*(3), 380–383. https://doi.org/10.2105/ajph.93.3.380

LoBiondo-Wood, G., & Haber, J. (2014). *Nursing research: Methods and critical appraisal for evidence-based practice* (8th ed., p. 171). Elsevier.

Magnan, S. (2017). *Social determinants of health 101 for health care.* National Academy of Medicine. NAM.edu/Perspectives.

McGuire, M. (2016, May). *Program design & development resources.* United Way of Toronto and York Region.

Mulley, A. G. (1989). E. A. Codman and the end results idea: A commentary. *Milbank Quarterly, 67*(2), 257–261. https://doi.org/10.2307/3350140

Nanda, V. (2017). 7 types of evaluation you need to know. https://humansofdata.atlan.com/2017/04/7-types-of-evaluation/

National Academy of Medicine. (2020). The future of nursing 2020-2030. https://nam.edu/publications/the-future-of-nursing-2020-2030/

National Center for Health Statistics. (2020). *Healthy People 2030: NCHS fact sheet, August 2020.* https://www.cdc.gov/nchs/about/factsheets/factsheet-hp2030.htm

National Patient Safety Foundation's Lucian Leape Institute. (2015). *Shining a light: Safer health care through transparency.* Author.

National Research Council of the National Academies. (2005). *Advancing the nation's health needs: NIH research training programs.* National Academies Press.

Nelson, E. C., Batalden, P. B., & Godfrey, M. M. (Eds.). (2007). *Quality by design: A clinical microsystems approach.* Jossey-Bass.

Nelson, E. C., Batalden, P. B., Godfrey, M. M., & Lazar, J. D. (Eds.). (2011). *Value by design: Developing clinical microsystems to achieve organizational excellence.* Jossey-Bass.

Nightingale, F. (1859). *Notes on nursing: What it is, and what it is not.* Compass Circle.

Ogrinc, G. S., Headrick, L. A., Barton, A. J., Dolansky, M. A., Madigosky, W. S., & Miltner, R. S. (2018). *Fundamentals of health care improvement: A Guide to improving your patients' care* (3rd ed.). The Joint Commission Resources.

Porter, M. E. (2010). What is value in health care? *New England Journal of Medicine, 363,* 2477–2481. https://doi.org/10.1056/NEJMp1011024

Rickert, J. (2012). Patient-centered care: What it means and how to get there. http://healthaffairs.org/blog/2012/01/24/patient-centered-care-what-it-means-and-how-to-get-there/

Robert Wood Johnson Foundation. (2013). Quality/equality glossary. http://www.rwjf.org/en/library/research/2013/04/quality-equality-glossary.html

Rossi, P. H., Lipsey, M. W., & Henry, G. T. (2019). *Evaluation: A systematic approach* (8th ed.). Sage.

Rossouw, J. E., Anderson, G. L., Prentice, R. L., LaCroix, A. Z., Kooperberg, C., Stefanick, M. L., Jackson, R. D., Beresford, S. A. A., Howard, B. V., Johnson, K. C., Kotchen, J. M., Ockene, J., Writing Group for the Women's Health Initiative Investigators. (2002). Risks and benefits of estrogen plus progestin in healthy postmenopausal women: Principal results from the women's health initiative randomized controlled trial. *JAMA, 288*(3), 321–333. https://doi.org/10.1001/jama.288.3.321

Royal College of Nursing. (2020). What person-cantered care means. Retrieved February 24, 2020, from http://rcnhca.org.uk/sample-page/what-person-centred-care-means

Saba, V. K., & McCormick, K. A. (2015). *Essentials of nursing informatics* (6th ed.). McGraw-Hill.

Salmond, S. W., & Echevarria, M. (2017). Healthcare transformation and changing roles for nursing. *Orthopedic Nursing, 36*(1), 12–25. https://doi.org/10.1097/NOR.0000000000000308

Scriven, M. (1991). *Evaluation thesaurus* (4th ed.). Sage.

Scriven, M. (1993). *Hard-won lessons in program evaluation* (New Directions for Program Evaluation, No. 58). Jossey-Bass.

Shook, L. L. (2011). An update on hormone replacement therapy: Health and medicine for women: A multidisciplinary, evidence-based review of mid-life health concerns. *The Yale Journal of Biology and Medicine, 84*(1), 39–42. https://www.ncbi.nlm.nih.gov/pmc/articles/PMC3064244/

Sidani, S., & Braden, C. J. (2011). *Design, evaluation, and translation of nursing interventions.* Wiley-Blackwell.

Spiegelhalter, D. J. (1999). Surgical audit: Statistical lessons from Nightingale and Codman. *Journal of the Royal Statistical Society A, 162*(Pt. 1), 45–58. https://www.jstor.org/stable/2680466

Starfield, B., Hyde, J., Gervas, J., & Heath, I. (2008). The concept of prevention: A good idea gone astray? *Journal of Epidemiology & Community Health, 62,* 580–583. https://doi.org/10.1136/jech.2007.071027

Suñol, R. (2000). Avedis Donabedian. *International Journal for Quality in Health Care, 12*(6), 451–454. https://doi.org/10.1093/intqhc/12.6.451

U.S. Department of Health and Human Services. (2020). *Healthy People 2030: Building a healthier future for all.* https://health.gov/healthypeople

Wikipedia. (2020a). Evaluation. Retrieved April 1, 2020, from https://en.wikipedia.org/wiki/Evaluation#cite_ref-2

Wikipedia. (2020b). Problem statement. Retrieved March 17, 2020, from https://en.wikipedia.org/wiki/Problem_statement

World Health Organization. (2019a). WHO definition of health. Retrieved March 31, 2020, from https://www.google.com/search?ei=tZuDXraQGILIsAWnxJOACA&q=who+definition+of+health+2019&oq=WHO+definition+of+health&gs_lcp=CgZwc3ktYWIQARgAMgQIABBHMgQIABBHMgQIABBHMgQIABBHMgQIABBHMgQIABBHMgQIABBHUABYAGC5WmgAcAJ4AIABAIgBAJIBAJgBAKoBB2d3cy13aXo&sclient=psy-ab

World Health Organization. (2019b). What are the social determinants of health? Retrieved March 24, 2020, from https://www.who.int/social_determinants/sdh_definition/en/

TWO

THE NATURE OF EVIDENCE AS A BASIS FOR EVALUATION

Joanne V. Hickey

It ain't so much what you don't know that gets you into
trouble, it's what you know for sure that just ain't so.
—*Mark Twain*

INTRODUCTION

Evaluation is based on collecting, analyzing, organizing, and critically reviewing evidence to make a judgment or decision about value. This chapter defines evidence from a generic perspective and discusses the sources and classification of evidence in its many forms. It describes how evidence is organized and ranked, addresses evidence integrity, and examines how evidence is used and interpreted for evaluation. This information provides a basis for exploring how Doctor of Nursing Practice (DNP) graduates acquire and use evidence for evaluation. This chapter is organized around a broad discussion of evidence and then focuses on the use of evidence by DNP-prepared nurses. Evidence, within the context of evidence-based practice in patient-centered clinical practice, is discussed in Chapter 10.

EVIDENCE

The word *evidence* comes from Middle English via Latin (*evidentia*— obvious to the eye or mind) and Old French (*evidence*— appearance from which inferences may be drawn). Evidence, as a broad and generic concept, is information presented to support or dispute an assertion. This support may be strong or weak. The strongest type of evidence is that which provides direct proof of the truth of an assertion. At the other extreme is evidence that is merely consistent with an assertion but that does not rule out other, contradictory assertions. The presence of bias often influences the credibility of how evidence is perceived. Further discussion of the strength of evidence is found later in this chapter.

The word *evidence* can be a noun or a verb. For the purposes of this discussion, only *evidence* as a noun is addressed. According to Webster's Dictionary, evidence is "a condition of being evident; something that makes something else evident; and something that tends to prove or to provide grounds for belief." Evidence is a single fact or collection of facts believed to be true. Evidence is that which is accepted as conclusive (e.g., clear, obvious, acceptable, confirmed) support of a statement (Angeles, 1992, p. 97). To have evidence is to have some conceptual warrant for belief or action (Goodman, 2003, p. 2).

Evidence has also been defined as:

- Facts or physical signs that help to prove or disprove something.
- The basis of belief; the substantiation or confirmation that is needed in order to believe that something is true or false (Pearson et al., 2005).
- The available facts and circumstances supporting or refuting a belief or proposition or indicating whether something is true or valid (Pearsall & Trumble, 1995).

From a clinical practice perspective, evidence can also be viewed as external and internal evidence.

External evidence is generated through rigorous research (e.g., randomized controlled trials [RCTs], observational studies) and is intended to be generalized to and used in other settings (Melnyk & Fineout-Overholt, 2015). By comparison, *internal evidence* is generated through practice initiatives, such as quality improvement and evidence-based practice projects, that use internal evidence generated from patient, provider, and organizational data within an organization to improve clinical care. Internal evidence can also be viewed as *local evidence*, that is, evidence generated as a result of the interaction of contextual, organizational, microsystem, community, provider, and patient population characteristics. Although internal evidence is not generalizable, it is transferable to other settings.

Empirical Perspective of Evidence

When health professionals talk about evidence, they are generally referring to empirical evidence. *Empirical evidence* (also known as scientific evidence) is information ascertained by *observation* and *experimentation* that serves to support, refute, or modify a scientific hypothesis or theory when collected and interpreted in accordance with the scientific method. The scientific methods follow systematic, logical, and specific principles that guide the pursuit of knowledge from problem identification, to development of a plan for investigation, to deliberate collection of selected data through a variety of measurement methods (e.g., observation, instrumentation, and experimentation), to formulation and testing of hypotheses, to analysis of data to formulate data-based conclusions. Through the investigation of a phenomenon, new knowledge, or connection or integration of previously known knowledge, occurs to further expand knowledge in a given area. *Data integrity* refers to the accuracy and consistency (validity) of data over their life cycle. The term *data integrity* may be confusing because it may refer to either a state or a process. *Data integrity as a state* defines a data set that is both valid and accurate. However, *data integrity as a process* describes measures used to ensure validity and accuracy of a data set or all data contained in a database or other construct. For example, error checking and validation methods may be referred to as data integrity processes (Brook, 2019).

The scientific method is generally synonymous with the acquisition of credible knowledge through various research designs and methods. The following briefly describes qualitative, quantitative, and mixed methods design for generation of knowledge.

Quantitative Research Methods

Quantitative research is the systematic empirical investigation of observable phenomena via statistical, mathematical, or computational techniques (Given, 2008). The focus of quantitative research is to develop and employ mathematical models, theories, and/or hypotheses pertinent to the phenomena. The measurement process is central to quantitative research because it provides the fundamental connection between empirical observation and mathematical expression of quantitative relationships (Given, 2008). Quantitative data are any data that are in numerical form, such as counts or percentages. This means that the quantitative investigator asks a specific, narrow question and collects a sample of numerical data from observable phenomena, study participants, or instruments/scales/surveys. The investigator analyzes the data using statistics. The findings may be generalized to some larger population. Quantitative methodologies have been the dominant approach to empirical research recognized for methodological rigor, and the RCT is still considered the gold standard for high-quality research.

Qualitative Research Methods

An appreciation of the value of qualitative methodologies has been recognized in knowledge development. By comparison to quantitative research, *qualitative research* addresses broad questions and collects word data about phenomena or from participants. The investigator searches for themes and describes the information in themes and patterns exclusive to that set of participants so that generalizability of research findings is not an expectation. Qualitative methods are often used when there is little known about a phenomenon in order to define the dimensions or domains of the concept for further clarification and concept development.

Mixed Method

A *mixed methods* design has gained favor as a research methodology that involves collecting, analyzing, and integrating quantitative (e.g., experiments, surveys) and qualitative (e.g., focus groups, interviews) research. It is a mix of including both qualitative and quantitative methodologies to answer a research question in order to provide a comprehensive answer to the research questions that would not be possible in using only one methodology. The overall goal of mixed methods research is to expand and strengthen a study's conclusions and, therefore, contribute to the published literature. A mixed method design should contribute to answering research questions that could not be answered by the use of either qualitative or quantitative designs exclusively.

Technology and Statistical Methods for Generation of Evidence/Knowledge

The phenomenal and rapid advances in technology, computational and statistical methods, and informatics have had a profound impact on health care and its ability to collect, warehouse, and analyze huge amounts of data to inform practice and clinical care. Medical devices with computer applications, also known as apps, are revamping health care services by integrating data from remote health monitoring systems such as wearables to monitor and manage patient care. We now live in a world consisting of cloud storage, the Internet of Things (IoT), 5G speed, and artificial intelligence (AI), designed to enable connectivity of huge amounts of data for deep analysis to uncover patterns and knowledge previously unavailable and do it in unbelievably compressed time frames. Basic descriptions of these terms are provided as a basis for discussion.

Cloud storage is a cloud computing model in which data are stored on remote servers accessed from the Internet or "cloud." It is maintained, operated, and managed by a cloud storage service provider; data are stored on storage servers that are built on virtualization techniques (Techopedia, 2020a). This means large amounts of data can be stored, and qualified users can access the data.

The *IoT* is a network of physical devices and other items, embedded with electronics, software, sensors, remote monitoring devices, and network connectivity, which enable these objects to collect and exchange data (Zanella et al., 2014). The advent of electronic medical records (EMR) has ushered in the convergence of health care, which is being transformed by information technology. One of the major challenges to the implementation of the IoT is communication among the many devices, some of which have proprietary protocols so that sensors from different manufacturers can't necessarily speak with each other. This fragmented software environment, coupled with privacy concerns and the bureaucratic tendency to hoard all collected information, frequently stifles valuable information on data islands, undermining the fundamental purpose of the IoT (Kruse et al., 2016). However, as these issues continue to be addressed and resolved, the potential future for IoT in health care is revolutionary.

The term *5G* is the 5th generation mobile network released in 2019. It is a new global wireless standard after 1G, 2G, 3G, and 4G networks. 5G enables a new kind of network that is designed to connect virtually everyone and everything together, including machines, objects, and devices. 5G wireless technology offers higher speed than 4G, ultralow latency, increased reliability, massive network capacity, increased availability, and a more uniform user experience to more users. Higher performance and improved efficiency empower new user experiences and connect new industries (Qual Communications, 2020).

AI, also known as machine intelligence, is a branch of computer science that creates software that can analyze data sets using either predetermined rules and search algorithms or pattern recognizing machine learning models and then make decisions on the basis of those analyses. AI attempts to mimic human intelligence to allow the software application or system to act with varying degrees of autonomy, thereby reducing manual human intervention for a wide range of functions. AI does its work at lightning speed and can manage complex data sets that humans could not address (Techopedia, 2020b).

The convergence of these and other technological innovations provides a platform for the generation of huge amounts of data as a source of new knowledge development and learning to improve health care for populations and individuals. Two examples of approaches to uncover new information and knowledge used in health care are big data and data mining.

BIG DATA

The remarkable rapid development of computer technology capacity that can support exabytes (2.5×10^{18}) of data has made it possible to work with huge data sets. The concept of big data is deceiving in that it appears to relate only to volume of data when, in fact, it also reflects the technology (e.g., tools and processes) required to manage and work with the large amounts of data and its storage. The term *big data* is relative and represents a massive volume of both structured, semistructured, and unstructured data that is so large that it is difficult to process using traditional database and software techniques. The sheer volume of data and the ongoing rapid addition to a database often exceed current processing capacity. Although big data currently does not refer to any specific quantity, the term is often used when speaking about petabytes and exabytes of data (De Mauro et al., 2015). A big data set might be exabytes (1,024 petabytes) of data, consisting of billions of data elements from records of millions of people, all from different sources. The data are typically loosely structured and often incomplete and inaccessible. Magaoulas and Lorica (2009) note that the term *big data* is relative and that it depends on the capabilities of the users and their tools. What is considered big data today will become ordinary data in the not-too-distant future.

In health care, big data refers to collecting, analyzing, and leveraging consumer, patient, physical, and clinical data that are too vast or complex to be understood by traditional means of data processing. An example of a big data set is the Healthcare Effectiveness Data and Information Set (HEDIS), a data set used by most American health care plans to measure performance on dimensions of care and service. Big data might consist of millions of data elements from diverse sources such as EMR, diagnostics, laboratory data, monitoring data, medical histories, and outcomes. These data come in both structured and unstructured forms. Big data in health care is important because it can be used in the prediction of outcome of diseases, prevention of comorbidities, mortality, effectiveness of treatments, prognosis, and cost of treatment. *Health care data management* is the process of storing, protecting, and analyzing data extracted from diverse sources. Managing the wealth of available health care data allows health systems to create holistic views of patients, personalize treatments, improve communication, and enhance health outcomes.

A common definition of big data is based on the three Vs of volume, velocity, and variety, to which have been added variability, veracity, and complexity. A consensual definition states that "big data represents the information assets characterized by a high volume, velocity, and variety to require specific technology and analytical methods for its transformation into value" (De Mauro et al., 2015, p. 156). The following describes the three Vs (i.e., volume, velocity, and variety) plus other characteristics (i.e., variability, variability, and complexity) addressed in the consensual definition.

Volume addresses the quantity of generated data and is important to the context of big data, the bigness of data, and its potential usefulness. Multiple factors have contributed to the increase in data volume, including accumulating previously collected stored data, unstructured data from social media, and increasing use of new sources of data collection and storage such as EMR. A substantial decrease in the cost of data storage has supported further increases in the volume of data and has precipitated issues about the determination of relevance within large data sets and how to use analytics to create value from relevant data. The term *velocity* refers to the speed of generation of data. The amount of data generated each day is unprecedented and will only increase in the future. How to organize and access these data streams for added value is challenging. *Variety* addresses the types of data and format of data, including structured, semistructured, and unstructured forms. The challenge is to manage, merge, and administer their use according to ethical and constructive practices.

The term *variability* refers to the inconsistency that can be evident in the data at times, thus hampering the process of being able to handle and manage the data effectively. *Veracity* refers to the quality of the data and recognizing that the data being captured can vary greatly. Statistical techniques are used to examine data quality before data analysis. Verification of the "cleanliness" of data is critical because it directly affects the analytical accuracy of the data set. Finally, the notion of *complexity* must be considered. Data management can become a very complex process, especially when large volumes of data come from multiple sources. These data need to be linked, connected, and correlated in order to be able to grasp the comprehensive information that is supposed to be conveyed by these data.

DATA MINING

Data mining is briefly mentioned as a way of extracting patterns from data sets that may include big data as well as smaller data sets that can be managed by more conventional technology and statistical methods.*Data mining* is defined as a method of querying large databases in order to discover patterns within the data to generate new information. The term "data mining" is deceiving because the goal of data mining is the extraction of patterns and knowledge from large amounts of data, not the extraction (*mining*) of data itself (Han et al., 2012). Data mining involves effective data collection and warehousing as well as sophisticated computer processing such as machine learning and statistical modes to uncover patterns in large data sets. *Knowledge discovery in data (KDD)* is another term used for data mining. Although the statistical techniques used for data mining are beyond the focus of this chapter, what can be underscored is the nurse–statistician collaboration. Nurses provide the clinical questions that need to be answered in clinical practice, including its context, and the statistician provides the statistical expertise to help answer the question.

We live in a world where vast amounts of data are collected daily in clinical practice. These data are a gold mine of information to be examined to determine patterns that can inform practice. Analyzing such data is important to inform and improve health care. Big data have the potential to influence health care in five ways—reducing cost, increasing access to complete information, supporting better preventive care, personalizing diagnosis and care, and improving evaluation (Dimitrov, 2016).

Evidence-Based Practice Perspective of Evidence

Evidence-based practice is defined as the conscientious and judicious use of current best evidence in conjunction with clinical expertise, patient values, and circumstances to guide health care decisions (LoBiondo-Wood et al., 2019). Although there are many definitions of evidence-based practice, the key components include best scientific evidence, expert opinion, and patient preference. In evidence-based practice, the term *evidence* is used deliberately instead of *proof* to note important differences. Evidence can be so weak that it is not convincing, and thus has little or no value, or it can be so strong that no one doubts its correctness. Therefore, it is important to be able to determine the quality and strength of evidence to determine its value. A number of levels of evidence pyramids have been developed for this purpose and specify a hierarchical order based on various sources of evidence such as research designs and their internal validity (Center for Evidence-Based Management, n.d.). Methods to evaluate the quality of evidence are addressed later in this chapter.

Data, Information, Knowledge, and Wisdom Model

Evidence that takes the form of data, information, knowledge, and wisdom requires some discussion. The data, information, knowledge, and wisdom (DIKW) model, also known as the DIKW hierarchy, has evolved over time from a five-level model (i.e., data, information, knowledge, understanding, and wisdom) to a four-level model, which is described here. Data, information, and knowledge are sometimes used interchangeably in practice and evaluation. Therefore, clear definitions are essential to understand the model (Bellinger et al., 2004).

- *Datum* (singular; plural: *data*) is a single discrete element or symbol that has been described objectively but has not been interpreted. It is an individual fact, figure, or measurement. An example of datum is a single blood pressure reading, a numerical value without any interpretation, meaning, or context.
- *Information* is defined as data that have been organized, linked, interpreted, structured, and categorized (American Nurses Association, 2015). It provides *context* to data. Ackoff (1989) noted that information is data that are processed to be useful; it provides answers to "who," "what," "where," and "when" questions.
- *Knowledge* includes ideas, notions, concepts, synthesis, comparison, learning, and discussion, and thus provides *meaning*.
- *Wisdom* is defined as evaluated understanding, integration, application, reflection, and understanding of principles, patterns, and evaluation of the accumulated knowledge. It provides *insight* and suggests application of knowledge, including new and innovative ways.

Ackoff (1989) noted that the first three categories (i.e., data, information, knowledge) relate to the past and what has been or what is known. However, wisdom is focused on the future because it deals with visioning and designing the future. Note that the original Ackoff model included understanding along with data, information, and knowledge. In the current four-level models, understanding is considered part of wisdom. See Table 2.1.

In summary, it is clear that evidence is all around you, but it comes in various forms that provide some direction to the evaluation of the strength and value of the evidence.

FOUNDATIONS OF THOUGHT

The next section examines the origins of Western thinking and the philosophical underpinnings of thought to better understand the foundations and models on which evidence has developed.

TABLE 2.1   Data, Information, Knowledge, and Wisdom (DIKW) Model

Term	Definition/Description	Example
Data	Symbols; elements Exist in and of themselves and have no significance beyond existence Do not have meaning by themselves Exist in both usable and nonusable forms	Single blood pressure, pulse, or serum glucose reading Overall budget amount
Information	Data that are processed and have been given meaning by connecting them to something The meaning provided may or may not be useful Provides answers to "who," "what," "where," and "when" questions	Notice trend regarding decrease in satisfaction score after elimination of receptionist in clinic
Knowledge	Application of data and information Collection of information organized to be useful It is not at the level of integration Provides answers to how something works Answers "how" questions	Recognizing the fit of using complexity science as a framework to understand implementation of electronic medical records in a health care organization
Wisdom	Evaluates understanding based on an integration and synthesis of cumulative knowledge and experience and inclusion of a moral and ethical context to provide insight and high-level understanding to complex and not easily answered questions From knowledge, a cognitive and analytical process of applying and appreciating relationships Process by which knowledge can be synthesized into new knowledge by combining other knowledge with current knowledge to create something new	Ability to appreciate the ethical and moral impact of providing access to care for all members of a society

Western Models

Western models of thinking can be traced back to ancient Greek–Roman times and the development of what we now call philosophy, knowledge, and science. *Philosophy* is defined as the pursuit of wisdom, a search for meaning, and represents a perspective and set of beliefs and understandings about reality and values. The word *science,* which comes from the Latin word "scientia," means knowledge. It refers to both the processes and outcomes of general laws and observations. General laws are bases of nature that guide physical life, such as the laws of gravity and motion. These laws are used in a systematic way to create a body of knowledge about a specific topic. What developed was a scientific method or systematic process that proves a set of data (evidence) supported by propositions about an area of study (Polifroni, 2018, p. 4). *Knowledge* is the theoretical or practical understanding of a subject. This began the development of ways of viewing and thinking about the world.

Philosophical Foundations

In ancient times, the concept of philosophy included not only what philosophers today would consider philosophy, but also advanced studies such as physics, math, biology, psychology, and political science. As these fields developed a body of knowledge and distinct methodologies, they separated from philosophy and became independent disciplines. For example, epistemology is the branch of philosophy that investigates the origin, nature, methods, validity, and limitations of human knowledge. It also addresses related notions of truth, belief, and justification. Logic is the branch of philosophy that focuses on valid reasoning and dates back to Aristotle. The root of the word *epistemology* comes from the Greek words *epistême* (knowledge) and *logos* (study of).

Roots in Logic

Logic focuses on valid reasoning. A number of terms from logic are threaded into the discussion about evidence such as proposition, inference, premise, induction, deduction, and conclusion. A *proposition* is a statement or declarative sentence that may be true or false. *Inference* is a logical or conceptual process of deriving a statement from one or more other statements (Angeles, 1992, p. 145). For example, because large organizations are complex and the organization under review is large, it is reasonable to assume that the organization under review is complex. A *premise* is defined as a statement that is true or that is believed to be true; it is any statement that serves as the basis for an argument or inference (Angeles, 1992, p. 240). A premise is composed of propositions; when taken together, they form a conclusion. For example, intensive care units within the same facility often have different lengths of stay. Yet these units are part of the same organization. One can surmise that patient acuity and practice patterns must play some part in variation of length of stay.

Inductive reasoning is the process of reasoning from a part to a whole, from a particular instance of something to a general statement, or from particular to universal (Angeles, 1992, p. 144). For example, if using a particular patient-turning device on one unit of a facility is effective in reducing pressure ulcers, then using the device on all other units in the facility should also be effective in reducing pressure ulcers throughout the facility. This statement may or may not be true for a variety of reasons such as variations in patient populations and acuity. *Deductive reasoning* is the process of reasoning from a general truth to a particular instance of a truth, from the general to the particular, or from the universal to the particular. For example, all men have two feet and two arms; John is a man; therefore, John has two feet and two arms. *Deduction* is a form of logical inference that proceeds from observation to a hypothesis that accounts for the reliable data (observation) and seeks to explain relevant evidence. A *conclusion* is a statement that has been inferred from other statements. It is the logical consequence or implication of the premises of an argument (Angeles, 1992, p. 51). In summary, understanding the origins of knowledge, science, and scientific methods helps us to understand the concept of evidence.

Empiricism

Historically, evidence has its roots in empiricism and positivism, a philosophical view that has greatly influenced the perceptions of knowledge in nursing for decades (Billay et al., 2007). *Empiricism* is a branch of philosophy that ties knowledge to experience. It states that all ideas are abstractions formed by combining and recombining what is experienced. Experience is the sole source of knowledge, and all that we know is ultimately dependent on data from the senses. Information provided by the senses serves as the basic building block for all knowledge. *Positivism* is an outgrowth of traditional empiricism attributed to Comte, the 19th century French philosopher, and is based on the belief that the highest or only form of knowledge is the description of sensory phenomena. Comte expounded three stages of human belief: the theological, the metaphysical, and the positive. From a positivist perspective, knowledge is equated to truth that can be discovered.

From an empirical framework, all evidence comes exclusively from one's experiences. What one sees, hears, smells, tastes, and feels through touch are interpreted; that interpretation is one's source of knowledge and the evidence for making sense of everything. Yet an empirical approach to evidence and knowledge is dependent on a number of interrelated factors that include what one experiences as one lives; awareness of those experiences; how one processes and thinks about the experiences (perception); how one talks about those experiences; and how we diagram or sketch the experiences in our minds, thus creating a mental model. Therefore, the sources of evidence based on empiricism are personal observations and experiences along with one's interpretation of those observations or experiences. An example of current work grounded in the empirical tradition is exemplified by the definition of evidence provided by Guyatt et al. (2008), who have published extensively about evidence-based practice. They define *evidence* as an empirical observation that constitutes potential evidence, whether systematically collected or not. Copi and Cohen (2009), in their classic book on logic, note that evidence ultimately refers to experience.

Many would argue that this definition of evidence is a narrow perspective of evidence for the 21st century and one that is prone to bias, which is discussed later in this chapter. Goldberg (2006) argues that rather than empirical evidence, which increases certainty by factoring out the subjective and contextual components of everyday experience that bias understanding, empirical evidence obscures the subjective elements that inescapably enter all forms of human inquiry. From this perspective, evidence is not objective or neutral but rather part of a social system of knowledge production. Although health professionals have been taught to value empirical knowledge above all forms of knowledge, new paradigms are challenging these beliefs and are redefining how health professionals think about the bases of health care and practice.

Critics of empiricism and positivism began with philosophers such as Dewey and others who believed that knowledge was not something that must correspond to some antecedent truth, superimposed reality, or predefined description of the world; rather, knowledge is something emergent and is always interactive with experience and action and, as such, requires continuous interpretation or revised description (Mantzoukas, 2007). Mantzoukas goes on to say that knowledge is inextricably linked with action and is specific. Good action is described as that which works and is effective. Knowledge and advancement of knowledge emerge from interpretive descriptions of the effectiveness or noneffectiveness of one's experiences and actions (Gallagher, 1964). Building on the concept that knowledge emerges from actions and practice experiences, Schön (1983) proposed the concept of *reflection* as a means of acquiring and developing professional knowledge. Schön (1983, 1987) reasoned that research-based knowledge driven by theory resulted in linear, certain, and clear-cut solutions. By comparison, practice is nonlinear, uncertain, complex, and conflicting. Therefore, positivism-based research knowledge does not provide all of the answers to practitioners and does not guarantee best practice. The messy world of practice is often nonlinear and is better understood from the perspective of nonlinear complexity science and models.

NURSING MODELS

Although nursing has embraced empiricism and scientific methods, it has also incorporated other methods to uncover evidence and knowledge for practice. Two important models that have influenced nursing practice are fundamental patterns of knowing and reflective thinking.

Fundamental Patterns of Knowing

Another approach to evidence is to examine how we know. In a seminal article Carper (1978) described four fundamental patterns of knowing in nursing. The first pattern of knowing is *empirical knowing*. The basis of this pattern is positivism, "which believes that objective data, measurement, and generalizability are essential to the generation and dissemination of [nursing] knowledge" (Streubert-Speziale & Carpenter, 2003, p. 4). An example of empirical knowing is knowledge from the physical and biological sciences that helps nurses to understand laws of movement and human physiology. The second pattern of knowing is *aesthetics*. It involves the subjective experience and the creative aspect of nursing care. Although this concept is more difficult to define, Fawcett et al. (2001, p. 6) proposed that aesthetic knowing is "the 'artful' performance of manual and technical skills." It answers the question of "how" a nursing act is performed rather than the key elements of the act. Aesthetic knowing has to do with style and delivery, which is personalized by the nurse for a particular patient. The third way of knowing is *personal knowing*, which involves the nurse as a person. The nurse is present or connects with others, a process often referred to as the therapeutic nurse–patient relationship (Fawcett et al., 2001) or intersubjectivity, the subject-to-subject relationship involving true presence (Parse, 1981, 1992). Presence refers to being totally focused and "being there" with authenticity and honesty in open, honest, and genuine communications. The fourth pattern of knowing is *ethical knowing*, which addresses the ethical and moral component of practice. It guides the nurse about how to behave in a given situation and emanates from an individual's sense of right and wrong. It requires the nurse to understand various philosophical perspectives and accepted standards of conduct and practice regarding what is good, right, and desirable (Billay et al., 2007).

Other scholars have added to Carper's work, including White (1995), who suggested that the fifth way of knowing is *sociopolitical knowing*. This form of knowing relates to how nurses address cultural differences of patients, political awareness, and policy issues and adds to the contextual component of individualized care.

What is clear from this brief overview of knowing is that no single pattern of knowing should be used in isolation from the others because the practice of nursing relies on an integration of all five ways of knowing to provide quality care. Knowing is a form of the stream of evidence that guides practice, including the dimension of evaluation.

Reflective Thinking

Another perspective of evidence is practitioner generated and is called *reflective knowledge*. *Reflection* is described as a process of transforming unconscious types of knowledge and practices into conscious, explicit, and logically articulated knowledge and practices that allow for transparent and justifiable clinical decision-making (Freshwater et al., 2008; Johns & Freshwater, 2005; Mantzoukas, 2007). Two types of reflection are addressed: reflection-in-action and reflection-on-action. *Reflection-in-action* is a cognitive process of observing how we think in the conduct of an action or experience and of adapting our thoughts to the requirement of the change we are trying to achieve. It is real-world management in real time of the approach we are taking to analyze the situation, the assumptions we are making, and the key characteristics of our mental model as it applies to the problem that we are addressing. By comparison, *reflection-on-action* occurs after an activity or experience is completed, in which one reconstructs the activity or experience based on recall. *Reflection-on-action* is an effort to relive the experience, explore memory to retrieve the fragmented elements of the experience for the purpose of understanding the meaning of what has happened, and draw lessons learned from the experience (Ferreira, 2020).

The fundamental basis of reflection is primarily the experiences of the practitioner and the conscious effort of the practitioner to link reflective knowledge with other types of knowledge to be applied to the current situation of interest. Understanding reflective knowledge and how it is used in practice and evaluation is complex and evolving. Practitioners can use reflective techniques to identify and frame unique problematic situations and find workable unique solutions. By consciously and methodically analyzing the problematic situation and action taken, lessons learned can inform future practice regarding what works and what is more effective. Reflection offers a means for explicating practice, analyzing decision-making processes, and ensuring individualized and unique best practice and care.

Nursing's thought leaders have built on the concept of reflection in many ways, including elucidating intuitive knowledge in nursing practice. Mitchell (1994) defines *intuition* as the instant understanding of knowledge without evidence of sensible thought. In addressing clinical intuition, Benner and Tanner (1987) write that intuition is understanding without rationale. Intuition is a process of arriving at accurate conclusions based on relatively small amounts of knowledge and/or information (Westcott, cited in Benner & Tanner, 1987). In the renowned book, *From Novice to Expert: Excellence and Power in Clinical Nursing Practice* (1984), Benner reports on research that investigated how nurses make clinical decisions on the basis of different levels of experience. The levels of nursing practice are novice, advanced beginner, competent, proficient, and expert. Inherent in the notion of the expert nurse is intuitive knowing, which is also called intuitive knowledge. It is intuitive knowledge and judgment that separate expert judgment from that of a beginner (Benner & Tanner, 1987, p. 23). According to Benner and other nurse scholars, intuition is a source of knowledge in nursing to be valued and embraced. Some authors refer to intuition as tacit knowledge. *Tacit knowledge* is that which is difficult to express but inferable from a subject's actions (Blackburn, 2008, p. 358). Blackburn (2008, p. 358) also defines *tacit communications* as the unexpressed recognition of the position of others that leads to strategies from common activity. It is knowledge that is so embedded and integrated into one's thinking that there may not even be conscious awareness of its presence.

In summary, reflection provides structure and guidance to transpose unconscious and intuitive types of knowledge to conscious knowledge and allows for linkages to be developed with previous knowledge and experience, formal theories, and research knowledge to provide the best sources of evidence for professional practice and care.

SOURCES OF EVIDENCE

In order to consider the credibility of evidence, the sources of evidence and how evidence is generated must be considered. To answer the question "where does evidence come from?" there are many ways to think about the sources of evidence. Classification of the sources of evidence and knowledge includes a variety of lenses to think about evidence and is discussed in this section.

Classification of Sources of Evidence

Published Sources

Primary Sources
Primary sources of published evidence refer to information in its original form, that is, information that has not been interpreted, condensed, or evaluated. It is the original thinking, reports, discoveries, or shared new insights. Primary sources represent the first time the material has been released in physical, print, or electronic format. Examples of primary sources include journal articles of original research published in peer-reviewed journals; survey results; proceedings of meetings, conferences, or symposia; newspaper or electronic media postings; patient medical records; and data sets, such as national census descriptive statistics (University of Maryland Libraries, 2006).

Secondary Sources
Secondary sources of published evidence are accounts that are removed from the event or information and are provided after the fact. They describe, interpret, analyze, or evaluate information provided from primary sources. Examples of secondary sources are biographies, commentaries, monographs, textbooks, review articles, critiques, or opinion articles.

Tertiary Sources
Tertiary sources of published evidence are works that include both primary and secondary resources in a special subject area that have been synthesized, reformatted, and condensed to a convenient and easy-to-read format. It may also include compilations of primary and secondary sources of information that recommend how to use the information. Other examples of tertiary sources are clinical guidelines, manuals, handbooks, and practice protocols. These forms of evidence fall under the heading of gray literature, which will be discussed in what follows.

Gray Literature
Gray (or grey) literature are materials and research produced by organizations outside of the traditional commercial or academic publishing and distribution channels. It includes unpublished research reports, government reports, evaluations, theses, dissertations, webcasts, poster sessions, presentations, conference proceedings, PowerPoint presentations, textbooks, fact sheets, standards, newsletters, technical documents, white papers, and other unpublished works (DeBellis, 2020). The fact that the strength and quality of gray literature sources of evidence will vary needs to be incorporated into the decision to use gray literature.

Scientific Sources

There are many ways to think about the sources of evidence in addition to sources that have been described earlier in this chapter. One needs to consider the validity, reliability, and application of scientific sources as well. The following perspectives are included when discussing classification of sources: external and internal sources; real-world data and real-world evidence; and research sources.

External and Internal Sources

Evidence can come from external and internal sources. *External evidence* is generated through rigorous research such as RCTs and can be generalized to other settings. Melnyk and Fineout-Overholt (2015) point out that an important question to consider when applying external evidence to a project is whether the same results can be achieved in a different setting. In other words, does the research evidence translate and transfer to a real-world setting and project? By contrast, *internal evidence* is evidence generated through practice initiatives such as outcomes management and quality improvement projects that were conducted to improve care or outcomes in the setting in which the change was initiated.

Real-World Data and Real-World Evidence

According to the Food Drug Administration (2020), *real-world data* (RWD) and *real-world evidence* (RWE) are playing an increasing role in health care decisions. RWD are the data relating to patient health status and/or the delivery of health care routinely collected from a variety of sources, including EMRs, claims databases, product and disease registries, patient-generated data from electronic devices and software applications (or apps), and social media. These sources can provide new insight into health status and illness. RWE is the clinical evidence about the usage and potential benefits or risks of a medical product derived from analysis of RWD. RWE can be generated by different study designs or analyses, including prospective and retrospective observational studies, large simple trials, and pragmatic trials (https://www.fda.gov/science-research/science-and-research-special-topics/real-world-evidence). Sherman et al. (2016) point out that clinical trials continue to be necessary powerful tools for developing scientific evidence about safety and efficacy of medical products and informing an understanding of the biological mechanisms supporting the therapeutic action. There is no substitute for this robust research, resulting in evidence that suggests that a treatment is effective. However, the controls included in robust research strongly support internal validity at the expense of generalizability, especially because the characteristics of the sample enrolled in the study may differ significantly from those patients seen in real-world practice.

RWE can be viewed as a means of incorporating diverse types of evidence into information on health care. One caution is the quality of the RWD because of unclear methodological approaches and the settings in which evidence is generated by those without research expertise. However, RWE can inform therapeutic development (e.g., drugs and devices, outcomes research, patient care, research on health care systems, quality improvement, safety surveillance, and well-controlled effectiveness studies [Sherman et al., 2016]). A primary distinguishing characteristic of RWE as opposed to research is setting. RWE is gathered in clinical care and home or community settings as compared with research that is conducted in research-intensive or academic environments (Sherman et al., 2016). In an era of COVID-19, marked by an urgency to develop a vaccine, RWD and RWE are being used along with RCTs to develop a vaccine in a contracted time frame.

Research Methodologies

Another way to think about the sources of evidence is based on qualitative and quantitative research methods discussed earlier in this chapter. *Qualitative methods* are used to investigate a phenomenon or area of interest through the collection of (non-numeric) narrative materials using a variety of methods to collect the data. By comparison, *quantitative methods* are used to collect data in a quantified (numeric) form; the focus of the investigation lends itself to precise measurement and quantification. This raises the question of value. Is evidence from one method of investigation better when conducting an evaluation? The response to that question is "it depends." It depends on the elements of the evaluation and what evidence you are trying to collect. Some questions are answerable by qualitative methods. For example, if the evaluator wishes to determine how staff nurses feel about a seminal event in a clinical unit, then qualitative methods such as semistructured interviews are appropriate to tap into those personal responses. However, if the evaluator wishes to determine the demographic characteristics of the nursing staff employed in a cardiovascular service, then a quantitative method such as a forced-choice questionnaire is appropriate. In most evaluations, both qualitative and quantitative methods are needed to collect all of the evidence necessary to complete a comprehensive evaluation.

QUALITY OF EVIDENCE

Quality is a notion that has to do with value to the beholder, thus suggesting a degree of subjectivity. The quality of evidence can be examined from a number of perspectives. Because evaluation is based on the accumulation and organization of evidence, examining the quality of evidence is briefly addressed in this section. Melnyk and Fineout-Overholt (2015) note that the level of evidence plus the quality of evidence equals the strength of the evidence, which provides a level of confidence to act on the evidence to change practice.

There are various forms of evidence, and methods for evaluation of the quality of evidence vary. For example, when published research is being considered as evidence in an evaluation, there are a number of critical appraisal tools that are specific for the type of research reported for both quantitative and qualitative studies. Using these tools helps the evaluator determine the quality of research design and the findings reported and whether the findings are applicable for use as evidence to the evaluation. Other forms of evidence require a different approach to determine quality. For example, testimony of individual interviews for credibility and motivation of the respondent need to be evaluated. Although evidence in this form is classified as opinion, and placed on a lower hierarchical level, this form of evidence is often included in the course of the conduct of an evaluation.

Strength of Evidence and Evidence Hierarchies for Research

An important distinction is made between strength of evidence systems and evidence hierarchies. Evidence hierarchies focus on the study design, with meta-analysis and systematic reviews of RCTs positioned at the highest level. By comparison, strength of evidence systems incorporate not only study design, but also other components such as presence or absence of bias, quality of the evidence, and precision of estimates (Owens et al., 2010). Yet the domains included in the strength of evidence systems are not uniform, thus contributing to the confusion of grading evidence. See Table 2.2 for an example of levels of evidence based on a hierarchy of evidence for intervention/treatment questions. Burns et al. (2011) provide examples of hierarchies developed by several professional organizations.

TABLE 2.2 Rating System for the Hierarchy of Evidence for Intervention/Treatment Questions

Level of Evidence	Description
Level I	Evidence from a systematic review of all relevant RCTs, or evidence-based clinical practice guidelines based on systematic reviews of RCTs (includes meta-analysis)
Level II	Evidence obtained from at least one well-designed RCT
Level III	Evidence obtained from well-designed controlled trials without randomization, quasi-experimental
Level IV	Evidence from well-designed case-control and cohort studies
Level V	Evidence from systematic reviews of descriptive and qualitative studies
Level VI	Evidence from a single descriptive or qualitative study
Level VII	Evidence from the opinion of authorities and/or reports of expert committees

RCT, randomized controlled trial.

Source: From Melnyk, B., & Fineout-Overholt, E. (2015). *Evidence-based practice in nursing and healthcare* (3rd ed.). Lippincott Williams & Wilkins.

Given the movement in the last 30 years to evidence-based practice, several evidence hierarchies have been developed by a number of scholars and organizations to grade scientific evidence according to the quality and strength of the empirical evidence for clinical practice. These hierarchies are specifically designed for scientific evidence, most often from publications reporting systematic reviews, RCTs, quasi-experimental designs, qualitative studies, case reports, and other forms of research. These hierarchies are further discussed in Chapter 10. Hierarchies are helpful when a review of the literature is conducted to determine the state of the science about a particular area of interest addressed through RCTs or to understand the constructs of interest. Not all questions lend themselves to be investigated through RCTs. When considering evidence for evaluation, the evaluator is confronted with several questions, such as: What is the strength of the evidence? What is the value of the evidence? How confident are you about the validity of the evidence? Can you trust the evidence?

Level I evidence is the highest level of evidence. Strength has to do with the capacity to exert influence. In the case of evaluation, it is the strength of the evidence that informs the evaluator about the focus of interest. Strong evidence is compelling, whereas weak evidence contributes little or nothing to the evaluation process. Primary evidence is viewed as stronger than secondary evidence. The value of evidence requires judgment by the evaluator, is subject to bias, and often depends on the purpose for which the evidence is to be used. Purpose helps the evaluator decide what kind of evidence is needed, in what form, and in what amount.

The value of evidence also depends on the context and environment in which it will be used. Some evidence will be critically based on the context of an evaluation, whereas other information may be helpful but not critical. Evidence is used to inform decision-making and judgment so that the evaluator must determine whether the evidence collected is appropriate, useful, credible, accurate, and trustworthy. It may take some investigation to verify that these characteristics of evidence are present. The legitimacy of evidence is always linked to purpose. The evaluator makes a judgment on a continuous series of questions throughout the evaluation process. The evaluator's goal is to access the best available evidence possible.

The evaluator is challenged to search for the best evidence important to the project. This requires comprehensive knowledge about collecting targeted data through a variety of sources, such as electronic databases, other repositories of information, and expert consultation. In the pursuit of the "best evidence" to evaluate anything—a program, practice change, or published guidelines—evaluation is a high-level, complex process that involves an understanding of the nature of evidence and how it is collected, used, and evaluated as a basis for decision-making. In evaluation, evidence can be considered as clues or pieces of a puzzle that contribute to creating an accurate picture of the focus of evaluation. It is a process to search for truth as a basis for evaluation.

Finding and Evaluating Credible Evidence

The premise for credible evidence is based on transparency and a commitment to being open without a preconceived conviction of the answers or outcomes of the evaluation. Follow the evidence, and it will take you to the truth. It is also reflective of ethical practice. With preconceived ideas, evidence will be ignored or distorted to fit a preconceived result, and a fair and balanced result will not be achieved. This sounds simple but needs to be monitored carefully because there are many opportunities for bias to influence the conduct of an evaluation. Discussion of bias is discussed further in the next section.

What should the evaluator do if the desired evidence is not available? There are times when the evaluator does not have access to the evidence that they would like to collect, or it may not exist. This may be because evidence has not been recorded, the informant is unavailable, or access is limited owing to the confidential nature of some information or other reasons. In such a situation, the evaluator must decide how critical the information is to the evaluation process. Often, some evidence is nice to have but is not critical; in other instances, certain evidence may be critical to the evaluation. The evaluator must determine whether there is other available evidence that can substitute or be a proxy for the desired evidence. It may be possible to infer from other pieces of evidence about the area of interest. If the evaluator determines that missing evidence is indeed very important in the evaluation process and is unattainable, then this information should be listed as a limitation of the evaluation.

BIAS, RELIABILITY, VALIDITY, AND APPLICATION OF EVIDENCE

In examining the quality of evidence in any evaluation, bias, reliability, validity, and application that influence evidence and its usefulness in the evaluation process must be considered.

Bias

For the purposes of this chapter, *bias* is defined as any influence that produces a distortion in the result of an evaluation. It can affect the quality of evidence in both qualitative and quantitative components of an evaluation (Polit & Beck, 2021). Bias can be further divided into bias related to the evaluator or observer and bias related to evidence and process.

Interviewer Bias

Interviewer bias can occur in a number of forms. If the evaluator interviews people in the course of the evaluation process, interviewer bias is possible. The ideal interviewer is a neutral agent through which evaluation-focused questions are passed and recorded. However, this seemingly simple notion is difficult to achieve. The respondents and interviewer interact on a human level that includes complex verbal and nonverbal communications and interaction (LoBiondo-Wood & Haber, 2018). These interactions can affect the interviewee's responses to questions. This means the quality of the information or evidence provided is inaccurate or incomplete, thus having a negative effect on the evaluation outcome. Interviewer bias may be communicated verbally or nonverbally, and the bias may be subtle. The basis of the bias may be personal preference for the outcome of the evaluation, allegiances to stakeholders who will be affected by the evaluation outcome, or a desire to validate previously articulated beliefs or experience.

A second potential source of bias is *observer bias*; that is, the evaluator collects evidence for an evaluation by observation. Observation is often an excellent alternative to self-reporting methods with subjects. Observation is useful to record characteristics and conditions of individuals, groups, and environments; verbal and nonverbal communications; activities and behaviors; and performance characteristics. Polit and Beck (2021) address the following factors that interfere with objective observations:

- Observer prejudices, attitudes, and values may result in faulty inferences.
- Personal commitment may distort observations in a preferred direction.
- Anticipation of what is to be observed may affect what is observed.
- Premature decisions before adequate information is collected may result in errors of classification or conclusions.

Although observational biases cannot be removed completely, they can be minimized through careful training of the observer and attention to bias in the study design. Structured observations help to control bias and to systematically record observations so that comparable evidence is collected for all subjects.

Participant Bias

As with evaluator bias, there is potential bias from the participants in an evaluation. In any evaluation, evidence is often collected from people either directly or indirectly involved in the evaluation process. Participants may be a source of evidence through input from interviews or from information provided through questionnaires, documents, reports, or other sources of evidence. Bias can be introduced in a number of ways, such as *nonresponse bias*, *selection bias*, and *attrition bias*. Individuals decide whether they wish to participate in an evaluation. It is important for the evaluator to determine whether there are any group differences between the responders and nonresponders such as demographic, socioeconomic, or other differences that could be a source of bias. This form of bias is called *nonresponse bias*. Another form of bias is *selection bias*. The evaluator must have a representative sample to collect evidence so that there is no segment of evidence excluded from the evaluation that could distort the findings. *Attrition bias* refers to participants who remove themselves from continuation in the process. The evaluator should determine whether there are any group differences between those that continue to participate and those who withdraw. The reasons for withdrawal may provide important insight into the evaluation or the evaluation process.

Participants who are directly interviewed by the evaluator may demonstrate social desirability response bias and extreme response bias. *Social desirability response bias* is noted when participants mask their true responses consistently and provide responses that are reflective of prevailing social values or professional expectations (Polit & Beck, 2021). Another form of social desirability bias occurs when the respondent knows or has a personal relationship with the evaluator. The respondent may not wish to offend the evaluator or may not wish the responses to seem critical or unappreciative of the evaluator's efforts and may therefore answer in a way that they believe will please, or at least not offend, the evaluator. *Extreme response bias* is demonstrated by participants who distort their opinions and respond such that everything is reported as very positive or very negative. In designing an evaluation, the evaluator should take into consideration all possible sources of bias and attempt to find ways to control or minimize their influence.

Reliability

Simply stated, *reliability* is the ability of an instrument to measure the attribute or a variable or construct consistently (LoBiondo-Wood & Haber, 2018). In conducting an evaluation, the evaluators want to be sure that any instruments that they are using are reliable and consistent. The instruments developed for an evaluation must reflect the purpose of the evaluation and the specific area of interest. That means the instrument must be carefully crafted to be useful and valuable to the conduct of the evaluation. One specific type of reliability that is particularly important to evaluation is interrater reliability, also known as interobserver reliability. *Interrater reliability* measures the degree of agreement between different people (observers) observing or assessing the same thing. The observers may be assigning ratings, scores, or categories to one or more variables, or they may be tasked with identifying and describing elements critical to the evaluation. People see things differently and are therefore subjective, so different observers' perceptions of situations and phenomena naturally differ. Depending on the scope of the evaluation, there may be more than one person collecting data. Regardless of the number of observers, to support and maintain a high level of interrater reliability, initial training and assessing for a high level of reliability among observers is necessary. To improve interrater reliability, common sense strategies that the evaluation leader can implement to support reliability include (a) clearly defining the variables and the methods that will be used to measure them; (b) developing detailed, objective criteria for how the variables will be rated, counted or categorized, or captured; and (c) if multiple researchers are involved, ensuring that they all have exactly the same information and training.

Cohen's kappa (k) coefficient is a statistic used to measure interrater reliability between two independent raters that expresses the level of agreement observed beyond the level that would be expected by chance alone (LoBiondo-Wood & Haber, 2018; McHugh, 2012). Kappa scores range from +1 (total agreement) to 0 (no agreement). A *k* of 0.80 to 1.00 indicates good interrater reliability. *k* between 0.80 and 0.68 is considered acceptable/substantial agreement; <0.68 allows tentative conclusions to be drawn at times when lower levels are acceptable (LoBiondo-Wood & Haber, 2018). What is considered an acceptable score is a judgment of the evaluation leader. However, a score in the 0.90s range is considered desirable by most evaluators. Once a satisfactory kappa score has been achieved after initial training, periodic assessment should be conducted to verify maintenance of required interrater levels. If the interrater reliability is slipping, it suggests the need for more education to achieve the desired levels of performance.

Validity

Validity is the extent to which an instrument measures the attributes of a concept accurately (LoBiondo-Wood & Haber, 2018). Validity can be divided into internal and external validity. *Internal validity* concerns the validity of inferences that there truly is an empirical relationship or correlation between the presumed cause and the effect (Polit & Beck, 2021). Internal validity means that the independent variable, rather than something else, causes the outcome. The justification is based on the extent to which a study minimizes systematic error (or bias). *External validity* is the extent to which the results of a study can be confidently generalized to other situations and to other people. There are a number of threats to internal validity; these include temporal ambiguity, selection, history, maturation, mortality/attrition, and testing/instrumentation. These concepts are well described in a number of research texts and are not addressed in this chapter.

Evaluation can be a form of research, especially when it is conducted with the rigor of a scientific investigation. Many concepts addressed in research texts are applicable to evaluation. From the perspective of research design, Shadish et al. (2002, p. 34) define *validity* as "the approximate truth of an inference." Polit and Beck (2021) note that validity is not an absolute value but, rather, a matter of degree. Moving from a perspective of validity in research to evidence, validity of evidence is the degree to which the evidence is justified, supported, and founded on truth. Therefore, the validity of evidence is critical when considering design, conduct, and analysis in evaluation.

Construct Validity

A special form of validity, called *construct validity*, is an important consideration in evaluation. A *construct* is an abstract (nonobservable) entity, the existence of which is postulated and explained by the use of observable phenomena (Angeles, 1992, p. 55). *Construct validity* involves the validity of inferences. It is the extent to which an instrument is said to measure a theoretical construct or trait (LoBiondo-Wood & Haber, 2018). The concept of construct validity can also be applied to evaluation. Constructs link the methods used in the evaluation to the higher order concept of interest and to the ways the resulting evidence is translated into knowledge to make decisions related to that concept. A construct in an evaluation must be defined and operationalized before the evaluator can determine the key characteristics of interest and the best way to measure those characteristics. For example, if the focus of the evaluation is to examine interprofessional collaboration on a unit, the evaluator must first describe and operationalize the concept of interprofessional collaboration by establishing an operational definition. What are the key characteristics to examine? A review of the literature might reveal that interprofessional collaboration is based on mutual respect, transparency, open and honest communications, and a common goal. The evaluator would then focus on ways to collect evidence about these attributes from the team that is being evaluated. Because there are a variety of methods of eliciting the evidence related to a construct, the evaluator would have to decide what methods would provide the best evidence to address the question. The evaluator may use more than one method to collect evidence, which is often necessary to provide information about different aspects of a construct.

Threats to construct validity, defined as erroneous inferences from the particular evaluation study to the higher-level abstract concept, must be considered. Threats can occur if there is a mismatch between the higher-level concept of interest, for example interprofessional collaboration, and how the evaluator has operationalized the concept for the purpose of the evaluation. Threats to construct validity can also occur if irrelevant evidence is collected and included in the evaluation process. Although the evidence may be accurate, it is irrelevant to the focus of the evaluation. Other forms of threats to construct validity include evaluator bias and participant bias, both of which were discussed earlier in this chapter. In thinking about validity, it is never a determination of either validity being present or not present; validity is always a determination of the degree of validity.

Application

Application refers to the practical issue of how the evaluation can be used in the real world to address important problems and provide information for decision-making. In requesting an evaluation, there must be a clear purpose for how the findings will be used. Concurrently, in the design and implementation of an evaluation, the purpose of the evaluation must be kept in mind as a key driver of the evaluation to provide a practical outcome of usable information for the stakeholders requesting the evaluation.

Contextual and Environmental Dimensions of Evidence

In conducting any evaluation, the context and local environment in which the evaluation takes place are important. Stetler (2003) described this evidence source as "internal evidence," which she says comes primarily from local systematically collected information, including data about local performance, planning, quality, and outcomes; knowledge about the culture of the organization and the individuals in it; and local and national policy. The focus of the evaluation, be it an organization, a group, or an individual that is being evaluated, has to be appreciated within the context of the environment in which it operates. There may be special contextual and environmental characteristics unique to the focus of the evaluation that must be taken into consideration. For example, if an evaluator is assisting an organization to determine its readiness to apply for the Magnet® Recognition Program offered by the American Nurses Credentialing Center (ANCC), the mission, size, and community in which the organization is located should be considered. A 75-bed, acute care facility located in a rural setting may not have the infrastructure to meet the research expectations of the Magnet criteria. Such a facility may be better positioned to apply for the Pathway to Excellence Program, which is also administered by ANCC, with criteria that focus on the use of evidence-based practice rather than the generation of new knowledge. An evaluation is designed to examine the situation or program as it exists against some form of criteria in order to provide information that will be useful for understanding and decision-making.

DOCTOR OF NURSING PRACTICE NURSES AND EVALUATION

The interest in evidence by health professionals is related to their need to substantiate the worth of a wide variety of activities and interventions (Pearson et al., 2007). Basing all beliefs and practices strictly on evidence allegedly separates science from other activities (Husserl, 1982; Kuhn, 1996). The type of evidence sought by the evaluator varies according to the focus of the evaluation, which might be a clinical question or a question about the nature of an intervention, activity, or focus of interest. The previous discussion provided a background for the evaluation in a generic sense to assist the DNP nurse in thinking about evidence. In this final section, the evaluation process focuses on the role of the DNP nurse in evaluation.

Roles of Doctor of Nursing Practice Nurses in Evaluation

DNP nurses often assume responsibility and accountability for evaluation. Evaluation of care for individual patients and populations is an integral part of professional practice. However, DNP nurses may be asked to evaluate any number of practices, interventions, products, programs, and policies either as an individual evaluator or as part of a team of evaluators. Additionally, evaluation in the digital age offers new dimensions for sources of evidence as well as the collection, storage, and organization of evidence. The following provides examples of common types of evaluations that DNP nurses may conduct.

Practice

For DNP nurses, the word *evidence* is usually synonymous with evidence-based practice. Clinical practice and the practices or processes involved in providing care are exceedingly complex. For example, the DNP nurse may be asked to examine the hand-off practices by nurses and physicians on a unit or service line. In thinking about this request, the DNP nurse considers the many forms of hand-offs in health care. There are nurse-to-nurse hand-offs between shifts, at mealtime, and during transfer to another unit. Physician-to-physician hand-offs occur when a patient is transferred to another unit or another hospital. In a model where physicians are employed by a health care facility to work shifts, such as a hospitalist or resident, there is physician-to-physician hand-off between shifts. The DNP nurse evaluating hand-off practices would most likely begin with focusing on the overall evaluation and then conducting a review of the literature to understand the state of the science related to hand-offs. In the process of review, the DNP nurse would identify key variables to address and might also find instruments useful for collecting and measuring variables of interest. The literature is often a good guide for developing a protocol for the evaluation.

Another example of practice evaluation is one that examines the effectiveness of interprofessional teams for their impact on core measures and patient or organizational outcomes. Although it is generally believed that high-performance, interprofessional teams have better patient and provider outcomes, teasing out the contributions that each team member contributes to outcomes may be difficult. This is an example of a complex evaluation focus that might be conducted by a team that includes an expert consult to guide the process. Sources of evidence might include review of the literature, observation, semistructured interviews, questionnaires, and mining of patient outcome data related to practice processes, cost analyses, and core measures data.

Interventions

Although providers like to think that their practice is evidence based, it is clear that more than half of what is done in practice has no scientific basis. DNP nurses understand the processes of care and how to examine processes of care with such tools as process mapping and review of the literature for best practices. For example, the nursing practice of turning a patient every 2 hours has no scientific basis. The focus of the evaluation could be to examine the practices of turning patients and the incidence of pressure ulcers in a facility. This information could be of value to a nursing practice committee charged with reviewing patient-turning protocols in a long-term care facility. Sources of evidence are similar to practice inquiry and might include review of the literature, observation, semistructured interviews, questionnaires, mining of patient outcome data related to team performance, cost analyses, and core measures data.

Products

Health care facilities must make decisions on all products, from beds to dressings to educational materials. The decision may be about including new products in a facility or replacing a newer product with an established product. The DNP nurse is often asked to evaluate a new product and compare it with current products. The evaluation is based not only on cost, but also on achievement of stated outcomes, user friendliness, time required by the care provider to use the product, and acceptability by the patient. Because products and equipment are a big part of the operating budget, decisions on product evaluation have ramifications for the cost of health care. Helpful sources of evidence might include the literature on comparative effectiveness with other similar products, interviews with current users to determine how it is used, ease of use, reliability, cost, maintenance requirements, contribution to patient care, and return on investment.

Programs

Another type of evaluation that DNP nurses might conduct is that of program evaluation. The program could be a clinical program such as a community-outreach stroke prevention program, an established comprehensive heart failure program within a hospital or system, or an orientation program for newly hired registered nurses on a specialty unit such as an orthopedic service. All programs should first be effective. It is important to understand the purpose of the evaluation. Is the purpose of the evaluation for feasibility, impact on a community, or cost? The purpose will determine what evidence will need to be examined. The findings of a program evaluation may lead to a quality improvement project. In the current cost-conscious environment of quality and safety, much emphasis is being placed on comparative effectiveness evaluation to guide decision-making. Sources of evidence to evaluate a program might include the literature; descriptions of characteristics of effective high-performance programs for purposes of focused data collection and comparison; interviews with a broad range of stakeholders, including providers, administrators, and recipients about effectiveness and meeting of recipients' needs; patient/client outcome data; cost analysis; analysis of return on investment; projected changes in the program for the future, including need for additional resources and cost; and observations of program processes.

Policies

Policies and procedures that guide practice and care must be evaluated and updated on a regular basis to stay current and in compliance with regulatory bodies and professional standards. The DNP nurse is often responsible for evaluating and updating policies and procedures as an individual evaluator or as part of a committee or other group advising decision makers. For example, a policy that requires 10 units of continuing education for all nursing staff may be scheduled for review in light of changes made by the state board of nursing for relicensure. The number of continuing education units may need to be increased because of new mandatory continuing education required by the State Nurse Practice Act. The evaluation process might include current policy, mandatory changes, financial impact on the health care facility to support the continuing education requirements, and methods of communicating the change to staff. Sources of evidence to evaluate policies include a review of the literature, interviews with stakeholders affected by the policy or policies, policy analysis with local and national compliance imperatives, potential consequences of policy change or lack of change, cost implications of policy decisions, and the social environmental impact of the policy. Much of the evidence can be collected from internal sources, including people and databases, and then applied to the local and national imperatives and standards required by the organization.

COMMON SOURCES OF EVIDENCE USED BY DOCTOR OF NURSING PRACTICE NURSES

Common sources of evidence used by DNP nurses when conducting an evaluation are included in Table 2.3.

In planning any evaluation, regardless of whether it appears simple or complex, careful attention must be paid to models and design. Models for evaluation provide a framework for the evaluation. Design includes thinking prospectively of all possible factors that could undermine the quality of the evaluation, including bias and validity. Although evaluation is generally considered at the end of many processes, it should be integrated early into the planning stage of any new project. The steps in conducting an evaluation are discussed in Chapter 1.

TABLE 2.3 Common Sources of Evidence for DNPs

Source	Examples
Print and electronic sources, including data mining from internal and external databases	Journals, websites, electronic databases, books, survey data, dashboards, minutes of meetings, patient medical records, internally developed databases
Guidelines, protocols, and authoritative publications of professional organizations and state and national reports	American Heart Association clinical practice guidelines and Institute of Medicine reports
Forums and consensus standards for performance, which are considered the gold standard for evidence	National Quality Forum
Real-world evidence	EHRs; claims databases; product and disease registries; patient-generated data from electronic devices and software applications (or apps); and social media
Gray literature	Unpublished research reports, government reports and evaluations, theses, dissertations, webcasts, poster sessions, conference presentations and proceedings, PowerPoint presentations, textbooks, fact sheets, standards, newsletters, technical documents, white papers, and other unpublished works
Observations	Physical examination, participatory interactions (attending meetings, demonstrations)
Interviews	Individuals, groups
Surveys/instruments	Conducted electronically (e.g., SurveyMonkey) or in paper format; reported as aggregate data
Experiments/comparisons	Use of comparison groups or products
Personal experiences	Composite of clinical, professional, and personal experiences gained in a variety of ways Practice knowledge (what is learned in practice)
Reflections	Linking knowledge learned from patient care or other experiences with other forms of knowledge to provide best practice Seeing similarities in a new patient situation with previously accumulated knowledge from other cases

DNP, Doctor of Nursing Practice; EHRs, electronic health records.

SUMMARY

Evaluation is based on the collection, organization, and critical review of evidence to make decisions about value. Evidence comes from many sources and is found in many forms. The evaluator must not only understand the overall process of evaluation, but must also be able to identify and collect the necessary evidence for the particular focus of the evaluation. The quality of the evidence must be constantly considered, including bias and validity of evidence that will lead to the best possible evidence that can be trusted for evaluation and decision-making.

REFERENCES

Ackoff, R. L. (1989). From data to wisdom. *Journal of Applied System Analysis, 16*(1), 3–9.

American Nurses Association. (2015). *Scope and standards of nursing informatics practice* (3rd ed.). American Nurses Publishing.

Angeles, P. A. (1992). *The HarperCollins dictionary of philosophy* (2nd ed., p. 85). HarperCollins.

Bellinger, G., Castro, D., & Mills, A. (2004). Data information, knowledge, and wisdom. http://www.systems-thinking.org/dikw/dikw.htm

Benner, P. (1984). *From novice to expert: Excellence and power in clinical nursing practice.* Addison-Wesley.

Benner, P., & Tanner, C. (1987). Clinical judgment: How expert nurses use intuition. *American Journal of Nursing, 87*(1), 23–31. PMID: 3642979.

Billay, D., Myrick, F., Luhanga, F., & Yonge, O. (2007). A pragmatic view of intuitive knowledge in nursing practice. *Nursing Forum, 42*(3), 147–155. https://doi.org/10.1111/j.1744-6198.2007.00079.x

Blackburn, S. (2008). *Oxford dictionary of philosophy.* Oxford University Press.

Brook, C. (2019). What is data integrity: Definition, best practices & more. Retrieved April 20, 2020, from https://digitalguardian.com/blog/what-data-integrity-data-protection-101

Burns, P. B., Rohrich, R. J., & Chung, K. C. (2011). The levels of evidence and their role in evidence-based medicine. *Plastic Reconstructive Surgery, 128*(1), 305–310. https://doi.org/10.1097/PRS/0b013e318219c17

Carper, B. (1978). Fundamental patterns of knowing in nursing. *Advances in Nursing Science, 1*(1), 12–23. https://doi.org/10.1097/00012272-197810000-00004

Center for Evidence-Based Management. (n.d.). What are the levels of evidence? http://www.cebma.org/frequently-asked-questions/what-are-the-levels-of-evidence/

Copi, I. M., & Cohen, C. (2009). *Introduction to logic* (13th ed.). Pearson Prentice Hall.

DeBellis, N. (2020). Grey literature: Gray literature. https://csulb.libguides.com/graylit

De Mauro, A., Greco, M., & Grimaldi, M. (2015). What is big data? A consensual definition and a review of key research topics. *AIP Conference Proceedings, 1644*(1), 97–104. https://doi.org/10.1063/1.4907823

Dimitrov, D. V. (2016). Medical internet of things and big data in healthcare. *Health Informatics Research, 22*(3), 156–163. https://doi.org/10.4258/hir.2016.22.3.156

Fawcett, J., Watson, J., Neuman, B., Hinton-Walker, P., & Fitzpatrick, J. J. (2001). On nursing theories and evidence. *Journal of Nursing Scholarship, 33*(2), 115–119. https://doi.org/10.1111/j.1547-5069.2001.00115.x

Federal Drug Administration. (2020). Real-world evidence. https://www.fda.gov/science-research/science-and-research-special-topics/real-world-evidence

Ferreira, S. (2020). Reflecting in and on action. Retrieved May 1, 2020, from http://web.mit.edu/cil/web_scripts/www/work/Reflecting%20in%20and%20on%20Action%20CoLab.pdf

Freshwater, D., Taylor, B. J., & Sherwood, G. (Eds.). (2008). *International textbook of reflective practice in nursing.* John Wiley & Sons.

Gallagher, T. K. (1964). *The philosophy of knowledge.* Sheed and Ward.

Given, L. M. (2008). *The Sage encyclopedia of qualitative research methods.* Sage.

Goldberg, M. J. (2006). On evidence and evidence-based medicine: Lessons from the philosophy of science. *Social Science and Medicine, 62*(11), 2621–2632. https://doi.org/10.1016/j.socscimed.2005.11.031

Goodman, K. W. (2003). *Ethics and evidence-based medicine: Fallibility and responsibility in clinical science.* Cambridge University Press.

Guyatt, G., Rennie, D., Meade, M. O., & Cook, D. (2008). *Users' guide to the medical literature* (2nd ed.). McGraw-Hill.

Han, J., Kamber, M., & Pei, J. (2012). *Data mining: Concepts and techniques* (3rd ed., pp. 1–6). Elsevier.

Husserl, E. (1982). *Ideas pertaining to a pure phenomenology and a phenomenological philosophy: First book: General introduction to a pure phenomenology.* F. Kersten (Trans.). Nijoff.

Johns, C., & Freshwater, D. (2005). *Transforming nursing through reflective practice* (2nd ed.). Blackwell.

Kuhn, T. (1996). *The structure of scientific revolutions.* University of Chicago Press.

Kruse, C. S., Kothman, K, Anerobi, K., & Abanaka, L. (2016). Adoption factors of the electronic health record: a systematic review. *Journal of Medical Internet Research, 4*(2), e19. https://doi.org/10.2196/medinform.5525

LoBiondo-Wood, G., & Haber, J. (2018). *Nursing research: Methods and critical appraisal for evidence-based practice* (9th ed.). Elsevier Mosby.

LoBiondo-Wood, G., Haber, J., & Titler, M. G. (Eds.). (2019). *Evidence-based practice for nursing and healthcare quality improvement.* Elsevier Mosby.

Magaoulas, R., & Lorica, B. (2009). Introduction to big data. Released 2.0. O'Reilly Media.

Mantzoukas, S. (2007). A review of evidence-based practice, nursing research, and reflection: Leveling the hierarchy. *Journal of Clinical Nursing, 17*(2), 214–223. https://doi.org/10.1111/j.1365-2702.2006.01912.x

McHugh, M. L. (2012). Interrater reliability: The kappa statistic. *Biochemical Medica, 22*(3), 276–282. https://doi.org/doi:10.11613/bm.2012.031

Melnyk, B., & Fineout-Overholt, E. (2015). *Evidence-based practice in nursing and healthcare* (3rd ed.). Lippincott Williams & Wilkins.

Mitchell, G. J. (1994). Intuitive knowing: Exposing a myth in theory development. *Nursing Science Quarterly, 7*(1), 2–3. https://doi.org/10.1177/089431849400700102

Owens, D. K., Lohr, K. N., Atkins, D., Treadwell, J. R., Reston, J. T., Bass, E. B., Chang, S., & Helfand, M. (2010). AHRQ series paper 5: Grading the strength of a body of evidence when comparing medical interventions–Agency for Healthcare Research and Quality and the Effective Health-Care Program. *Journal of Clinical Epidemiology, 63*(5), 513–523. https://doi.org/10.1016/j.jclinepi.2009.03.009

Parse, R. R. (1981). *Man-living-health: A theory of nursing.* John Wiley & Sons.

Parse, R. R. (1992). Human becoming: Parse's theory of nursing. *Nursing Science Quarterly, 5*(1), 35–42. https://doi.org/10.1177/089431849200500109

Pearsall, J., & Trumble, B. (Eds.). (1995). *The Oxford encyclopedia dictionary* (2nd ed.). Oxford University Press.

Pearson, A., Wiechula, R., Court, A., & Lockwood, C. (2005). The JBI model of evidence-based healthcare. *International Journal of Evidence-Based Healthcare, 3,* 207–215. https://doi.org/10.1111/j.1479-6988.2005.00026.x

Pearson, A., Wiechula, R., Court, A., & Lockwood, C. (2007). A re-consideration of what constitutes "evidence" in the health care professions. *Nursing Science Quarterly, 20*(1), 85–88. https://doi.org/10.1177/0894318406296306

Polifroni, E. C. (2018). Philosophy of science: An introduction and a grounding for your practice. In J. B. Butt & K. L. Rich (Eds.), *Philosophies and theories for advanced nursing practice* (3rd ed., pp. 3–19). Jones & Bartlett Learning.

Polit, D. F., & Beck, C. T. (2021). *Nursing research: Generating and assessing evidence for nursing practice* (11th ed.). Wolters Kluwer/Lippincott Williams & Wilkins.

Qual Communications. (2020). What is 5G? Retrieved May 21, 2020, from https://www.qualcomm.com/invention/5g/what-is-5g

Schön, D. (1983). *The reflective practitioner.* Temple Smith.

Schön, D. (1987). *Educating the reflective practitioner.* Jossey-Bass.

Shadish, W. R., Cook, T. D., & Campbell, D. T. (2002). *Experimental and quasi-experimental designs for generalized causal inference.* Houghton Mifflin.

Sherman, R. E., Anderson, S. A., Dal Pan, G. J., Gray, G. W., Gross, T., Hunter, N. L., LaVange, L., Marinac-Dabic, D., Marks, P. W., Robb, M. A., Shuren, J., Temple, R., Woodcock, J., Yue, L., & Califf, R. M. (2016). Real-world evidence—What is it and what can it tell us? *New England Journal of Medicine, 375*(23), 2293–2297. https://doi.org/10.1056/NEJMsb1609216

Stetler, C. (2003). The role of the organization in translating research into evidence-based practice. *Outcomes Management for Nursing Practice, 7*(3), 97–103. PMID: 12881970

Streubert-Speziale, H. J., & Carpenter, D. R. (2003). *Qualitative research in nursing: Advancing the humanistic imperative* (2nd ed.). Lippincott.

Techopedia. (2020a). Cloud storage. https://www.techopedia.com/definition/26535/cloud-storage

Techopedia. (2020b). Artificial intelligence. https://www.techopedia.com/definition/190/artificial-intelligence-ai

University of Maryland Libraries. (2006). Primary, secondary, and tertiary sources. http://www.lib.imd.edu/guides/promary-sources.html

White, J. (1995). Patterns of knowing: Review, critique, and update. *Advances in Nursing Science, 17*(4), 73–86. https://doi.org/10.1097/00012272-199506000-00007

Zanella, A., Bui, N., Castellani, Vangelista, L., & Zorzi, M. (2014). Internet of things for smart cities. *IEEE Internet of Things Journal, 1*(1), 22–32. https://doi.org/10.1109/JIOT.2014.2306328

THREE

MODELS FOR EVALUATION IN ADVANCED NURSING PRACTICE

Joanne V. Hickey

> *Do not go where the path may lead, go instead*
> *where there is no path and leave a trail.*
> —*Ralph Waldo Emerson*

INTRODUCTION

The profession of nursing has a unique paradigm and view of health care delivery and professional practice, just as other disciplines have their unique paradigms. Foundational to professional nursing practice is the nursing process. The nursing process includes six sequential and interrelated steps that include assessment, diagnosis, outcomes identification, planning, implementation, and evaluation (American Nurses Association [ANA], 2015, p. 88). The nursing process is foundational for professional nursing practice and a critical thinking model used by nurses to integrate singular and concurrent actions into a comprehensive and integrated approach to patient care (2015, p. 88). The purpose of the nursing process is to identify a client's/patient's health care status, including actual or potential health problems, establish a plan to meet the identified needs, deliver specific nursing interventions to address those needs, set expected outcomes of care, and evaluate achievement of the expected outcomes. Students are introduced to the nursing process in fundamental nursing courses within basic undergraduate programs, and the nursing process framework influences all levels of nursing education, including graduate and doctoral education.

Evaluation is part of the nursing process and is defined as "the process of determining the progress toward attainment of expected outcomes, including the effectiveness of care" (ANA, 2015, p. 87). What is clear is that the definition of evaluation is discipline specific for nursing and reflective of the nursing paradigm as compared with other definitions of evaluation that are broader in scope and application. The operational definition of evaluation and the criteria used for evaluation are also discipline specific.

In the discussion of evaluation in this book, the definition of evaluation extends beyond discipline-specific definitions and takes the nurse into evaluation science that is multidisciplinary and broad in scope. The evaluation models that will be discussed in this chapter originate from a variety of theoretical roots, sources, and disciplines but are also adaptable to a variety of other settings and purposes. In order for advanced practice nurses and doctor of nursing practice (DNP) nurses to work collaboratively as equal team members as well as leaders, knowledge of evaluation models beyond nursing is necessary to demonstrate quality and effectiveness in a broader arena of health care. The DNP nurse may be invited to participate in the evaluation of technologies, programs, guidelines/protocols, information systems, health education programs, and policies. Depending on knowledge, experience, and skill set for the particular project, the nurse may be a team leader or a member of an interdisciplinary evaluation team. In this book, the terms program and project are used interchangeably.

Terminology can be confusing. Terms such as theoretical foundation, framework, and model have different meanings. Theories provide a systematic guide for understanding events or behaviors by providing interrelated concepts, definitions, and propositions that explain or predict outcomes by specifying relationships among variables (Glanz & Bishop, 2010). Theories are abstract and broadly applicable, although they are not content or topic specific (Green & Krenter, 2005). A *framework* is a structure that provides a systematic way of organization that is useful to develop, manage, and evaluate interventions by helping to focus interventions on the essential processes of change (Tabak et al., 2012). Models are a physical and conceptual representation of a system of ideas, events, or processes; they describe theories and frameworks collectively (2012). In this chapter, models and frameworks are used interchangeably. In examining the origins of the models, the theoretical bases of the model are noted. For example, the theoretical basis of some evaluation models is social–ecological, based on the social and ecological sciences. Understanding the basis of a model is helpful in appreciating how the concepts are defined and the interrelatedness of the concepts.

CLASSIFICATION OF MODELS

The DNP nurse is confronted with a myriad of conceptual and theoretical models, many of which have an evaluation component, adding to the confusion regarding classification of models and their uses. For purposes of this discussion it is useful to differentiate evaluation models from those designed to translate evidence into practice or to guide change. The following discussion attempts to unravel the boundaries of these classifications.

The English word *translation* derives from the Latin word *translatio*, which comes from *trans*, "across," plus *ferre*, "to carry" or "to bring." The ending "-latio" comes from *latus*, the past participle of *ferre*. Thus, *translatio* is "a carrying across" or "a bringing across something" (https://en.wikipedia.org/wiki/Translation). *Translation* is moving something from one source to another target. In evidence-based practice translation, the sources for translation emanate from the literature, expert opinion, or experience and are applied to improving a clinical or health-related problem for an individual or group of patients. The purpose of translation is to convey the original intent of a source and interpret it to fit another target, while taking into account contextual differences between the source and the target that can alter some of the original meaning for fit with the new setting and context.

Keep in mind that *evidence-based practice* is defined as the conscious and judicious use of the current "best" evidence in the care of patients and delivery of health care services (LoBiondo-Wood & Haber, 2018, p. 394) and implies a translation. There are several models for translating evidence into practice, such as the *Iowa Model of Evidence-Based Practice to Promote Quality Care*, which has evolved over the years (Titler et al., 2001). Evaluation of the literature, expert opinion, and other sources of evidence for application to a current clinical problem are part of translation, but the primary goal of evidence-based practice and related translation is to improve practice by incorporating the best scientific and other knowledge available to address a clinical problem for an individual or group of patients.

The word *change*, as a noun, is defined as the act or instance of making or becoming something different. The definition of change as a verb is to make or become different. A number of change models are used in health care such as Kotter's *Model of Change* (Kotter, 2012), which is an eight-step process for leading change. Another example is Rogers's *Diffusion of Innovation* model (Rogers, 2003). This theory explains how, why, and at what rate new ideas and technology spread. Rogers's premise is that diffusion is a process by which an innovation is communicated over time among participants of a social system to support change (https://en.wikipedia.org/wiki/Diffusion_of_innovations). Again, there are components of evaluation in creating change such as evaluating an organization's readiness for change or the organizational structure or processes of care as a means of visioning a better organization or processes or evaluating the speed of change. However, the primary purpose of change models is to guide the change process of becoming something different, that is, change.

By comparison, evaluation models are designed for the primary purpose of evaluating selected characteristics or elements of a program, policy, guideline, workflow, or other entity and comparing those elements with specific and established criteria. In addition, the evaluation is conducted by a neutral evaluator or team of evaluators with established competency in evaluation. Donahue and vanOstenberg (2000) point out two common characteristics of all evaluation models. The first characteristic is that explicit criteria or standards are a pre-established set of expectations stated as standards or evaluation criteria that are reviewed, approved, and accepted to guide the evaluation. The standards or evaluation criteria may originate from a respected organization or may be criteria developed and approved by the organization requesting the evaluation. The second characteristic common to all evaluations is that the evaluation is conducted by external reviewers or surveyors/evaluators dispatched from an established, sanctioned entity authorized to provide an assessment or survey against a pre-established or explicit set of criteria or standards. Further, the reviewer may be a consultant or neutral person invited into the organization on an informal basis to apply the evaluation criteria desired by the organization (2000, p. 244). The evaluator is expected to have the competencies and a neutral mindset to conduct the evaluation according to ethical standards.

OVERVIEW OF APPROACHES TO EVALUATION

The conceptual/theoretical foundation that supports the expanded scope of evaluation is interdisciplinary and continues to evolve. This chapter describes a number of models and approaches for evaluating the quality of health care. The models are different in their approach or focus on conceptual elements important in the evaluation of health care. Some models useful in health care evaluation are discussed in this chapter, but there are other models that may be of value that will not be addressed.

The first approach to evaluation is Donabedian's conceptual model, which was introduced in the first chapter and is discussed here in more depth. Not only is his model applied directly in health care evaluation, but also his concepts of structure, process, and outcomes (S–P–O) have been adapted for use in the development of alternative evaluation models of various scopes (Donabedian, 1988). The second evaluation model is the effectiveness–efficiency–equity conceptual approach developed by Aday et al. (2004). It has application across a variety of settings and perspectives and is particularly relevant to the evaluation of policies affecting populations.

Logic models, the third approach, provide a blueprint to guide the planning, implementing, and evaluating process and illustrate how the components of the evaluation process relate to each other. Logic models are popular, particularly among funding agencies, because they provide a comprehensive view of what is being proposed. They are useful for both small and large evaluation projects.

The fourth approach, monitoring and evaluating health systems strengthening, is a conceptual framework developed by the World Health Organization (WHO) and other international organizations (Boerma et al., 2009). The framework is especially useful for the evaluation of very large health care systems, such as those at the national level. Finally, the Triple Aim framework has gained widespread acceptance because it is a comprehensive approach to evaluate the effectiveness and efficiency of care provided to both individuals and populations (Berwick et al., 2008).

With so many approaches and models available, choosing the best model for a particular evaluation project can be daunting. This requires knowledge about the purpose, scope, key conceptual elements, and the pros and cons of various models. In addition, some models are designed to evaluate large entities such as organizations and systems, whereas others are designed to work well for smaller scale projects. Some models that were originally designed for large-scale evaluation have evolved over time and have the flexibility of being adaptable to either large- or small-scale evaluation projects. One example of such a flexible model is Donabedian's S–P–O model. The goal of selecting the most appropriate model is to match the purpose and scope of the project to be evaluated with the best model available.

MODELS FOR EVALUATION

The discussion of evaluation models is approached from the perspective of models designed for both large-scale and smaller scale evaluations. This is an artificial view of evaluation because models originally designed for larger scale evaluation have also been adapted for smaller scale evaluations such as DNP projects. As noted previously, the focus of large-scope evaluation projects may include the organization, system, state, national, or international level. For example, an 800-bed acute care facility may wish to evaluate factors influencing nosocomial infections within the organization, which includes all of the individual care units, to see how they compare with other facilities within a major health care system. Selected areas for evaluation may include team collaboration at all 10 clinical facilities within their system. An example at the state level is a state such as Texas, which may wish to evaluate the effectiveness of diabetes prevention in all state-funded agencies. The same focus on diabetes prevention could also evaluate federally funded programs in all 50 states. Finally, WHO evaluates the achievement of individual countries with reference to multiple factors: infant mortality, suicides, diabetes prevention, and a host of other health-related indicators. Examples of a smaller scale project, such as a DNP quality improvement project, could include implementation of a change in practice to decrease falls in a nursing home (NH) setting or pressure ulcers within an acute care clinical unit (e.g., microsystem). The versatility of models will be noted as they are explained in what follows.

Donabedian's Conceptual Model: Structure, Process, Outcomes Model

Donabedian's contribution to developing a systematic and objective method of ensuring the quality of health care evolved over four decades, beginning in 1966, when he first introduced his model for evaluating quality. He observed that quality means different things to different people: "The definition of quality may be almost anything anyone wishes it to be, although it is, ordinarily, a reflection of values and goals current in the medical care system and in the larger society of which it is a part" (Donabedian, 1966, p. 167). He suggested that one could evaluate quality using three approaches individually or in combination. Evaluation could focus on the structure of care, the process of care, or the outcome of care.

Donabedian identified basic problems in successfully conducting systematic and objective evaluations regardless of approach. These include (a) a lack of valid and reliable measures, (b) the limitations of data sources and standards of measurement, (c) inadequate measurement scales, and (d) difficulty in establishing the link among each of the three approaches (S–P–O). Donabedian spent his professional career (and his life) examining these concerns and their relevance to improving the health of patients.

Health and Health Care

At the most basic level, health focuses on biophysical status (Donabedian, 1987). Practitioners assess the baseline health status of a patient, diagnose the condition, develop a plan of care, and intervene with evidence-based treatment. Outcome evaluation focuses primarily on the positive or negative changes in health status that result from the treatment provided. For example, in evaluating the outcome of individual care, a practitioner might measure the change in temperature and laboratory values after an acutely ill pediatric patient diagnosed with H3N2 influenza is treated appropriately with medication and IV fluids. In evaluating a program, a practitioner may measure the change in the number of cases of H3N2 diagnosed in a community as a result of a vaccine program. In evaluating population health, a practitioner may measure the change in the number of deaths caused by H3N2 in a city among individuals who did receive the vaccine and those who did not.

Evaluation functions occur at the macro-, meso-, and microlevels. Evaluating quality measures at all three levels provides the most comprehensive analysis of a system (Donabedian, 1987). Macro level evaluation occurs when there is a need to examine the totality of care provided by a nation (macrolevel) or regional health system (mesolevel) to meet the health care needs of a population. Care provided to individual patients and groups of patients at the microlevel should be monitored more frequently. If health care at the microlevel is found to be less than optimum, practitioners can make appropriate changes that will theoretically impact care at the macro- and mesolevels.

DNPs who participate in monitoring activities can use Donabedian's framework as a method for deciding what indicators to monitor (Donabedian, 2003). Some indicators are externally imposed, such as those required by regulatory organizations and agencies in order to maintain accreditation or to establish a unique status. The Joint Commission, Centers for Medicare & Medicaid Services, and the American Nurses Credentialing Center Magnet® Recognition Program are examples of external influences on monitoring health care.

Defining the Pathways to Quality: Structure, Process, and Outcome

At the most fundamental level, quality is an assessment of the "technical performance of individual health care practitioners" (Donabedian, 1987, p. 75). An expanded description provides contextual components of the interaction between patient and practitioner. Contextual components include patient adherence to practitioner recommendations, the barriers and facilitators to obtaining health, and the hospital or clinic environment.

Donabedian's S–P–O model lays out three approaches or pathways to evaluating health care: structure, process, and outcome. *Structure* refers to the administrative support provided for quality care and the environment in which health care occurs. Adequacy of supplies and equipment, number and proficiency of health care personnel, the hospital environment, and barriers and facilitators to access are structural components (Donabedian, 1987, 2003). Tarlov et al. (1989) also included patient characteristics such as age, comorbidity, risk, and beliefs under the category of structure.

Process comprises practitioner–patient interactions and the practitioners' technical proficiency in their therapeutic relationships with patients. Process indicators offer a direct approach to evaluating health care quality because health care that meets best practice standards in a specific time and place is quality care. Inherent in the selection of process criteria is the assumption that a strong link exists between how providers interact with patients and the outcomes of care (Donabedian, 1966, 1978, 2003). The type and number of diagnostic tests ordered, differential diagnoses listed, interpretation of test results, treatment prescribed, and type of patient education are all process characteristics (Donabedian, 2003; Tarlov et al., 1989). Process indicators reflect current standards of practice and, as a result, evolve over time (Larson & Muller, 2002).

Outcomes refer to a measurable change in patient health status that results from the delivery of health care (Donabedian, 1988, 2003). While measuring outcomes does not provide as direct a path as process in evaluating quality, outcomes are "the ultimate validators of the effectiveness and quality of medical care" (Donabedian, 1966, p. 169). An advantage of measuring outcomes is that both practitioners and patients can recognize results. Practitioners can objectively measure treatment effects, and patients can report whether a treatment made them feel better or worse. Another advantage is that desired outcomes can be standardized across settings. For example, a 10% reduction of nosocomial infections in a hospital is an outcome that can be compared with infection rates in other hospitals and national benchmarks regardless of geographic location.

Outcomes may be generic or specific to a disease (Donabedian, 2003). Generic outcomes such as mortality and life expectancy are generally influenced by more than disease and reflect the culture and values of family and society. Disease-specific outcomes provide a better link to the quality of health care provided. For example, a practitioner determines that mortality among a group of patients with atherosclerosis is higher than among patients without atherosclerosis (a generic outcome). Unless investigated further, the practitioner cannot conclude that the higher mortality is a direct result of atherosclerosis because it could have been caused by other factors common to the age group at risk for atherosclerosis, such as cancer, accidents, pneumonia, and so on. On the other hand, an evaluator might audit clinic records to determine the range of high-density lipoprotein (HDL) and low-density lipoprotein (LDL) cholesterol values in patients with atherosclerosis and hyperlipidemia (a disease-specific end point). Determining that 90% of patients have cholesterol values within a normal range after 1 year of treatment provides evidence that intervention has been effective in lowering cholesterol.

When we focus on only one path to quality, we assume that there is a strong correlation among structure–process–outcome (Donabedian, 1987; Larson & Muller, 2002). If we evaluate only outcome, we may assume that the change in health status was a result of the structure and/or process of care. For example, a practitioner presumes that a decrease in blood pressure in a hypertensive patient indicates that the treatment prescribed was correct. However, in actuality, the patient stopped taking the prescribed medication because of the unpleasant side effects associated with it. The patient's blood pressure decreased after the patient resigned from a stressful job. In this case, the practitioner wrongly assumed that there was a link between the medication (process) and improved health status (outcome).

Establishing links among and between S–P–O can be challenging, although a valid and reliable link must be demonstrated if the evaluation is to be trusted (Donabedian, 1978). Over time, evaluators have found a stronger correlation between process and outcome indicators than between structure and process or between structure and outcome indicators. This may be attributable to a lack of research in establishing the effect of structure on quality. It does not mean that structural indicators should be ignored; rather, each approach should be viewed as providing unique and complementary information. Taken together, S–P–O provide the most comprehensive evaluation of quality care (Donabedian, 1978, 2003).

Criteria and Standards

Criteria, standards, and norms are key components in Donabedian's framework, yet their definition and application often lack clarity and consistency across evaluations (Donabedian, 1981, 1982). Donabedian addressed this problem by comparing and contrasting the terms. He described *criterion* as "an attribute of S–P–O that is used to draw an inference about quality" (Donabedian, 2003, p. 60). He defined a *standard* as a "specified quantitative measure of magnitude or frequency that specifies what is good or less so" (Donabedian, 2003, p. 60).

Criteria and standards acting together are the means by which evaluators actualize the conceptual model of S–P–O. For example, a structural criterion for providing quality care in a nursing home might be the number of registered nurses who staff the facility, whereas the associated standard might be that the facility will not have less than one registered nurse on each shift (Table 3.1). A process criterion might be the number and percentage of patients assessed for decubitus ulcers; the associated standard might be that 100% of patients will be assessed daily for pressure ulcers. An outcome criterion might be the number of patients with pressure ulcers; the associated standard might be that no patient will develop a pressure ulcer.

TABLE 3.1 Examples of Criteria and Standards

Approach	Criterion	Standard
Structure	RNs staffing a nursing home Protocol for screening patients with diabetes mellitus	No less than one RN on each shift Protocol will include measuring HbA1c and blood pressure at each clinic visit
Process	Patients assessed for pressure ulcers Patients tested for HbA1c and high blood pressure	100% of patients will be assessed daily for pressure ulcers 100% of patients will have HbA1c and blood pressure measured
Outcomes	Patients diagnosed with pressure ulcers Level of HbA1c and blood pressure	No patient will develop a pressure ulcer 80% of patients will have HbA1c <7 and blood pressure <140/80

Role of Patient/Consumer

Patients play a vital role in evaluating the quality of health care. As one-half of the practitioner–patient dyad, they are well qualified to provide certain input about their care. Patients are qualified to rate the amenities of care that form the contextual and environmental experience (structure). For example, patients are qualified to assess whether the room was clean and odor free, whether the food was tasty and delivered promptly, and whether parking was available and affordable.

Patients also provide a unique perspective in rating the technical proficiency and interpersonal skills of their practitioners (process). Did the practitioner explain the problem and interventions clearly? Did the practitioner appear caring? Did the practitioner spend time answering questions? Was the staff pleasant and respectful? Although they may not understand the intricacies of technology, patients do know whether a procedure made them feel better or worse (an outcome). Patients can determine whether a treatment improved their ability to perform activities of daily living or enabled them to return to work (Donabedian, 1980, 1992, 2003).

Evaluators must bear in mind that, for a variety of reasons, patients are not always the best judges of quality. The amenities that please one patient may cause distress in another. For example, one patient's hospital experience may be improved by having a roommate, whereas another patient prefers to be alone. Some patients focus on interpersonal relationships, whereas others are more concerned with technical performance. Expectations of a successful outcome may or may not be realistic. Regardless of limitations, patient input is an essential component in determining quality of care (Donabedian, 1987, 1992, 2003; Larson & Muller, 2002).

Application of the Structure, Process, and Outcome Conceptual Model

From a practical perspective, the most important attribute of the Donabedian S–P–O model is how useful it has proven to be over time. The S–P–O concepts are so universally accepted that practitioners may assume that the categories of S–P–O have always been part of quality evaluation. In fact, the model has evolved and adapted as practitioners increasingly apply it in innovative and novel ways. Three studies that illustrate how Donabedian's model adapts to a variety of settings and clinical specialties are presented in Table 3.2 and discussed in the following text.

TABLE 3.2 Examples of Evaluative Studies Using Structure–Process–Outcome

Study	Structure	Process	Outcome	Findings/Conclusions
Kilbourne et al. (2010)				
Developed a framework to measure quality of care in patients with mental disorders and comorbidities	Number of general practitioners available Percent of mental health practitioners with knowledge of substance abuse Number of dual-diagnosis beds available Compliance with evidence-based care	Percent of patients receiving recommended screening for lipids and hypertension Percent of patients who had ocular and foot assessments Percent of patients with substance use screening Percent of patients receiving substance use care	Percent with acceptable screening results Patient satisfaction Mortality Addiction severity index changes Percent going back to work	Authors plan to use the framework and evaluate results
Shield et al. (2014)				
Developed a model to represent the effect of medical staff on the quality of care in nursing homes	Type of staffing—open versus closed Number of staff attendance	Communication Coordination Presence at staff meetings	Emergency visits Readmission Pain control	Donabedian's model clarified variable interactions and advanced research
Holt et al. (2014)				
Integrative review assessed the characteristics of NMHCs	Holistic care Facilities Faculty providers Grants Vulnerable population	Health education programs Screening programs Chronic disease care Midwifery care Referral care	Patient satisfaction Increased detection of disease Increased vaccines Better birth outcomes	Donabedian's model proved valuable in evaluating quality of care and in developing an evidence-based description of NMHCs

NMHC, nurse-managed health center.

Kilbourne et al. (2010) were concerned that patients with major mental health disorders frequently receive less than optimal care when they are diagnosed with accompanying substance abuse and medical problems. Using Donabedian's model, they sought to develop a method to identify S–P–O measures with the goal of improving quality of care. They identified structural measures, including the availability of medical care practitioners, practitioners with substance abuse knowledge, readiness of hospital beds for patients with dual diagnoses, and patient compliance with evidence-based treatment protocols. Process measures focused on screening and treatment for substance abuse and diagnosis of problems related to diabetes mellitus, hypertension, and comorbidities common in this patient population. Process measures were linked to outcomes that included patient satisfaction, morbidity, and mortality data. The authors noted that it was not difficult to obtain data about structural measures because there was no need to rely on patient records but that it was difficult to establish the link between structure and process and between structure and outcome. They determined that the comprehensiveness of the S–P–O model was an advantage in successfully evaluating care provided to this patient population and resolved to apply and assess the validity of Donabedian's model in future studies.

Shield et al. (2014) evaluated the structure of care and its link to process and outcome in a series of interrelated studies focused on the effectiveness of medical staff in nursing homes. Physicians, nurse practitioners (NPs), and physician assistants were categorized as medical staff. Using data from studies and surveys that they had conducted, the authors adapted Donabedian's model to interpret interactions in the clinical setting of a nursing home. Based on the results, the authors concluded that regulating the frequency and length of attendance by the medical staff (e.g., in a closed staff model) increases medical presence in the nursing home. Medical presence was associated with better communication and coordination of care. They also noted that geriatric NPs were perceived to provide higher quality care than physician assistants or other types of NPs. The authors concluded that this study enabled them to more clearly define links among the variables in their model, to ascertain which interactions increased quality of care, and to determine future research topics.

Holt et al. (2014) applied Donabedian's model to guide an integrative review of the literature that examined the characteristics of nurse-managed health centers (NMHCs) within the context of health care quality. Their review yielded 59 articles that were included in the study. The authors then used qualitative analysis to categorize the articles under the classifications of S–P–O. As a result of the review, the authors were able to develop an evidence-based description of NMHCs that would facilitate the continuing examination of this model of care and its comparison with other health care models.

Although these examples represent disparate uses of Donabedian's S–P–O model, all have in common a precise identification of the aspects of S–P–O as they relate to the study. In each case, the S–P–O model facilitated an objective and systematic assessment of health care quality and a direction for future evaluations.

Effectiveness–Efficiency–Equity Model

Aday collaborated with economists, physicians, and other health service researchers in developing an integrated and comprehensive framework that evaluates health policies on the basis of three principles: effectiveness, efficiency, and equity (Aday &

Andersen, 1974; Aday et al., 1999, 2004). Aday's framework is eclectic, integrating some of Donabedian's concepts with other constructs from epidemiology, sociology, ethics, economics, and the behavioral sciences. The framework addresses the interactive nature of policy and health care quality by providing practitioners with methodologies to measure the impact of policy and the skills to influence policy changes. Depending on the goal, evaluation may be at the microsystem, mesosystem, or macrosystem level.

In the effectiveness–efficiency–equity framework, health care policies are viewed from the perspective of the practitioner or researcher who seeks to understand the intricacies and variety of policies at the local, state, and federal levels and their impact on practice and achievement of health outcomes (Aday et al., 2004). The practitioner examines the positive and negative ways that policy affects the health status of individuals, communities, and populations and compares and contrasts the impact of alternate health care programs and offers recommendations to administrators and lawmakers who ultimately make health care policy decisions (Aday & Andersen, 1984; Phillips et al., 2000; Quill et al., 1999).

Aday and colleagues adapted Donabedian's S–P–O Model to categorize the components of their framework and to provide an approach for evaluation. The system for delivering health care, the population projected to need health care, and the setting in which the population lives comprise the structure of care. The attained access to health care and the health risks of the patients seeking care comprise the process of care. The health status of individuals and populations comprises the outcome of care, with effectiveness, efficiency, and equity in health care serving as the criteria against which these outcomes are evaluated.

Aday et al. (2004, p. 57) defined *effectiveness* as "the degree to which improvements in health now attainable, are, in fact, attained." In analyzing effectiveness, the practitioner includes not only improvements resulting from the health services provided, but also improvements associated with the familial, cultural, and environmental settings. Effectiveness can further be evaluated at the micro (clinical) and macro (population) levels. Clinical effectiveness relates primarily to changes in the health status of individuals through the health care provided. Population effectiveness relates to changes in the overall health status of populations achieved through health care and environmental factors (Aday et al., 2004).

Efficiency refers to both the production and allocation of health care services. Aday et al. (2004, p. 121) refer to *production efficiency* as "producing a given level of output at a minimum cost." They refer to allocative efficiency as the "attainment of the 'right,' or most valued, mix of outputs" (Aday et al., 2004, p. 121). Efficiency can be viewed from a macro- or microperspective (2004). The DNP nurse may or may not be involved in evaluating efficiency at the macrolevel but may collaborate with other health professionals in conducting microlevel evaluations. For example, the practitioner may be asked to determine the best combination of supplies, equipment, and human resources (the inputs) needed to efficiently produce a health care service (2004). A practitioner may also be part of a team conducting a cost-effectiveness, cost-benefit, or cost-utility analysis of a technology, service, or program.

Equity refers to "maximizing the fairness in the distribution of health care (procedural equity) and minimizing the disparities in health across groups (substantive equity)" (Aday et al., 2004, p. 189). Indicators of procedural equity include equality of input into policy decisions, types of facilities and providers available, payment sources, number of services provided, and patient satisfaction. Indicators of disparity in health groups include inequalities with regard to clinical indicators and to population rates of morbidity and mortality. A DNP nurse may be called upon to collect information about one or more of these indicators in order to determine the equity of current health policies in an agency, community, or population. In evaluating equity, the practitioner examines factors that facilitate and factors that hinder the fair and just distribution of health care across all demographic and clinical groups (Aday et al., 1999, 2004).

Centers for Disease Control and Prevention Model

The Centers for Disease Control and Prevention (CDC) provides a generic framework for evaluating large programs such as community-based or population-based systems (see Figure 3.1). According to the CDC, the following framework is a practical nonprescriptive tool that logically summarizes the important elements of program evaluation. It contains two related dimensions of steps in the evaluation process and sets standards for a "good" evaluation. The following six connected steps of the framework are components of any evaluation, both large or small. There are many options at each step and a large number of potential ways to gather evidence.

- Engage stakeholders—to include those involved in program operations, those served or affected by the program, and primary users of the evaluation.
- Describe the program—to include the need, expected effects (outcomes), activities, resources, stage, context, and logic model.
- Focus the evaluation design—to assess the issues of greatest concern to stakeholders while using time and resources as efficiently as possible. Consider the purpose, users, uses, questions, methods, and agreements.

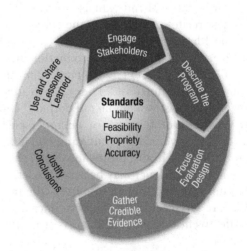

Figure 3.1 CDC evaluation model.
Source: Centers for Disease Control and Prevention. (2016). *A framework for program evaluation.* http://www.cdc.gov/eval/framework/.

- Gather credible evidence—to strengthen evaluation judgments and the recommendations that follow. These aspects of evidence gathering typically affect perceptions of credibility: indicators, sources, quality, quantity, and logistics.
- Justify conclusions—to link conclusions to the evidence gathered and judge those conclusions against agreed-upon values or standards set by the stakeholders. Justify conclusions on the basis of evidence (data) using these five elements: standards, analysis/synthesis, interpretation, judgment, and recommendations.
- Ensure—to use and share lessons learned—developing evaluation reports requires design, preparation, feedback, follow-up, and dissemination.

In general, activities flow according to a sequence of logical activities, although in practice the steps may be encountered slightly out of order. Following the sequence is useful because earlier steps provide the foundation for subsequent progress, although the built-in flexibility is acknowledged. Decisions about conduct of a given step should not be finalized until prior steps have been thoroughly addressed (CDC, 2011).

Standards

Intrinsic to the framework is the application of each of four groups of evaluation standards that are used as a "lens" to help isolate the best approaches at each step. The CDC offers 30 standards that are organized into the four groups. These standards help answer the question, "Will this evaluation be a 'good' evaluation?" The set of 30 standards assesses the quality of evaluation activities, determining whether a set of evaluative activities are well designed and working to their potential. These standards, adopted from The Joint Committee on Standards for Educational Evaluation, answer the question, "Will this evaluation be effective?" The standards are recommended as criteria for judging the quality of program evaluation efforts in public health.

The four groups of standards are:

- Utility standards—ensure that an evaluation will serve the information needs of intended users.
- Feasibility standards—ensure that an evaluation will be realistic, prudent, diplomatic, and frugal.
- Propriety standards—ensure that an evaluation will be conducted legally, ethically, and with due regard for the welfare of those involved in the evaluation, as well as those affected by its results.
- Accuracy standards—ensure that an evaluation will reveal and convey technically adequate information about the features that determine the worth or merit of the program being evaluated.

The steps and standards are used together throughout the evaluation process. For each step, there is a subset of standards that are most relevant to that aspect of the appraisal and are available at the CDC website (www.cdc.gov/eval/steps/index.htm). There is broad applicability of this model to various size evaluations from the perspectives of both scope and complexity of the evaluation undertaken.

The Triple Aim Framework

In 2007, a group of researchers sponsored by the Institute for Health Improvement (IHI) developed the Triple Aim framework, an ambitious attempt to guide the work of organizations and other entities seeking to improve the quality of health care (IHI, 2015a; Lewis, 2014; Whittington et al., 2015). Simply stated, the Triple Aim seeks to improve the health of populations, enhance the experience of care for individuals, and reduce the per capita cost of health care. This framework continues to be a viable and useful framework for evaluating health care.

The first aim is to *advance population health*. In many instances, this can be accomplished through public health activities, such as providing nutrition education and increasing the number of individuals who are immunized. These interventions may not involve expensive high-tech procedures but can have a large impact on the health of communities. Another example is educating people about prevention of COVID-19 using CDC guidelines. The second aim is to *improve the health experiences of individuals*. In defining health experience, the architects of the Triple Aim referred to the six dimensions of quality described by the Institute of Medicine (IOM). These quality dimensions are safety, effectiveness, patient-centeredness, timeliness, efficiency, and equity (IOM, 2001). The third aim is to *decrease the per person cost of health care*. The United States' low position among developed countries ranked on the basis of health care indicators is incongruent with the cost of health care, which surpasses the spending of all other developed countries. There are many reasons for this paradox, including excessive administrative costs, extensive use of expensive high-tech interventions, greater charges for health products and services in the United States compared with those in other countries, and the prevalent perception among health care providers that they must practice "defensive medicine" (Reinhardt, 2008). Concerns with health care include overutilization, underutilization, and wrong health care services.

Berwick et al. (2008) stressed that the position of "integrator" is essential to the success of the Triple Aim framework. The integrator is a recognized group responsible for coordinating all health care activities of the organization as well as implementing the components of the Triple Aim strategy. These components include encouraging individuals and families to become more engaged in their own health care, changing the way primary care is delivered, controlling the delivery of resources to populations, educating the population about the cost of healthcare, and providing a link between the organization and the larger health care system. The authors cited Kaiser Permanente as an example of a noteworthy integrator.

Many recent discussions have been on revising the Triple Aim to the Quadruple Aim by adding a fourth aim of attaining joy in work for caregivers. Some organizations have added other priority aims. For example, the Military Health System has added readiness as their fourth aim (Feeley, 2017). In addressing the issue of adding a fourth aim, Feeley (2017) points out the following: the Triple Aim is solely about patients; the original Triple Aim has not been accomplished to date; don't lose focus on achieving the Triple Aim by diluting the focus; and stay true to measuring what matters to patients. Although joy in the workplace is important in delivery of care, it detracts from the focus on patients. He further points out that raising joy in the workplace is a strategy in the pursuit of the Triple Aim. Finally, he notes that organizations should feel free to interpret the Triple Aim in a way that makes sense to them, but that this should be done deliberately and strategically.

An Organized Approach to Improving Quality

The IHI uses the phrase "science of improvement" to describe the steps in a process designed to move organizations and communities toward achieving their objectives. To be successful, organizations should have the following: well-defined goals; an appropriate rubric for measuring success; an explanation of how the concepts they develop will result in desired change; a plan that directs activities; a commitment to implementing the plan on a small scale to determine its impact; a method to represent systems interactions; and the ability to learn through experimentation (IHI, 2015b). One key to successful implementation of the model of improvement is the use of valid and reliable measures. The IHI urges organizations to include process, balancing, and outcome measures. Balancing measures are used to ensure that one activity does not offset the desired effect of another by having a negative impact in another area within the organization.

The IHI also developed metrics, referred to as "whole system measures," which are linked to each of the aims and may be added to the existing metrics of an organization. Thus, progress toward achieving the three aims can be compared across organizations and populations. For example, patient experience is measured through surveys and indicators linked to the IOM's six dimensions of quality. Population health is quantified using functional health status, risk status, disease burden, and mortality. Per capita cost is calculated using patient cost and hospital utilization rates (Nelson et al., 2007).

Application of the Triple Aim Framework

The Triple Aim has become widely accepted as a guide to evaluating performance quality. In 2007, the IHI invited national and international participation to evaluate the performance of the framework (Whittington et al., 2015). A total of 141 entities took part, including hospitals, insurance companies, and public health agencies. Some of these organizations were successful in applying the framework, whereas others did not meet the mark. The investigators observed that organizations had difficulty achieving all three aims and that the greatest challenge was decreasing health cost, largely because of the reluctance of organizations to eliminate sources of revenue. The investigators concluded that the following principles increased the chances of success: a solid foundation, services appropriate for the population; and a long-term educational program about Triple Aim strategies.

In 2010, Dr. Donald Berwick, Administrator for Medicare and Medicaid Services (CMS), recommended using the framework to improve the quality of health care for Medicare and Medicaid enrollees (Fleming, 2010). His recommendation, along with the passage of the Affordable Care Act, encouraged organizations to apply the framework in a variety of health care settings. Ouslander and Maslow (2012) discussed the importance of developing valid measures that are aligned with the Triple Aim for patients in long-term care. Potter et al. (2013) used the framework to create a research protocol to support quality care for patients with inborn errors of metabolism. Christopher (2014) discussed the relevance of the Triple Aim to the Visiting Nurse Services of New York.

One article has particular relevance to DNP nurses. Hoyle and Johnson (2015) discussed the impact of health care reform on the nursing profession and the related requests from organizations such as the American Association of Colleges of

Nursing (2006) for educational initiatives to develop increased leadership abilities among advanced practice nurses. These recommendations provided the impetus for faculty at the University of Washington, School of Nursing, to offer DNP students the education and experience to increase their proficiency in quality improvement activities. The authors described a DNP–family nurse practitioner curriculum that is aligned with the goals of the Triple Aim. Students were introduced to quality improvement strategies, tools, and processes that they then applied in the clinical setting. Ongoing evaluation was conducted using a clinical evaluation instrument, along with peer, faculty, and agency feedback.

In another example of the flexibility of the Triple Aim framework, Prior et al. (2014) observed that children with chronic diseases frequently have a difficult time transitioning from pediatric to adult clinical settings. The authors utilized the Triple Aim framework to conduct a systematic literature review designed to examine measures associated with the transition process. A total of 33 studies were included in the final review, of which 12 focused on diabetes mellitus. Other conditions included were transplants, sickle cell disease, cystic fibrosis, and HIV. Health care measures were classified using the Triple Aim. The authors concluded that studies examining transition care often employ methodologies and tools that are inconsistent and whose validity and reliability have not been established. They recommended that experts in the field work together to create measures that are applicable across a wide variety of chronic disease states.

Logic Models

Logic models can be used for both large-scale and small-scale evaluations. Many DNP students have found the logic model a valuable tool for the planning, implementation, and evaluation of their DNP projects because a logic model maps the key elements of the project and how various components relate to each other. Similarities of the logic model are noted with other models. Logic models have components similar to the S–P–O model. However, logic models provide a more detailed blueprint of how to plan, implement, measure, and evaluate performance. Emphasis is placed on first defining end points and then determining what activities and inputs are needed to achieve the desired outcomes. Each component of a logic model is connected to and is a consequence of a prior component. The approach is iterative because activities may be modified if end points are not attained. For example, logic models are frequently used by health professionals who are concerned with evaluating mission-motivated rather than profit-motivated end points of the organization (Chen, 2005; Fitzpatrick et al., 2004). A logic model may be applied at the macrosystem, mesosystem, or microsystem level.

Logic models focus on the *inputs* (also called resources), activities, and end points of a program or project. *End points* may be referred to as *outputs, outcomes,* or *impact.* Figure 3.2 presents an example of a logic model used by the CDC Division for Heart Disease and Stroke Prevention (2011) to evaluate a large-scale project. *Inputs* refer to structural components such as the organizational framework, administrative guidelines and protocols, number of health care providers, health care environment, and financial resources. Project activities are the processes that take place as a program is implemented. These may include health care interventions, educational activities, or technological services.

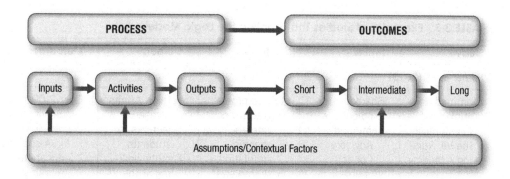

Figure 3.2 Layout of general logic model.
Source: Centers for Disease Control and Prevention Division for Heart Disease and Stroke Prevention. (2011).
State heart disease and stroke prevention program. Evaluation guide: Developing and using a logic model.
http://www.cdc.gov/DHDSP/index.htm. Reprinted with permission.

Logic models use distinct end points defined by scope and time (Fitzpatrick et al., 2004). Although the number of end points may vary, there are generally three types of end points described in a logic model. The first end point is output. *Outputs* are immediate consequences of activities; for example, the number and types of patients receiving a particular health care intervention, the quantity of health education pamphlets delivered to patients, or the total number of hours of screening dedicated to community-outcomes provide evaluators with a specific timeline to measure program performance. End points may be short term, intermediate, or long term depending on the project. *Outcomes* focus on improvements in health status, including cognitive, behavioral, and attitudinal change. In some logic models, the term *impact* is used to represent a long-term end point such as a change in policy or population health. There are a number of guidelines available online that facilitate the creation of logic models, including those developed by the Kellogg Foundation (2004) and the CDC Division for Heart Disease and Stroke Prevention (2011).

Application of Logic Models

Logic models have been used extensively in a variety of health care programs, including a statewide heart disease and stroke prevention program (Sitaker et al., 2008), a teenage pregnancy prevention program (Hulton, 2007), the creation of a DNP orthopedic clinical specialty (Instone & Palmer, 2013), and the collaboration of a school of nursing and a Veteran Affairs (VA) Medical Center to develop a VA Nursing Academy (Harper et al., 2015). Two examples along with selected variables are provided in the following text and in Table 3.3.

Harper et al. (2015) described the collaboration between the Birmingham VA Medical Center and the University of Alabama at Birmingham School of Nursing (SON) to form the Birmingham VA Nursing Academy. Formation of the Academy was part of a 5-year grant funded by Veterans Affairs. The objectives of this alliance between academia and service included the recruitment of graduates from the SON to work at the VA Medical Center, the integration of veteran-related content into the curriculum at the SON, and improvement in the quality of care delivered to

TABLE 3.3 Examples of Studies That Applied the Logic Model

Study	Inputs	Activities	Outputs	Outcomes
Harper et al. (2015)				
Examined a joint effort to establish the VA Nursing Academy	Shared objectives Combined Advisory Council VA nurses SON faculty	Create programs for: veteran-specific simulation, shared staff between the VA, and the SON Formative evaluation	Veteran Affairs focused lectures to students Faculty working at the VA VA staff teaching at SON Summative evaluation plan	Over 2,000 BSN students participated in VA-specific educational programs Increased support for veteran students Increased quality of care for veterans
Instone and Palmer (2013)				
Developed a plan to include orthopedic content into a DNP program	Orthopedic certification DNP programs Experienced faculty	Administrative approval Local resources Program personnel Potential students	Didactic orthopedic course Clinical practice	Graduation rates Certification exam pass rates Faculty and student satisfaction Orthopedic nursing employment Increased number of low-income clients receiving care from DNPs

DNP, Doctor of Nursing Practice; SON, School of Nursing; VA, Veterans Affairs.

veterans. The authors applied the logic model to provide organization and direction for both institutions as they continue their partnership.

Instone and Palmer (2013) observed that an aging population and an insufficient supply of orthopedic surgeons resulted in an unmet need among practitioners with the education and experience to provide quality care to patients with orthopedic problems. NPs educated in this specialty at the master's level currently provide care to this population; however, the emergence of the DNP nurse presents an opportunity to expand the number and expertise of orthopedic providers. The authors asserted that a realistic solution is to place orthopedic content and practice into the DNP program as a specialty area. They applied the logic model to provide a blueprint for action. In order to be eligible to take the orthopedic nursing certification examination, students must have accrued at least 2,500 hours of clinical training. Some or all of this training may fit into the clinical concentration of the DNP educational program. They concluded that increasing the number of DNP nurses trained as orthopedic specialists allows nurses to collaborate with physicians in a partnership to improve the quality of care for all patients with orthopedic problems, particularly those from vulnerable populations who have historically lacked access to care.

Monitoring and Evaluation of Health Systems Strengthening Framework

National and international leaders have long recognized the need to measure the health status of citizens and the benefit of comparing standard health outcomes in one nation with those of other nations. The framework for monitoring and evaluation of health systems strengthening was developed in response to this need through the collaborative efforts of several international organizations, including WHO, the World Bank, the Global Alliance for Vaccines and Immunization (GAVI), and the Global Fund (Boerma et al., 2009). This macrosystem level framework shares components with the basic logic model described previously. It also provides guidelines for standardizing terms, indicators, and methods with the goal of improving the quality and comprehensiveness of health care evaluation within and among individual countries. Although it is recommended for use at the national or international level, the framework is also suitable for use at a regional or state level.

The monitoring and evaluation of health systems strengthening framework (M&E framework) consists of four main indicator domains: inputs and processes, outputs, outcomes, and impact. The *inputs and processes* domain contains governance, health financing, infrastructure, workforce, and supplies. The *outputs* domain contains services readiness and access, as well as intervention quality, safety, and efficiency. The *outcomes* domain contains coverage of interventions and risk behaviors and factors. The *impact* domain contains improved health outcomes and equity; social, financial risk protection; and responsiveness.

An important component of the M&E framework is the use of valid and reliable core indicators across the domains. The authors recommended that evaluators not only develop indicators relevant to their own target population, but also avail themselves of internationally accepted indicators when appropriate. As in every evaluation, sources for data collection should be relevant and feasible. Such sources include, but are not limited to, surveys, clinical trials, large national databases, registries, and hospital records. Once collected, data are analyzed using a variety of statistical tests. Results are first reported to the decision makers who requested the information and then disseminated to a wider audience in the form of oral presentations and publications. The ultimate benefit of many nations using the same framework, definitions, indicators, and methods and then sharing their results is an increase in the validity of the findings and a better chance that health care programs will be effective, efficient, and equitable.

Application of the Monitoring and Evaluation Framework

As an example, a DNP nurse may be a member of an evaluation team that is asked to examine the quality of newborn care in a southwestern region of the United States (Table 3.4). One of the initial decisions that the team makes is to choose indicators and sources to evaluate the four domains (i.e., inputs and processes, outputs, outcomes, and impact). Under the domain of *inputs and processes*, indicators might include hospital expenditures (health financing), number of registered nurses (workforce), neonatal intensive care unit beds (infrastructure), and average cost of ventilators and incubators (supplies). National health databases, registries, surveys, and assessments of clinical and hospital facilities are good sources of these data.

TABLE 3.4 An Example of the Monitoring and Evaluation Framework: Indicators and Sources for Evaluating Quality of Newborn Care

Domain	Indicators	Sources
Inputs and process	1. Expenditures for hospital newborn facilities 2. Number of registered nurses per 10,000 population 3. Number of neonatal intensive care units per 10,000 population 4. Average cost for ventilators and incubators	1. National health databases 2. National nurse registries 3. Hospital surveys 4. Hospital surveys and facility assessment
Outputs	1. Utilization of registered nurses 2. Geographic location of newborn facilities in relation to population 3. Neonatal case fatality	1. Survey 2. Survey 3. Hospital records and national databases
Outcomes	1. Neonatal aftercare home coverage 2. Immunization coverage 3. Newborn screening for hearing coverage 4. Breastfeeding for 6 months	1. Survey 2. Medical records 3. National registries 4. Medical records
Impact	1. Child mortality (under 5 years) 2. Hearing disabilities diagnosed in children under 5 years	1. Vital statistics 2. Survey and medical records

In the *output domain*, indicators might include utilization of registered nurses (service readiness), location of facilities (access), and neonatal case fatality (quality and safety). Surveys, registries, hospital records, and national databases are generally used as sources for these types of indicators. In the *outcome domain*, indicators might include use of aftercare home coverage, immunization coverage, and newborn screening for hearing cost (coverage of interventions), and breastfeeding for 6 months (risk factors and behaviors). Data could be collected through surveys and medical record review. Impact indicators include child mortality and hearing disabilities diagnosed. Information related to these impact indicators might be obtained from vital statistics, surveys, and health records. See Table 3.4.

Kirkpatrick's Four Levels of Learning Evaluation Model

Many DNP projects include some form of educational intervention that requires evaluation. The Kirkpatrick model is one of the best known models for evaluating the results of training and educational programs. It takes into account both informal formats and a variety of styles of training/educating to determine aptitude based on criteria at four levels. Developed by Dr. Donald Kirkpatrick in the 1950s, it has withstood the test of time as a useful evaluation model for a variety of businesses. The model has great flexibility in that it can be implemented before, throughout, and following training to show the value of training. *Level 1: Reaction* measures how participants react to the training (e.g., satisfaction with the training).

Level 2: Learning analyzes whether the participants truly understood the training (e.g., increase in knowledge, skills, or experience). *Level 3: Behavior* tries to ascertain whether participants are utilizing what they learned at work (e.g., change in behaviors), and *Level 4: Results* determines if the material had a positive impact on the organization (clinical facility) or its practices (e.g., team effectiveness). See Table 3.5 for further discussion of the Kirkpatrick model. Figure 3.3 shows the sequential steps of the model.

The Kirkpatrick model is a linear model that proceeds from step one through four hierarchical steps. Data collected from all of the previous levels can be used as a foundation for analysis at the following levels. As a result, each subsequent level provides a clearer and more accurate measurement of the usefulness of the training course but also suggests a need for more detailed evaluation (Kirkpatrick model, https://educationaltechnology.net/kirkpatrick-model-four-levels-learning -evaluation/; Kirkpatrick, 1994; Kurt, 2016). Figure 3.4 shows the hierarchical organization of the Kirkpatrick model.

TABLE 3.5   Description of Levels in the Kirkpatrick Model

Level	Purpose/Description	Evaluation Questions and Methods
Level 1 Evaluation-Reaction	• Evaluate the individual's reaction to the training; ask questions to determine if participants enjoyed/were happy with the experience and if the content was useful for their work	• Did the training meet participants' needs? • Were the teaching methods used (PowerPoint, Canvas, etc.) helpful and acceptable? • Methods: interviews, online questionnaire
Level 2 Evaluation-Learning	• Designed to gauge the level of expertise, knowledge, or mindset that participants have developed • Generally easy to measure	• Observations, pre/post examination (printed format), interviews • Clear scoring to determine level of achievement; may use comparison groups
Level 3 Evaluation-Transfer (Was the learning being applied by participant?)	• Occurs 3–6 months post training • Analyze differences in participants' behavior at work after completing program • Focus on relation of behavioral change in knowledge, skills, or mindset related to program content	• Evaluator observations, interviews, surveys, supervisor observations, and others • Were the learned knowledge and skills used? • Takes more time to notice changes
Level 4 Evaluation-Results	• Review of overall training objectives and if they were achieved (e.g., decreased number of medication errors)	• Evaluate impact on organization's scorecard or other identified criteria • Report of change from participants and supervisors (e.g., yearly employee evaluation)

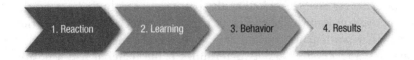

Figure 3.3   The Kirkpatrick model.

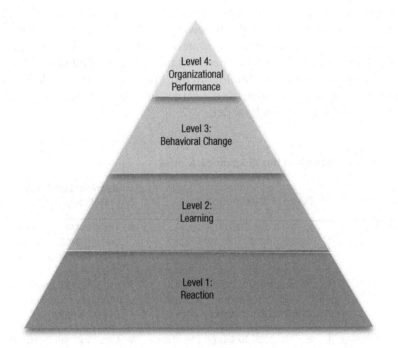

Figure 3.4   Hierarchical levels of the Kirkpatrick model.

USE OF MODELS BY DOCTOR OF NURSING PRACTICE NURSES

In this discussion of models for evaluation, there are similarities in the structure and domains of the models, in that they are all based on some established criteria that are known to both the project evaluator and the project or program being evaluated to support transparency and clarity. It is also implied that the evaluator is conducting the evaluation with an open mind and is focused on the criteria without preconceived opinions or bias. As one considers the various evaluation models presented in this chapter and available from other sources, many models are versatile in that they can be used for both large-scale evaluation projects as well as small-scale evaluations. For DNP students conducting their DNP projects, models such as the logic model are particularly valuable in that the logic model can be customized to the focus of the project as a useful blueprint for planning, implementing, and evaluating their DNP project. It can also be revised as conditions of the project change over time. In addition, we have found that Donabedian's S–P–O model has been a good evaluation model, particularly for DNP nurse executive students whose DNP projects often focus on organizational change issues. However, other models are also useful, so it is important to find the most appropriate models for the project at hand.

MODELS FOR OVERALL EVALUATION OF A PROJECT OR PROGRAM

DNP projects and evaluation can be considered on the basis of two aspects. The first is whether the specific *project outcomes* were achieved as a result of the planning and implementation of the project. The second aspect concerns what to do with the impact of the project (e.g., how to address the impact of the project) after project evaluation findings conclude that the project met its stated outcomes. Further questions have to consider whether the project targeted the correct stakeholders and whether the outcomes/findings were meaningful for the organization or stakeholders requesting the evaluation. Two high-level robust evaluation models are discussed that link program evaluation findings to decision-making, actions, adoption, and implementation of interventions that influence the usability and impact of the program or project: the context, inputs, process, and products (CIPP) model and the RE-AIM model.

Context, Inputs, Process, and Products Model

CIPP is a program evaluation model developed by Daniel Stufflebeam and colleagues in the 1960s to link evaluation with the needs of program decision makers to make decisions and act (Stufflebeam, 2003). Stufflebeam (2003) described the CIPP evaluation model as "a comprehensive framework for guiding evaluations of programs, projects, personnel, products, institutions, and evaluation systems." The CIPP evaluation model is used to guide program designers/creators to develop and implement projects (Stufflebeam, 2003). All parts of the project can be evaluated before, during, and after the project is completed. The CIPP model systematically collects information about a program to identify strengths and limitations in content or delivery, to improve program effectiveness, or plan for the future of the program (Zhang et al., 2011). The focus of the model is on continuous improvement by concentrating on four areas of a program, namely, the overall goals or mission (context evaluation), the plans and resources (input evaluation), the activities or components (process evaluation), and the outcomes or objectives (product evaluation), and are designed to judge a program's or project's value (Stufflebeam, 2003). Each component has a question associated with it that needs to be answered. The model is focused on using the evaluation process to identify problems with the processes and look for opportunities for improvement (Stufflebeam, 2003). The following briefly describes each of the four components of the model and the related question to be answered.

Context evaluation addresses the program's needs, problems, assets, and opportunities to help decision makers define goals, priorities, and outcomes. *Context evaluation* examines the purpose of a project, including assessment of the needs or problems to be solved, and then defines the goals used to target the problem (Zhang et al., 2011). Context evaluation can be achieved by answering the question, What needs to be done? The context evaluation often includes baseline audits and needs assessment.

The second component of the CIPP model is input evaluation. *Input evaluation* assesses the methods and work processes component of a project. It examines alternative approaches, competing action plans, staffing plans, and budget for their feasibility and potential cost-effectiveness to meet targeted needs and achieve goals. Input evaluation can be achieved by answering the question, How should it be done? With this information, decision makers can choose among alternate plans, funding proposals, allocation of resources, and other aspects of the program. At a later time, input evaluation can also assist others in judging the overall quality of the plan.

Process evaluation is the third component that monitors the project implementation processes, including implementation strategies, data collection, and feedback (Zhang et al., 2011). Process evaluation can be achieved by answering the question, Is it being done? It investigates the implementation plan so that decision makers can evaluate feasibility and flow as well as judge program performance. Process evaluation addresses fidelity, that is, is how consistently the implementation plan being followed. The evaluation includes documenting the project implementation process, which is valuable because it helps to identify areas for needed change during the implementation phase instead of evaluating the process after the result (Stufflebeam, 2003).

The fourth and last part of the CIPP model is *product evaluation*. This helps to identify the success or failure of a project's outcome or product (Stufflebeam, 2003). This component speaks to the value of the product. Product evaluations include identification of outcomes and their evaluation. Outcomes are classified broadly as intended and unintended, short term, intermediate, and long term. The evaluation that helps staff judge the success of the program in meeting its target needs can be achieved by answering the question, did the project succeed? Although the improvement may only achieve a short-term goal, achieving long-term success requires the completion of continued product evaluations.

In summary, the CIPP model is a process-based, thorough evaluation model that can be applied at any stage of project or program development such as planning a new program, assessing a mature program, or evaluating a program after its completion. The CIPP model is designed to assist decision makers in deciding to maintain, improve, or discontinue the program under review. According to Stufflebeam (1971) the purpose of evaluation is not to prove, but to improve. The model is applicable to both formative and summative program evaluation. An advantage of the CIPP model is that it is nonlinear and hence provides a dynamic framework for evaluating several aspects of a program to determine its value and allow for corrections to be made as necessary to meet the desired outcomes (https://en.wikipedia.org/wiki/CIPP_evaluation_model).

Reach, Effectiveness, Adoption, Implementation, and Maintenance Model

The acronym RE-AIM represents reach, effectiveness, adoption, implementation, and maintenance. The RE-AIM model was originally developed by Glasgow et al. (1999) as a framework for consistent reporting of research results and was later used to organize reviews of existing literature on health promotion and disease management in different settings (https://azhin.org/cummings/re-aim; Glasgow et al., 1999). More recently, RE-AIM has been used to translate research into practice, help programs improve their chances of working in "real-world" settings, and for evaluation. The goal of RE-AIM is to encourage stakeholders such as program planners, evaluators, and policy-makers to carefully examine key program components including external validity to improve the sustainable adoption and implementation of effective, generalizable, evidence-based interventions, and thus influence the impact and usability of the program or project (https://azhin.org/cummings/re-aim). This is an important point, especially for quality improvement initiatives, and the RE-AIM model has been useful in evaluating quality improvement projects.

The RE-AIM website (http://www.re-aim.org/about/what-is-re-aim/) provides excellent descriptive information about the model. The following is based on information from this website that includes the five steps involved in translating research into action but is also useful for evaluation.

- *Reach* asks, did you reach the target population that is willing to participate in the project?
- *Effectiveness* or efficacy examines whether the impact of an intervention on key outcomes includes possible negative effects.
- *Adoption* addresses the number of people (e.g., leadership, nursing staff) in the setting who are willing to adopt and use the new program or change.
- *Implementation* is defined as "at the setting level, implementation refers to the intervention agents' fidelity to the various elements of an intervention's protocol, including consistency of delivery as intended and the time and cost of the intervention. At the individual level, implementation refers to clients' use of the intervention strategies" (http://www.re-aim.org/about/what-is-re-aim). In other words, was the implementation delivered as planned?
- *Maintenance* refers to adoption, integration, and hardwiring of the program or policy into the organizational structure. Maintenance at the individual level is defined as "the long-term effects of a program on outcomes after 6 or more months after the most recent intervention contact" (http://www.re-aim .org/about/what-is-re-aim). See Applying the RE-AIM Framework on its website for answers to basic questions about the model.

In summary, review of the RE-AIM model shows that both individual-level impact and institutional or setting-level impact are addressed. RE-AIM is a useful and versatile model that considers impact at the micro-, meso-, and macrolevels. The model description notes its public health impact and speaks to both the macro-level impact and the individual level impact such as smaller projects (e.g., quality improvement projects). Although the outcomes of quality improvement projects are not considered generalizable in the same sense as research projects, processes and findings of quality improvement projects are considered transferable with the caveat of modification for contextual differences (American Association of Colleges of Nursing, 2015). Therefore, the RE-AIM model is useful for evaluating the overall impact of a quality improvement project and, in turn, DNP projects.

SUMMARY

This chapter explored models to comprehensively evaluate healthcare and to improve performance and outcomes. Evaluation is designed to support decision-making and action based on what is found from the evaluation process. Each of the approaches described has proven to be beneficial, and each provides the DNP nurse with options to systematically and objectively examine interventions, programs, projects, policies, and technologies that affect individuals, groups, and populations. As a member of an evaluation team, the DNP nurse contributes to the selection of the evaluation model that best fits the purpose of the evaluation to be conducted. Once the model is chosen, the team must address the challenges inherent in conducting evaluations. Methodological challenges involve selecting valid and reliable measures, establishing associations between the components of the model, and determining the most relevant data sources, data collection methods, and types of analyses. After the results of the evaluation are determined, the team must decide on an appropriate way to disseminate their findings. Team members should also be ready to report the strengths and weaknesses of the evaluation itself. A well-conducted evaluation provides a solid foundation of data and knowledge for decision-making and action designed to improve quality outcomes and performance in healthcare settings.

REFERENCES

Aday, L. A., & Andersen, R. (1974). A framework for the study of access to medical care. *Health Services Research*, 9(3), 208–220. PMID: 4436074.

Aday, L. A., & Andersen, R. (1984). The national profile of access to medical care: Where do we stand? *AJPH*, 74(12), 1331–1339. https://doi.org/10.2105/AJPH.74.12.1331

Aday, L. A., Begley, C. E., Lairson, D. R., & Balkrishnan, R. (2004). *Evaluating the healthcare system* (3rd ed.). Health Administration Press.

Aday, L. A., Begley, C. E., Lairson, D. R., Slater, C. H., Richard, A. J., & Menloya, I. D. (1999). A framework for assessing the effectiveness, efficiency, and equity of behavioral healthcare. *American Journal of Managed Care*, 5, SP25–SP44. PMID: 10538859.

American Association of Colleges of Nursing. (2006). *The essentials of doctoral education for advanced nursing practice*. Author.

American Association of Colleges of Nursing. (2015). *The Doctor of Nursing Practice: Current issues and clarifying recommendations. Report from the Task Force on Implementation of the DNP*. Author.

American Nurses Association. (2015). *Nursing: Scope and standards of practice* (3nd ed.). Author.

Berwick, D. M., Nolan, T. W., & Whittington, J. (2008). The triple aim: Care, health, and cost. *Health Affairs*, 27(3), 759–769. https://doi.org/10.1377/hlthaff.27.3.759

Boerma, T., Abou-Zahr, C., Bos, E., Hansen, P., Addai, E., & Low-Beer, D. (2009, November). *Monitoring and evaluation of health systems strengthening*. World Health Organization. http://www.who.int/healthinfo/HSS_MandE_framework_Nov_2009.pdf

Centers for Disease Control and Prevention Division for Heart Disease and Stroke Prevention. (2011). *State heart disease and stroke prevention program*. Evaluation guide: Developing and using a logic model. http://www.cdc.gov/DHDSP/index.htm

Chen, H. T. (2005). *Practical program evaluation*. Sage.

Christopher, M. A. (2014). The role of nursing and population health in achieving the triple aim. *Home Healthcare Nurse*, 32(8), 505–506. https://doi.org/10.1097/NHH.0000000000000130

Donabedian, A. (1966). Evaluating the quality of medical care. *Milbank Memorial Fund Quarterly*, 44(Suppl. 3), 166–206. https://doi.org/10.2307/3348969

Donabedian, A. (1978). The quality of medical care. *Science*, 200(4344), 856–864. https://doi.org/10.1126/science.417400

Donabedian, A. (1980). *Explorations in quality assessment and monitoring: Vol. I. The definitions of quality and approaches to its assessment*. Health Administration Press.

Donabedian, A. (1981). Criteria, norms and standards of quality: What do they mean? *AJPH*, 71(4), 409–412. https://doi.org/10.2105/AJPH.71.4.409

Donabedian, A. (1982). *Explorations in quality assessment and monitoring: Vol. II. The criteria and standards of quality*. Health Administration Press.

Donabedian, A. (1987). Commentary on some studies of the quality of care. *Health Care Financing Review*, 1987(Suppl), 75–85. PMID: 10312323.

Donabedian, A. (1988). Quality assessment and assurance: Unity of purpose, diversity of means. *Inquiry*, 25, 173–192. https://www.jstor.org/stable/29771941

Donabedian, A. (1992). The Lichfield lecture. Quality assurance in health care: Consumers' role. *Quality Health Care*, 1, 247–251. https://doi.org/10.1136/qshc.1.4.247

Donabedian, A. (2003). *An introduction to quality assurance in health care.* Oxford University Press.

Donahue, K. T., & vanOstenberg, P. (2000). Joint commission international accreditation: Relationship to four models of evaluation. *International Journal for quality in Health Care*, 12(3), 243–246. https://doi.org/10.1093/intqhc/12.3.243

Feeley, D. (2017). *The triple aim or the quadruple aim? Four points to help set your strategy.* http://www.ihi.org/communities/blogs/the-triple-aim-or-the-quadruple-aim-four-points-to-help-set-your-strategy

Fitzpatrick, J. A., Sanders, J. R., & Worthen, B. R. (2004). *Program evaluation: Alternative approaches and practical guidelines* (3rd ed.). Pearson Education.

Fleming, C. (2010, September 14). *Berwick brings the "Triple Aim" to CMS.* http://healthaffairs.org/blog/2010/09/14/berwick-brings-the-triple-aim-to-cms/.

Glanz K, & Bishop D. B. (2010). The role of behavioral science theory in development and implementation of public health interventions. *Annual Review of Public Health*, 31, 399–418. https://doi.org/10.1146/annurev.publhealth.012809.103604

Glasgow, R. E., Vogt, T. M., & Boles, S. M. (1999). Evaluating the public health impact of health promotion interventions: The RE-AIM framework. *American Journal of Public Health*, 89(9):1322–1327. https://doi.org/10.2105/AJPH.89.9.1322

Green, L. W., & Kreuter, M. W. (2005). *Health program planning: An educational and ecological approach* (4th ed.). McGraw-Hill.

Harper, D. C., Selleck, C. S., Eagerton, G., & Froelich, K. (2015). Partnership to improve quality care for veterans: The VA Nursing Academy. *Journal of Professional Nursing*, 31(1), 57–63. https://doi.org/10.1016/j.profnurs.2014.06.004

Holt, J., Zabler, B., & Baisch, M. J. (2014). Evidence-based characteristics of nurse-managed health centers for quality and outcomes. *Nursing Outlook*, 62(6), 428–439. https://doi.org/10.1016/j.outlook.2014.06.005

Hoyle, C., & Johnson, G. (2015). Building skills in organizational and systems changes. *Nurse Practitioner*, 40(4), 15–23. 10.1097/01.NPR.0000461948.38539.fc

Hulton, L. J. (2007). An evaluation of a school-based teenage pregnancy prevention program using a logic model framework. *The Journal of School Nursing*, 23(2), 104–110. https://doi.org/10.1177/10598405070230020801

Institute for Healthcare Improvement. (2015a). Initiatives. http://www.ihi.org/Engage/Initiatives/TripleAim/pages/default.aspx

Institute for Healthcare Improvement. (2015b). Science of improvement. http://www.ihi.org/about/Pages/ScienceofImprovement.aspx

Institute of Medicine. (2001). *Crossing the quality chasm: A new health system for the 21st century.* National Academies Press.

Institute of Medicine. (2010). *The future of nursing: Leading change, advancing health.* National Academies Press.

Instone, S. L., & Palmer, D. M. (2013). Bringing the Institute of Medicine's report to life: Developing a doctor of nursing practice orthopedic residency. *Journal of Nursing Education*, 52(2), 116–119. https://doi.org/10.3928/01484834-20130121-03

Kellogg Foundation. (2004). Logic model development guide. http://www.wkkf.org/resource-directory/resource/2006/02/wk-kellogg-foundation-logic-model-development guide

Kilbourne, A. M., Fullerton, C., Dausey, D., Pincus, H. A., & Hermann, R. C. (2010). A framework for measuring quality and promoting accountability across silos: The case of mental disorders and co-occurring conditions. *Quality and Safety in Health Care*, 19, 113–116. https://doi.org/10.1136/qshc.2008.027706

Kirkpatrick, D. L. (1994). Evaluating training programs: The four levels. Berrett-Koehler.

Kotter, J. P. (2012). *Leading change.* Harvard Business Review Press.

Kurt, S. (2016, October 24). Kirkpatrick model: Four levels of learning evaluation. In *Educational Technology*. https://educationaltechnology.net/kirkpatrick-model-four-levels-learning-evaluation/

Larson, J. S., & Muller, A. (2002). Managing the quality of health care. *Journal of Health and Human Services Administration*, Winter, 261–280. https://www.jstor.org/stable/25790644

Lewis, N. (2014, October 21). Re: A primer on defining the Triple Aim [Web log message]. http://www.ihi.org/resources/Pages/Publications/PrimerDefiningTripleAim.aspx

LoBiondo-Wood, G., & Haber, J. (2018). *Nursing research: Methods and critical appraisal for evidence-based practice*. Elsevier.

Nelson, M. L. A., Lloyd, R. C., & Nolan, T. W. (2007). *Whole system measures, IHI innovation series white paper*. Massachusetts Institute for Healthcare Improvement. http://www.ihi.org/resources/Pages/IHIWhitePapers/WholeSystemMeasuresWhitePaper.aspx

Ouslander, J. G., & Maslow, K. (2012). Geriatrics and the triple aim: Defining preventable hospitalizations in the long-term care population. *JAGS, 60*(12), 2313–2318. https://doi.org/10.1111/jgs.12002

Phillips, K. A., Mayer, M. L., & Aday, L. A. (2000). Barriers to care among racial/ethnic groups under managed care. *Health Affairs, 19*(4), 65–75. https://doi.org/10.1377/hlthaff.19.4.65

Potter, B. K., Chakraborty, P., Kronick, J. B., Wilson, K., Coyle, D., Feigenbaum, A., Geraghty, M. T., Karaceper, M. D., Little, J., Mhanni, A., Mitchell, J. J., Siriwardena, K., Wilson, B. J., & Syrowatka, A.; on behalf of the Canadian Inherited Metabolic Diseases Research Network. (2013). Achieving the "Triple Aim" for inborn errors of metabolism: A review of challenges to outcomes research and presentation of a new practice-based evidence framework. *Genetics in Medicine, 15*(6), 415–422. https://doi.org/10.1038/gim.2012.153

Prior, M., McManus, M., White, P., & Davidson, L. (2014). Measuring the "Triple Aim" in transition care: A systematic review. *Pediatrics, 134*(6), e1649–1661. https://doi.org/10.1542/peds.2014-1704

Quill, B. E., Aday, L. A., Hacker, C. S., & Reagan, J. K. (1999). Policy incongruence and public health professionals' dissonance: The case of immigrants and welfare policy. *Journal of Immigrant Health, 1*(1), 9–18. https://doi.org/10.1023/A:1022632029195

RE-AIM. (2020). What is RE-AIM. http://www.re-aim.org/about/what-is-re-aim/

Reinhardt, U. E. (2008, November 14). Why does U.S. health care cost so much? (Part I). http://www.blogs.nytimes.com/2008/11/14/why-does-us-health-care-cost-so-much-part-1/?

Rogers, E. (2003). *Diffusion of innovation* (5th ed.). Simon and Schuster.

Shield, R., Rosenthal, M., Wetle, T., Tyler, D., Clark, M., & Intrator, O. (2014). Medical staff involvement in nursing homes: Development of a conceptual model and research agenda. *Journal of Applied Gerontology, 33*(1), 75–96. https://doi.org/10.1177/0733464812463432

Sitaker, M., Jernigan, J., Ladd, S., & Patanian, M. (2008). Adapting logic models over time: The Washington State Health Disease and Stroke Prevention Program experience. *Preventing Chronic Disease, 5*(2), 1–8. https://www.cdc.gov/pcd/issues/2008/apr/07_0249.htm

Stufflebeam, D. L. (1971). *The relevance of the CIPP evaluation model for educational accountability*. Paper presented at the Annual meeting of the American Association of School Administrators (Atlantic City, N.J., February 24, 1971).

Stufflebeam, D. L. (2003). The CIPP model for evaluation. In T. Kellaghan & D. L. Stufflebeam (Eds.), *International handbook of educational evaluation* (p.31-62). Kluwer Academic Publishers.

Tabak, R. G., Khoong, B. S., Chambers, D., & Brownson, R. C. (2012). Bridging research and practice: Models for dissemination and implementation research. *American Journal of Preventive Medicine, 43*(3), 337–350. https://doi.org/10.1016/j.amepre.2012.05.024

Tarlov, A. R., Ware, J. E., Greenfield, S., Nelson, E. C., Perrin, E., & Zubkoff, M. (1989). The medical outcomes study. *JAMA, 262*(7), 925–930. doi: 10.1001/jama.1989.03430070073033

Titler, M. G., Kleiber, C., Steelman, V. J., Rakel, B. A., Budreau, G., Everett, L. Q., Buckwalter, K. C., Tripp-Reimer, T., & Goode, C. J. (2001). The Iowa model of evidence-based practice to promote quality care. *Critical Care Nursing Clinics of North America, 13*(4), 497–509. https://doi.org/10.1016/S0899-5885(18)30017-0

Whittington, J. W., Nolan, K., Lewis, N., & Torres, T. (2015). Pursuing the triple aim: The first 7 years. *Milbank Quarterly, 93*(2), 263–300. https://doi.org/10.1111/1468-0009.12122

Wikipedia. CIPP evaluation model. https://en.wikipedia.org/wiki/CIPP_evaluation_model

Wikipedia. Translation. https://en.wikipedia.org/wiki/Translation

Wikipedia. Diffusion of innovation. https://en.wikipedia.org/wiki/Diffusion_of_innovations

Zhang, G., Zeller, N., Griffith, R., Metcalf, D., Williams, J., Shea, C., & Misulis, K. (2011). Using the context, input, process and product evaluation model as a comprehensive framework to guide the planning, implementation, assessment of service-learning programs. *Journal of Higher Education Outreach and Engagement, 15*(4), 57–68. https://files.eric.ed.gov/fulltext/EJ957107.pdf

FOUR

EVALUATION AND OUTCOMES

Eileen R. Giardino

> *True genius resides in the capacity for evaluation of uncertain,*
> *hazardous, and conflicting information.*
> —*Winston Churchill*

INTRODUCTION

There are major issues driving health care evaluation in the United States and the context in which Doctor of Nursing Practice (DNP) nurses, advanced practice registered nurses (APRNs), and other health professionals seek to improve the quality of the care they provide. This chapter addresses the association between evaluation and outcomes, outcome measures, and measurement of outcomes; patient-centered outcomes; and provides sources for valid and reliable measures to assess the degree to which outcomes are achieved.

EXPECTATIONS OF THE DOCTOR OF NURSING PRACTICE GRADUATE FOR ADDRESSING OUTCOMES IN PATIENT CARE

The American Association of Colleges of Nursing (AACN) described the importance of the role of the DNP nurse in addressing patient outcomes in their document, *The Essentials of Doctoral Education for Advanced Nursing Practice* (2006). The original DNP Essentials document outlined curricular elements that should be present in DNP programs and competencies that the DNP nurse should put into practice in regard to outcomes of care (AACN, 2006). The AACN document entitled *The Essentials: Core Competencies for Professional Nursing Education* (AACN, 2021) addresses outcomes of care in a number of domains. Domain 2: Person-Centered Care addresses the competency of the DNP nurse to synthesize outcome data to inform evidence-based practice, while Domain 4: Scholarship for the Nursing Discipline addresses the role of the DNP nurse to guide improvements in practice and outcomes of care. Domain 3: Population Health addresses the need for collaborating interprofessionally to improve equitable population health outcomes. Interprofessional collaboration involves developing and sustaining partnerships with patients (individual, family, or group) and health professionals to promote optimal care and patient outcomes (AACN, 2021). Domain 5: Quality and Safety addresses the leadership of DNP nurses in systems and organizations to improve patient and health care outcomes while ensuring patient safety. It further describes DNP nurse competencies to monitor care outcomes, implement quality improvement initiatives to improve outcomes, and evaluate outcomes in systems of care (AACN, 2021).

QUALITY IMPROVEMENT AND OUTCOMES

During the past 60 years, health care professionals, health service researchers, consumers, and stakeholders have continued to work toward improving quality and safety in health care services. Researchers became increasingly interested in identifying clinical trials in which health-related variables could be compared across studies through either qualitative synthesis or statistical testing of aggregated data. Literature synthesis and meta-analysis studies now provide an evidence base for practice and for developing health care guidelines (Chassin & Loeb, 2011).

Utilization review committees and professional standards review organizations, which grew out of the Medicare legislation of 1965, came to be viewed as conduits for improving quality in participating hospitals (Chassin & Loeb, 2011). The Joint Commission (TJC), originally called The Joint Commission on Accreditation of Health Care Organizations, encouraged the use of evidence-based performance metrics and the application of Donabedian's structure–process–outcome indicators in evaluating hospital quality (Chassin & Loeb, 2011). In 1999, the Agency for Health Care Policy and Research, which is a part of the U.S. Department of Health and Human Services, was renamed the Agency for Healthcare Research and Quality (AHRQ) and charged with gathering and disseminating evidence on best health care practices. The National Quality Forum (NQF), a not-for-profit-organization formed in the same year, was tasked with supporting the application and dissemination of quality metrics (Sadeghi et al., 2013). In 2001, the report *Crossing the Quality Chasm* recommended redesigning the health care system with quality improvement in the forefront (Institute of Medicine [IOM], 2001). The Affordable Care Act of 2010 was instrumental in focusing on the improvement of care outcomes and contained major initiatives designed to improve health outcomes, along with incentives to help accomplish the goal.

There continue to be numerous governmental and nonprofit entities striving to construct the most direct path to quality improvement. Governmental entities such as the AHRQ, Centers for Medicare & Medicaid Services (CMS), and the National Quality Measures Clearinghouse (NQMC) contain sections devoted to reviewing and disseminating valid and reliable metrics. Nonprofit organizations, including the IOM, TJC, the National Committee for Quality Assurance, and the Institute for Health Improvement (IHI), offer guidance to providers, patients, and health care facilities on how to measure quality care and implement quality improvement initiatives that improve outcomes in health care organizations (Sadeghi et al., 2013).

The 1999 IOM report, *To Err Is Human: Building a Safer Health System*, identified the extent of poor health care outcomes within U.S. health care system. Health care providers in hospitals were responsible for medical errors that caused between 44,000 and 98,000 deaths and over one million injuries every year (IOM, 2000; Wakefield, 2008). Many hospital deaths were caused by preventable adverse events, and many injuries were sustained from medication-related errors.

To Err is Isuman (1999) noted that patient outcomes were rated as less than they should be or poor. Although the extensive report identified the high degree of errors that occurred in hospital systems, and extrapolated to ambulatory settings as well, most single events or errors resulted from multiple factors that converged into a major adverse event that caused injury or death (IOM, 2000). The message was clear: Improving safety and preventing errors requires a systems approach to address the conditions that contribute to errors. The more common approach of blaming those involved in causing the error was not an effective approach in dealing with professionals who are dedicated to helping those for whom they care. Blaming persons who might be responsible for a medical error did not prevent similar errors and did not change factors inherent in the systems that led to an adverse event (IOM, 2000).

DEFINING OUTCOMES

An *outcome* is a set of conditions, experiences, or behaviors that are the goal for an improvement or change. A *health care outcome* denotes a change in patient health status resulting from specific health care interventions, measures, or investments in health and results from care over time (Center for Assessment and Policy Development, 2013; Donabedian, 2003; Pantaleon, 2019; Porter, 2010a, 2010b). An outcome is a desired end state in which the status of change would end up or look like if the desired outcome were achieved. Donabedian stated that outcomes were "the ultimate validators of the effectiveness and quality of medical care" (Donabedian, 1966, p. 169). The goal of improving outcomes begins when a gap is identified between current outcomes achieved as compared with the acceptable rate determined for the outcome measure (Scoville, 2015). In health care, outcomes of care are evaluated using measures that indicate to what degree the outcomes are being achieved that indicate a level of quality.

In the realm of health outcomes and outcome measures, there are a number of terms that use similar words. Table 4.1 defines terms related to outcomes and outcome measures.

HEALTH OUTCOMES

Health outcomes are defined as events that occur as a result of an intervention or a change that results from antecedent health care (Donabedian, 1980) and are centered on the patient rather than the individual providers or specialty services providing the care (Porter, 2010b). Determining health outcomes involves measuring a change in an individual patient or patient population that is related to specific interventions (Edwards, 2016). Examples of health outcomes that a system might want to achieve include reducing missed appointments, medical errors, or hospital length of stay as well as avoidable readmissions, hospital-acquired infections, or mortality (Hostetter & Klein, 2020; Scoville, 2015).

TABLE 4.1 Definition of Terms

Term	Definition
Outcome	A set of conditions, experiences, or behaviors that are the goal for an improvement or change.
Health outcome	Denotes a change in patient health status resulting from specific health care interventions, measures, or investments in health and results from care over time and is a desired end state where the status of change would end up or would look like if the desired outcome were achieved (Center for Assessment and Policy Development, 2013; Donabedian, 2003; Pantaleon, 2019; Porter, 2010b).
Measure	A standard: A basis for comparison; a reference point against which other things can be evaluated.
Outcome measure	A "change in the health of an individual, group of people, or population that is attributable to an intervention or series of interventions." Captures how a system is performing in achieving end results or desired outcomes of care. Outcome measures (mortality, readmission, patient experience, etc.) are the quality and cost targets health care organizations are trying to improve. Identifies the degree to which a desired outcome has been achieved (Tinker, 2018).
Performance measures	Standardized and systematic methods to identify and improve suboptimal medical care and patient outcomes. Provide a way to assess health care against recognized standards (NQF, 2020a).
Quality measures	Tools that measure or quantify health care processes, outcomes, patient perceptions, and organizational structure and/or systems associated with the ability to provide high-quality health care and/or that relate to one or more quality goals for health care (CMS, 2020). A mechanism to assign a quantity to quality of care by comparison with a criterion (AHRQ, 2020a). May be useful for local quality improvement but are not yet appropriate for public reporting or pay-for-performance programs.
Benchmark in health care	Collaborative and continual process that measures and compares the results of key work processes with those of the best performers to evaluate an organization's performance. Measures of quality and safety use external benchmarks to track the progress of quality improvement initiatives or outcome measures (Hughes, 2008).
Quality indicators	Measures of health care quality that organizations can apply to inpatient hospital data to assess and improve health care quality, identify outcomes that need further evaluation, and track changes over time. Provide health care decision makers with tools to assess their data (AHRQ, 2018).

AHRQ, Agency for Healthcare Research and Quality; NQF, National Quality Forum.

QUALITY AND HEALTH OUTCOMES

The relationship between quality and health outcomes is that high-quality health care should produce positive and consistent health care outcomes. The IOM relates quality of health care delivered to health outcomes as the degree to which health care services for individuals and populations improve the likelihood that desired health outcomes will be achieved and that quality care is consistent with current evidence and professional knowledge (AHRQ, 2020a; IOM, 2001). The quality of patient outcomes for a particular health problem can vary across providers, institutions, regions, and countries. For example, the university hospital in one city may produce better patient outcomes for cardiac bypass surgery than the community hospital in the nearby town. High-quality health care provided to individuals or populations should produce better health outcomes than low-quality care. What, then, characterizes high-quality health care versus low-quality care? The IOM developed a framework that defined six properties or domains of quality health care that are the foundation on which all aspects of quality care are built. The six *characteristics that define quality care* are safe, effective, patient centered, timely, efficient, and equitable (IOM, 2001; Mitchell, 2008). High-quality care delivered to achieve any health care outcome should reflect the six domains. See Table 4.2 for the IOM Six Domains of Quality.

TABLE 4.2   Institute of Medicine Six Domains of Quality

Domain	Characteristics
Safe	Safety is inherent in the system; avoid harm to patients from care intended to help and heal
Effective	Health care should match scientific evidence-based knowledge neither overuse nor underuse best available techniques to all who could benefit
Patient centered	Address the patient's social context, culture, and specific needs; care provision is respectful and responsive to patient preferences; patients' values and preferences guide all clinical decisions
Timely	Prompt attention to patient is of benefit to patient and caregiver; unintended waiting for care or information is a system defect; delays in care may be harmful
Efficient	Consistent focus on reducing waste and cost of supplies, time, equipment, capital, space ideas, and opportunities
Equitable	The advances in health care delivery and benefits of medical science reach everyone equally; care provision is equal in quality for everyone regardless of race, ethnicity, gender, and socioeconomic status

Source: Adapted from Institute for Healthcare Improvement. (2020b). *Across the chasm: Six aims for changing the health care system.* http://www.ihi.org/resources/Pages/ImprovementStories/AcrosstheChasmSixAimsforChanging theHealthCareSystem.aspx; Agency for Healthcare Research and Quality. (2018). AHR Quality Indicators. Author. https://www.ahrq.gov/cpi/about/otherwebsites/qualityindicators.ahrq.gov/qualityindicators.html

Low-Quality Health Care and Outcomes

The opposite of high-quality care is care that does not produce consistent desired outcomes or meet criteria outlined in the six Domains of Quality (IOM, 2001) and that does not achieve high health care outcome measures when compared against benchmarks of quality (see Benchmarks section). Studies have found only a small to moderate association between cost and quality (Hussey et al., 2013; IOM, 2015). More expensive care does not necessarily equal higher quality care, because the cost of care is not an indicator of quality health care outcomes. The cost of health care services delivered varies significantly, and there is no correlation of quality care with specific regions of the country, states, localities, or providers practicing in the same practice. A high cost of treatment services and providers who charge high fees for services rendered do not guarantee that their care addresses the six domains of quality care.

OUTCOME MEASURES

An *outcome measure* is a "change in the health of an individual, group of people, or population that is attributable to an intervention or series of interventions" (Tinker, 2018, para. 5). Outcome measures capture how a system is performing in achieving end results or desired outcomes of care. Examples of outcome measures are mortality, patient experience, and successful treatment, as defined by the practice. Outcome measures can identify practices that need to be improved and the effectiveness of interventions in process improvement projects by determining the extent to which the outcomes compare with a desired goal or standardized outcome (Kleinpell, 2013).

The CMS analyzes hospital outcome measures annually to provide the public and institutions with greater insight into measurement trends and variation in outcomes as to hospital characteristics, location, cost, and patient disparities (CMS, 2020). The *Hospital Performance Reports: Chartbook Series,* which the CMS publishes on the web and is available to individuals and institutions reports outcome measures that individual hospitals across the country have achieved. Regarding outcome measures, the Chartbook (CMS, n.d.):

- Displays national trends and distributions of hospital performance on outcomes measures
- Highlights regional variation in performance on outcomes measures
- Examines how consistently hospitals perform on pairs of outcome measures
- Explores how a state's overall performance on measures relates to their performance for patients with and without social risk factors

Measuring performance is essential to improving performance (IOM, 2020). The quality of care delivered in places such as medical practices, hospital departments, and health care institutions is determined by the degree to which institutions have met desired outcomes. Tracking outcome measures is an important and essential step in identifying quality of care at the institutional level (CMS, n.d.). For example, when hospitals report their central line–associated bloodstream infection (CLABSI) rate in the ICU, it is then possible to compare which hospitals have the highest or lowest rates. Those hospitals with high CLABSI rates have a compelling incentive to improve their quality of care by decreasing or improving their rate of infection (IHI, 2015; Scheinker, 2020).

Many institutions report their outcome measures to commercial payers, government payers, and organizations that report on quality measures (Leapfrog Group, 2019). There are outcome measures that the CMS tracks, denying payment for the associated conditions that were acquired during the hospital stay. Those conditions, such as a hospital-acquired infection or hospital-acquired pressure ulcer (HAPU) are stated by the CMS to be preventable conditions that are expensive to treat and common causes of inpatient morbidity and mortality. In 2008, the CMS promulgated regulations that deny payment for selected conditions occurring during the hospital stay that were not present on admission, deemed preventable by the hospital, and caused by care or treatments that the hospital provided or failed to provide (Stone et al., 2010). The CMS payment policy is an example of how financial incentives drive hospitals to improve outcome measures related to specific quality indicators. The CMS payment policy is an example of the influence that financial incentives have on improving patient safety and care outcomes (Stone et al., 2010).

The Leapfrog Group is an example of a national nonprofit that evaluates and reports on U.S. hospital safety and quality performance to increase transparency of an institution's outcome measures so that the quality of care is clear to consumers (patients) and payers (CMS, private insurers). The need to be transparent and report the rate of poor outcomes (e.g., deaths related to surgical procedures, hospital-acquired pressure injuries [HAPIs], HAPUs) provides an incentive to improve outcomes and reduce deaths and morbidity that result from hospital errors, accidents, and injuries (Leapfrog Group, 2019). Knowing that an institution's results are public and able to be compared with other institutions is another incentive to improve outcomes.

The CMS and the Leapfrog Hospital Safety Grade collect and report on 28 national performance measures of patient safety to produce a single composite score that represents a hospital's overall performance in keeping patients safe from preventable harm and medical errors (Leapfrog Group, 2019). In addition, supplemental data from secondary data sources such as the American Hospital Association (AHA) and the Maryland Health Care Commission (for hospitals in Maryland only) are used to give hospitals as much credit as possible toward their Safety Grades.

HEALTH CARE QUALITY MEASURES

Quality measures are "tools that help us measure or quantify health care processes, outcomes, patient perceptions, and organizational structure and/or systems that are associated with the ability to provide high-quality health care and/or that relate to one or more quality goals for health care" (American Academy of Family Physicians [AAFP], 2020; CMS, 2020). Quality measures are used to identify opportunities to improve patient care (AAFP, 2020). *Health care quality measures* (HCQMs) focus on processes or structures of care that are under the auspices of the health care system and that have a demonstrated relationship to positive health outcomes. The AHRQ defines a *quality measure* as "a mechanism to assign a quantity to quality of care by comparison to a criterion" (AHRQ, 2020a, Section 2). HCQMs are used for three general purposes: quality improvement, accountability, and research (2020a). Donabedian provided a different perspective and categorized HCQMs as measures of structure, process, and outcome (SPO; Donabedian, 1966). More recently, cost and patient experience measures have been added as categories of HCQMs (AHRQ, 2016b).

The NQMC, which is part of the AHRQ, contains more than 2,000 quality measures that are currently used or have been recently tested. Quality measures focus on the effectiveness of clinical care and treatment. Institutions spend much time and financial resources on collecting and analyzing, validating, and maintaining the data. They report on 120 or more quality measures to an average of five regulators and payers at a cost to the institution of approximately 1% of their net patient service revenue (IOM, 2015). The identification of measures that need improvement leads to an increasing volume of improvement initiatives. The validation of outcome measures coupled with the proliferation of improvement initiatives are uncompensated activities that institutions must take on to improve quality of care and outcome measures (IHI, 2015).

For each HCQM, institutions collect their performance information and generate a score for each measure. To collect performance information, an institution asks patients (e.g., consumers of their services) to rate their services for a given quality measure. For example, for a quality measure such as "managing patients' pain on admission" or "the percent of patients whose pain was brought to a comfortable level within 48 hours of admission," patients complete a questionnaire after discharge that rates on a scale of 1 to 5 (or a similar scale) how well the institution managed their pain. The institution collects and analyzes the HCQM data and reports the results of the rating for that quality measure. The public can see Institution A's rating and compare it with Institution B's rating to determine which rating is better. The rating is considered a measure of quality. Comparing information on health care quality enables people to make informed decisions regarding choice of health care provider (AHRQ, 2016a).

TYPES OF HEALTH CARE QUALITY MEASURES

The three types of HCQMs used to assess and compare the quality of care provided by health care organizations are classified as either a structure, process, or outcome measure. Each type of measure addresses a specific aspect of how a health care system is performing and identifies strengths and weaknesses of the system to drive improvement (CMS, 2020).

Donabedian (1988a, 1988b) noted that quality of care was assessed through the constructs of SPO in that good structure should promote good processes, and good processes should, in turn, promote a good outcome (i.e., a unidirectional pathway; Donabedian, 1988a, 1988b). Donabedian defined *structure* as the organizational and professional resources associated with the provision of health care (e.g., availability of medicines/equipment and staff training). *Process* is things that are done to and for the patient (e.g., defaulter tracing and hospital referrals, counseling). An *outcome* is the desired end result of care as administered by the health provider (e.g., patient satisfaction with quality of care). Donabedian distinguished between two types of outcomes: (a) *technical outcomes*, which are the physical and functional aspects of care, such as absence of complications and reduction in disease, disability and death; and (b) *interpersonal outcomes*, which include patient's satisfaction with care and influence of care on patient's quality of life as perceived by the patient

(Ameh et al., 2017; Donabedian, 1988a, 1988b). The following further describes SPO measures and the focus of each measure.

Structure Measures

A structure measure assesses characteristics, infrastructure, or features of a health care organization relevant to its capacity to provide health care, such as equipment, personnel, or policies. Structure measures reflect the qualities of the service or provider (operating times of the service, staff-to-patient ratio; ACT Academy, n.d.) and describe whether clinical care has been provided appropriately (AHRQ, 2015).

Examples of structure measures include:

- Whether the health care organization uses electronic medical records or medication order entry systems
- The number or proportion of board-certified physicians
- The ratio of providers to patients
- Access to specific technologies (e.g., MRI scan)
- Access of specific units (e.g., cardiac care)
- Clinical guidelines revised every second year
- Convenience of accessing a pediatric practice

Process Measures

Process measures indicate what a provider does to maintain or improve health and reflect generally accepted recommendations for clinical practice (AHRQ, 2015) and address the processes in place to achieve or affect the outcome. If achieving a desired outcome requires clinicians to use the 2019 AHA/ACC Clinical Performance and Quality Measures for Adults with High Blood Pressure guidelines when treating patients in the practice with hypertension, it is not enough to tell clinicians to use the 2019 AHA/ACC guidelines. Processes must be put in place with clear expectations for the clinicians to follow in order to achieve the desired outcome of 80% of patients in the practice who will be treated for hypertension using the 2019 AHA/ACC guidelines.

Process measures can inform consumers about medical care they may expect to receive for a given condition or disease and can contribute toward improving health outcomes. The majority of HCQMs used for public reporting are process measures (AHRQ, 2020a). Process includes provider interactions, which are often easier to identify and describe than outcomes, and are also more apt to align with health care guidelines, which tend to focus on what a provider does. Sources of process measures may include documentation of the number of procedures billed, the number of patients who receive immunization for a particular disease, or the number of patients screened for hypertension. Porter (2010a) asserted that the majority of measures currently collected are process measures and that although they may reflect current quality standards, they do not necessarily correlate with patient health outcomes. Over time, experts in the field have reached the general consensus that more needs to be done to develop and use valid and reliable patient-centered outcome measures (Cassel et al., 2014; Lee, 2010; Porter, 2010a).

Examples of process measures include (AHRQ, 2015):

● The delivery of timely prophylactic antibiotics to reduce surgical site infection
● Patient admitted to a hospital with a myocardial infarction (MI) receives a prescription for a beta blocker when discharged
● The percentage of people in a population receiving preventive services (such as mammograms or immunizations)
● The percentage of people with diabetes in a specific population who had their blood glucose tested and controlled
● The percentage of people with diabetes who had their blood sugar tested and controlled

Outcome Measures

Outcome measures reflect the impact of the health care service or intervention on the health status of patients. There are hundreds of standardized outcome measures, ranging from changes in blood pressure in patients with hypertension to patient-reported outcome measures (PROMs). The CMS uses seven groupings of outcome measures to calculate hospital quality. They include mortality, safety of care, readmissions, patient experience, effectiveness of care, timeliness of care, and efficient use of medical imaging (CMS, n.d.).

From a practical perspective, outcome measures can be more difficult to develop and collect than process measures. Outcome is more patient centered than process and thus harder to identify and link with a specific treatment or intervention (Chin, 2014). Changes in health status often occur because of complex interactions and cannot always be attributed to a linear association of one provider to one patient. Donabedian discussed the concept of *attribution* and the possibility of weighting all factors that contribute to a change in health status. Thus, under certain circumstances, the contributions of physicians, nurses, therapists, pharmacists, families, and patients might be identified, measured, and analyzed to determine their impact on outcomes (Donabedian, 2003).

Examples of outcome measures include (AHRQ, 2015):

● The percentage of patients who died as a result of surgery (i.e., surgical mortality rates)
● HbA1c results for diabetics
● Blood pressure results for hypertensive patients
● Lipid profile results for patients with hyperlipidemia
● The rate of surgical complications or hospital-acquired infections

PATIENT-REPORTED OUTCOME MEASURES

PROMs are measures of health status and function and are a direct report by the patient that pertains to the patient's quality of life, health, or functional status associated with their health care treatment or delivery of their care (Weldring & Smith, 2013). Patient-related outcomes (PROs) enable health care providers to evaluate the patient's experience with health care treatment. PROs are usually measured in absolute terms, such as rating of pain severity, and can be used to report changes from a previous measure, such as an untoward effect following administration of a new drug. The evaluation of the quality of care delivery is enhanced by measuring PROs (Weldring & Smith, 2013). As in all outcome measures, patients (consumers) can compare the ratings of care providers and health care institutions on the degree to which they meet specific PROMs.

Patient experience is an essential aspect of quality care because *patient centered* is one of the IOM's six domains of quality (AHRQ, 2018; IHI, 2020b). A PROM may determine to what degree a patient's health care meets their personal and cultural expectations, was respectful and responsive to patient preferences, and considered personal values in care delivery. The assessment of PROMs is consistent with a patient-centered approach to care and necessary to adequately assess the impact of treatment and care.

PRO data to measure patients' perceptions of their functional well-being or health status may be collected using methods such as patient interviews, self-administered questionnaires, and standardized, validated instruments (National Health Service, 2009). Patients rate their health by scoring the severity or difficulty in completing certain tasks or routine activities. The measures assess the patient's perception of their health care experience and are in the category of the *patient experience* outcome measure. Information reported by the patient provides real-time information for local service improvement and gauges a patient's level of satisfaction with their health care experiences (Tinker, 2018).

A MAZE OF MEASURES

The U.S. health care system has made considerable progress in creating thousands of quality measures (Scott & Jha, 2014). Meyer et al. (2012) concluded that the proliferation of quality measures has become a costly endeavor that threatens to dilute their influence on health care. There are groups such as regulators and public and private payers that require an institution to provide their measures to them for the benefit of transparency of outcomes to consumers, patients, and payers. Although there are many benefits from the growth in measuring quality, the cost to institutions of determining the many measures needed to certify an institution's performance levels to judge quality and cost performance may cause institutions to shift their resources from improving quality to creating quality-performance metrics (Meyer et al., 2012). Although benefits have accrued from the growth in quality measurement, there is a move to require a more limited set of metrics that are balanced and targeted to provide information critical to quality improvement.

One way to control the growing maze of measures is to organize them into coherent and manageable domains. The quality domains described by the IOM in *Crossing the Quality Chasm* (2001) appear to meet this need. Safe, timely, effective, efficient, equitable, and patient-centered health care has become the sine qua non of quality improvement. The IOM domains are widely accepted by health care facilities, providers, governmental agencies, and consumers as theoretically sound and practical (Greenberg, 2015; Sadeghi et al., 2013). They have been incorporated into the Triple Aim framework (IHI, 2015) and serve as a framework for research.

SOURCES OF MEASURES

Numerous online resources provide valid and reliable quality measures that may be used in a variety of settings. Perhaps the most inclusive resource is the NQMC (www.qualitymeasures.ahrq.gov), which is an enterprise supported by the AHRQ and the U.S. Department of Health and Human Services. It provides a website with information, including tutorials, on such topics as establishing the validity of quality measures and deciding which outcome metrics are appropriate for specific health care settings (Sadeghi et al., 2013).

In describing the essential characteristics of quality measures, the NQMC recommended that they (a) respond to a situation that needs improvement, cover a variety of demographic groups, and be significant to stakeholders, providers, public health officials, and patients; (b) have a foundation in clinical evidence; (c) be valid, reliable, understandable, and permit case-mix adjustment; and (d) have available data sources and clear, precise methodologies. Data sources for measures include electronic health records, surveys, imaging and laboratory data, organizational protocols, provider attributes, public health, and registry information (Greenberg, 2015; NQMC, 2015).

QUALITY INDICATORS

Quality indicators are measures of health care quality that organizations can apply to inpatient hospital data to assess and improve health care quality, identify outcomes that need further evaluation, and track changes over time. A quality indicator uses available patient data to determine the incidence of specific phenomena within an institution, which can indicate the quality of care within the institution (AHRQ, 2018). Hospitals use quality indicators to determine to what degree they provide quality care to patients (AHRQ, 2017) and evaluate outcome performance in relation to self, peer institutions, and national benchmarks. Quality indicators highlight potential quality concerns, identify areas that need further study and investigation, and track changes over time. Hospital systems track and report on the incidence of quality indicators and measure the outcome rate to allow for comparison across clinic units or organizations. For example, CLABSI are often measured as infections per 1,000 line days, which can then be compared across institutions and against a national benchmark as well. By using rates of infection rather than actual numbers of infections, one can compare large units with small units and can compare their rate per 1,000 against national benchmarks (AHRQ, 2017, 2018).

Agency for Healthcare Research and Quality Quality Indicators

Between 1998 and 2002, the AHRQ contracted with an evidence-based practice center (EPC) to develop the quality indicators by reviewing evidence related to quality measurement based on data that are readily available from the billing or operational systems, do not require manual collection, and often lack the clinical details contained in progress notes (administrative data). Their purpose for developing quality indicators was to provide health care decision makers with tools to assess their outcome data (AHRQ, 2018). The EPC assessed the reliability and validity of the measures to identify the best indicators to be used (AHRQ, 2017).

The AHRQ developed four areas of quality indicators: prevention, inpatient, patient safety, and pediatric quality of care. The AHRQ quality indicators are standardized, evidence-based HCQMs that can be used with readily available hospital inpatient administrative data. There are 101 hospital inpatient setting quality indicators that measure quality associated with care delivery (AHRQ, 2020a). Currently, the AHRQ quality indicators are used only in acute care hospitals with administrative data and not in other settings (e.g., long-term care, outpatient, ambulatory, hospice, individual practice, emergency department, or diagnostic centers) or with other populations (e.g., mental health or substance abuse, emergency preparedness, patient falls, rehabilitation, readmission, surgery, heparin therapy, *Clostridium difficile*, or nursing quality; AHRQ, 2018, 2020a).

A HAPI is one example of an AHRQ inpatient quality indicator. The AQHR indicator, which is stated as Patient Safety Indicator 03 (PSI 03) Pressure Ulcer Rate, would include an institution's data for HAPI. The quality indicator has a specific description of the pressure ulcer as a Stage III or IV pressure ulcer or unstageable (secondary diagnosis) per 1,000 discharges among surgical or medical patients aged 18 years and older (AHRQ, 2020b). PSI-03 describes further characteristics of the pressure ulcer as well. The institution tracks the number of pressure ulcers that develop among inpatients and applies an analysis measurement to calculate the rate of HAPIs that occur in the hospital per 1,000 discharges (AHRQ, 2020b).

Hospitals strive to have low rates for quality indicator events that indicate poor outcomes (e.g., infection rates, mortality rates from surgical procedures, HAPIs). So, what does the quality indicator for pressure ulcers tell the institution? Quality indicators can tell the hospital what their rate of HAPIs is at given points in time, what their rate is compared with those of other hospitals, and what their quality indicator is in relation to national benchmarks.

The HAPI rate is a nursing quality indicator for a condition that is considered to be preventable (Rondinelli, 2018). When a HAPI reaches Stage III (full-thickness skin loss) or Stage IV (full-thickness skin loss and tissue loss), it becomes what is called a *never event* (i.e., an event that should not occur in the hospital). Institutions are required to report *never events* to the CMS. When the rate of a quality indicator falls below targeted performance, it may result in limited reimbursement from the payer to the institution.

The rate of pressure ulcer occurrences is a direct measure of how well the hospital is doing to prevent pressure ulcers. A low or decreasing rate indicates that the hospital is providing high-quality care or is on the path toward improvement, or is doing a good job in preventing pressure ulcers. On the other hand, a high or increasing rate indicates lower quality of care and a need for improvement (AHRQ, 2017).

MEASURING HEALTH CARE OUTCOMES AND MEASURES

Evaluators quantify health care outcomes using counts, means, proportions, percentages, or medians. For example, they may calculate the number of adverse events, the mean systolic and diastolic blood pressure, or the median length of hospital stay. Proportions are calculated by counting the number of persons with the outcome of interest and dividing that number by the number of all persons treated during a specified period (Romano et al., 2010). For example, 600 out of 1,000 patients (60%) surveyed during 2015 at a city hospital said they were satisfied with the care

---

TABLE 4.3 Selected Measures Used in Evaluating Treatment Outcomes

Measure	Description
Cumulative incidence	$$\frac{\text{Number of new occurrences in a population}}{\text{All individuals at risk in the population}}$$
Prevalence	$$\frac{\text{Number of persons who have an existing condition}}{\text{Entire population}}$$
All-cause mortality	$$\frac{\text{Number of persons who died from all causes}}{\text{All persons in the population}}$$
Cause-specific mortality	$$\frac{\text{Number of persons who died from a specific disorder}}{\text{Number of persons with the disorder}}$$
Case fatality rate	$$\frac{\text{Number of persons who died from a specific disorder}}{\text{Number of persons with the disorder}}$$
Relative risk	$$\frac{\text{Incidence among persons exposed}}{\text{Incidence among persons not exposed}}$$
Relative risk reduction	1 *minus* the relative risk
Absolute risk reduction	Incidence of outcome in the treated population *minus* the incidence of outcome in the untreated population
Number needed to treat	$$\frac{1}{\text{Absolute risk reduction}}$$
Number needed to screen	$$\frac{\text{Number needed to treat}}{\text{Disease prevalence}}$$

Source: Hennekens, C. H., & Buring, J. E. (1987). *Epidemiology in medicine.* Little, Brown and Company; Kendrach, M. G., Covington, T. R., McCarthy, M. W., & Harris, M. C. (1997). Calculating risks and number-needed-to-treat: A method of data interpretation. *Journal of Managed Care Pharmacy, 3*(2), 179–183; and Rembold, C. M. (1998). Number needed to screen: Development of a statistic for disease screening. *BMJ, 317,* 307–312.

they received during their hospital stay. Other outcomes associated with percentages include symptoms, pressure ulcers, falls, and readmissions within 30 days.

Rates, proportions, and ratios are used as measures of disease frequency and are often used to evaluate health outcomes, particularly in large health care facilities, communities, and populations. A description of commonly used frequencies is provided in Table 4.3. Two major types of frequency are prevalence and incidence. *Prevalence* refers to the proportion or percentage of the total number of individuals in a population who are known to have an existing condition at a particular point in time (Greenberg, 2015; Hennekens & Buring, 1987). Prevalence is useful in determining whether a chronic condition such as diabetes or cardiovascular disease is becoming more common and in estimating the total number of patients who need treatment.

Cumulative incidence refers to new events in a population at risk during a certain time interval. The population at risk is defined as all members of that population who are susceptible to the outcome of interest. For instance, a member of the population that is a prevalent case is not at risk of becoming an incident (i.e., new) case. *Incidence rates* are essential to studies of causes of disease because they are used to make inferences about risk or probability of disease (Greenberg, 2015; Hennekens & Buring, 1987).

Morbidity and mortality are particular types of incidence. Morbidity refers to the appearance of diagnosable disease, and mortality refers to death. All-cause mortality, cause-specific mortality, and case fatality provide different kinds of information. *All-cause mortality* includes everyone who died in a specific place during a specific time period divided by the total population. In *cause-specific mortality*, the numerator includes only those individuals dying from a particular disorder in the total population. In *case fatality*, the numerator includes the individuals who died from a certain disorder, and the denominator includes only those who have the disorder. When calculating the frequency of less common diseases, rates are often multiplied by 1,000, 10,000, or 100,000 so that they may be expressed as a whole number (Greenberg, 2015; Hennekens & Buring, 1987).

Measures of association compare rates in populations to estimate the probable amount of benefit or harm caused by an agent of interest. In *relative risk* (RR), the incidence of a studied event in an exposed population is divided by the incidence in an unexposed population. The exposure may refer to an environmental factor, disorder, diagnostic test, or treatment. A result less than 1 indicates lower risk (of harm or benefit), and a result greater than 1 indicates more risk (of harm or benefit) to the exposed population. A value of 1 indicates that the exposure had little or no effect. The result may be expressed as a percentage (Greenberg, 2015; Hennekens & Buring, 1987). For example, compared with a population of adults who were not exposed, a population exposed to a carcinogen over a 5-year period had an RR of 1.07 or a 7% greater risk of developing cancer than those never exposed to the carcinogen. In discussing a benefit of treatment, epidemiologists sometimes refer to *relative risk reduction* (RRR), which is 1 − RR (Kendrach et al., 1997). For instance, if 93 of 1,000 patients treated for hypertension go on to have strokes and 100 of 1,000 untreated patients have strokes, the RR of stroke is 0.93, and the RRR is 1 minus 0.93, which is 7%. This is the percentage of baseline risk that is reduced with treatment.

Absolute risk reduction (ARR) is obtained by subtracting the incidence of an outcome among untreated persons from the incidence among treated persons. ARR, which is generally expressed as a percentage, is a meaningful way to compare the results of randomized controlled trials (RCTs) because it estimates the actual benefit of the experimental treatment to a population. Its magnitude depends on the baseline risk that occurs in the absence of the experimental treatment (Greenberg, 2015; Kendrach et al., 1997). RRR compares only the numerators of risk, but ARR compares the denominators as well. RRR would be the same 7% if stroke decreased from 100 to 93 per 1,000 or from 100 to 93 per 100,000, but ARR would fall from 0.07% to 0.00007%.

A measure frequently used along with the ARR is the *number needed to treat (NNT)*. The NNT offers health care providers and decision makers an estimate of the total sum of individuals who must receive an intervention before obtaining a beneficial (or preventing a harmful) result. The NNT (Greenberg, 2015) is the inverse of the ARR (1 divided by ARR).

OUTCOME MEASUREMENT IN QUALITY IMPROVEMENT INITIATIVES

Measurement of outcomes is at the core of quality improvement projects because measurement helps to answer the question in the Model for Improvement of "How will we know a change is an improvement?" (Langley et al., 2009). Measurement has an essential role in effectively developing, testing, and implementing changes.

Measurement in quality improvement initiatives is the cornerstone of a successful improvement project because appropriate measurement of outcomes enables the quality improvement team to demonstrate current performance (or baseline data), set goals for future performance, and monitor the effects of changes as they are made. The key to knowing whether the changes or improvement plan implemented to achieve desired outcomes is working is to measure the outcomes that the initiative is aimed at achieving. Are the measured outcomes that the initiative is achieving moving in the direction of improvement that you want to achieve? It is always important to choose the right analytic measurement process so that the results of the change initiative are quantified (Health Quality Ontario, 2013; Langley et al., 2009).

Measuring outcomes shows how well you have achieved your desired goal and exchanges personal subjectivity as to how well you are doing for actual data to show if the changes you made are improving your current process. In quality improvement, the literature describes three types of measures that are linked to the aim and goals of your project.

CLABSI provide an example of how to differentiate between outcomes and measurement of outcome. In a quality improvement initiative, the desired outcome at the patient level may be to decrease the central line infections rate per 1,000 central line days by 30%. To determine whether the outcome is achieved, one must measure the rate of central line infection that occurs in the ICU at baseline prior to the start of the improvement initiative and then at regular intervals after the new protocol is introduced to determine whether the protocol is decreasing the CLABSI rate from the baseline. In order to determine whether the unit is moving toward or has achieved the desired outcome (decrease CLABSI rate by 30%), it is necessary to measure the CLABSI rate on an ongoing basis to determine to what degree the desired outcome has been achieved or maintained. The actual infection rate is measured and compared with the desired infection rate. In order to measure the CLABSI rate in a given ICU, the calculation would be: Number of CLABSI cases in each unit assessed × 1,000 Total number of central line – Days in each unit assessed (The Joint Commission, 2020). The measurement of the CLABSI rate over time and compared with the baseline rate and subsequent rates at regular time intervals is what determines whether the desired outcome is achieved.

CHALLENGES TO QUALITY MEASUREMENT

Developing HCQMs is a work in progress. While the Affordable Care Act and the Patient-Centered Outcomes Research Institute provided incentives to develop and use valid and reliable measures to improve health status, there is a long way to go before their recommendations are realized. Some of the biggest challenges are discussed here.

First, evaluators can lose their way amid the maze of measurements and methods. There are thousands of quality measures; some are valid, reliable, evidence based, and transparent, and some are not. Some measures evaluate quality improvement on the margins instead of measuring the total effect on health status (Cassel et al., 2014). Some measures overlap. At times, evaluators seem to miss the big picture of quality as a change in patient health status while focusing on the individual pixels of care (Sadeghi et al., 2013).

The sheer number of measures used internally by health care entities and mandated by external regulatory agencies, insurance companies, and other payers, has increased the cost of quality improvement activities. It is estimated that some systems spend 1% of net patient revenue on these activities. Administrators and policy makers have called for the development of a critical but limited cluster of quality measures for submission to external agencies. This would allow health entities to spend a larger proportion of their quality improvement budget on applying measures most specific to their current needs for quality improvement (Cassel et al., 2014; IOM, 2015; Meyer et al., 2012).

Second, the difficulty in linking SPO still exists, and as measures proliferate, the problem will only worsen. One cannot simply assume that a compliant administration policy or provider performance produces a good patient outcome unless the association is identified, described, and measured. If a linkage of SPO is established and the outcome is positive, the cause of the success can clearly be recognized. Conversely, if the outcome is not positive, one can trace back to process and structure to identify the problem (Donabedian, 2003).

A third challenge is the difficulty in attributing outcomes to particular activities or persons. Outcomes are not physician outcomes or nursing outcomes; they are patient outcomes. Today, health care is delivered by a system that includes administrators, health care professionals, ancillary health personnel, families, and patients (Sadeghi et al., 2013). Weighting the contribution of each of these entities is difficult. There have been attempts to use algorithms or modeling to weight each contribution to a patient outcome (Titler et al., 2011), but even if weighting could be apportioned, the attribution might still vary among individual providers, facilities, and geographic locations. So far, national guidelines for delineating attribution are not available (Romano et al., 2010).

The challenges are great, but DNP nurses and APRNs along with policy makers, patients, and other health professionals are making good strides toward quality improvement. And, as long as the focus remains on improving the safety and quality of the care provided in health care organizations, outcomes will continue to improve. As noted in *Crossing the Quality Chasm*, "Perfect care may be a long way off, but much better care is within our grasp" (IOM, 2001, p. 20).

PERFORMANCE MEASURES

How do we know if health care provided by hospitals and health care systems is quality care, and how do providers determine the steps in health care processes that need to be changed and improved to achieve better patient outcomes? Furthermore, how do insurers determine whether their care reimbursement is paying for the best care that providers can deliver?

Performance measures are used to quantify and measure outcomes, patient perceptions, health care processes, and organizational systems and/or structure that are associated with the ability to provide high-quality care. "Standardized performance measures are tools that assess the structure, process, outcomes, and patient perceptions of care; preferred practices that suggest a specific process that, when implemented effectively, leads to improve patient outcomes; and frameworks that provide a conceptual approach to organizing practices" (National Quality Forum [NQF], 2020b). Performance measures are used for quality improvement and public reporting of outcomes by health care systems, government agencies, and hospitals (CMS, 2020; NQF, 2020c).

Performance measures provide a way to assess health care against recognized standards and help ensure that patient care measures provided by health care providers are at the same high quality that nationally recognized standards recommend. The standardized and systematic performance measures identify and improve suboptimal medical care and patient outcomes (NQF, 2020a).

The NQF supports the Consensus Standards Approval Committee (CSAC) in its task of reviewing proposed standards (measures) for the purpose of either endorsing or declining to endorse the standards. The CSAC also advises on revisions to or enhancements of (NQF's) Consensus Development Process (CDP; NQF, 2020c). The NQF evaluates and endorses performance measures for the purpose of providing standards of care and process to improve the quality of health care that providers and institutions provide to patients (NQF, 2020b). Initiatives to improve the quality and outcomes of patient care often use standardized performance measures, which are tools that assess the SPO, and patient perceptions of care, and preferred practices that suggest a specific process that, when implemented effectively, leads to improved patient outcomes.

The NQF (2020b) describes uses of performance measures:

1. Institutions, providers, and health care consumers use performance standards to create reliable comparative performance information that consumers can use to make informed decisions about their care;
2. Hold practitioners and provider organizations accountable for the efficiency and quality of their performance; and
3. Support quality improvement activities.

Performance measures follow standards of design established by national organizations and have validated components that are precise, feasible, and actionable to achieve meaningful and desirable patient outcomes. They include the highest levels of evidence and recommendation from clinical practice guidelines, and their use can help improve gaps in care (Casey et al., 2019).

SUMMARY

This chapter explored the many types of outcomes and outcome measures used to evaluate the quality of health care delivered by providers and health care institutions. An understanding of the concepts of quality, quality measures, patient outcomes, and measurement of outcomes is essential to evaluating the performance of hospitals and health care institutions. Quality measures identify strengths and weaknesses of health care organizations and drive improvement initiatives so that the organization can achieve better organizational structures, care delivery processes, and safe and effective treatment and care outcome. The DNP nurse and APRNs are leaders of health care quality initiatives, understand the relationship of care processes to achieving outcomes that reflect high-quality care, and provide oversight to all aspects of quality in a health care organization. The DNP nurse leads evaluation efforts of health care organizations to meet quality benchmarks and ensure that the institution compares favorably with other high-quality institutions, because this is an indication of the quality care they provide.

REFERENCES

ACT Academy. (n.d.). *A model for measuring quality care*. https://improvement.nhs.uk/documents/2135/measuring-quality-care-model.pdf

Agency for Healthcare Research and Quality. (2016a). *Label health care quality measures in plain English*. https://www.ahrq.gov/talkingquality/translate/labels/measures.html

Agency for Healthcare Research and Quality. (2016b). *Organizing quality measures by type*. https://www.ahrq.gov/talkingquality/translate/organize/type.html

Agency for Healthcare Research and Quality. (2015). *Types of health care quality measures*. Author. https://www.ahrq.gov/talkingquality/measures/types.html

Agency for Healthcare Research and Quality. (2017). *Toolkit for using the AHRQ quality indicators*. Author. https://www.ahrq.gov/patient-safety/settings/hospital/resource/qitool/index.html

Agency for Healthcare Research and Quality. (2018). *AHRQuality indicators*. Author. https://www.ahrq.gov/cpi/about/otherwebsites/qualityindicators.ahrq.gov/qualityindicators.html

Agency for Healthcare Research and Quality. (2020a). *Understanding quality measurement*. https://www.ahrq.gov/patient-safety/quality-resources/tools/chtoolbx/understand/index.html

Agency for Healthcare Research and Quality. (2020b). *Patient Safety Indicator 03 (PSI 03) pressure ulcer rate*. Author. https://qualityindicators.ahrq.gov/Downloads/Modules/PSI/V2020/TechSpecs/PSI_03_Pressure_Ulcer_Rate.pdf

Ameh, S., Gómez-Olivé, F. X., Kahn, K., Tollman, S. M., & Klipstein-Grobusch, K. (2017). Relationships between structure, process and outcome to assess quality of integrated chronic disease management in a rural South African setting: Applying a structural equation model. *BMC Health Services Research, 17*, 229. https://doi.org/10.1186/s12913-017-2177-4

American Academy of Family Physicians. (2020). *Quality measures*. https://www.aafp.org/family-physician/practice-and-career/managing-your-practice/quality-measures.html

American Association of Colleges of Nursing. (2006). *The essentials of doctoral education for advanced nursing practice*. www.aacn.nche.edu

American Association of Colleges of Nursing. (2021). *The essentials: Core competencies for professional nursing education*. Author. https://www.aacnnursing.org/Portals/42/AcademicNursing/pdf/Essentials-2021.pdf

Casey, D. E., Thomas, R. J., Bhalla, V., Commodore-Mensah, Y., Heidenreich, P. A., Kolte, D., Muntner, P., Smith Jr, S. C., Spertus, J. A., Windle, J. R., Wozniak, G. D., & Ziaeian, B. (2019). 2019 AHA/ACC clinical performance and quality measures for adults with high blood pressure: A report of the American College of Cardiology/American Heart Association Task Force on performance measures. *Circulation: Cardiovascular Quality and Outcomes, 12*(11). https://doi.org/10.1161/HCQ.0000000000000057

Cassel, C. K., Conway, P. H., Delbanco, S. F., Jha, A. K., Saunders, R. S., & Lee, T. H. (2014). Getting more performance from performance measurement. *New England Journal of Medicine, 371*(23), 2145–2147. https://doi.org/10.1056/NEJMp1408345

Center for Assessment and Policy Development. (2013). *What is an outcome and what is an outcome indicator?* https://www.racialequitytools.org/resourcefiles/What_Is_An_Outcome_And_What_Is_An_Outcome_Indicator.pdf

Centers for Medicare and Medicaid Services. (n.d.). *Medicare hospital quality chartbook.* https://www.cmshospitalchartbook.com/

Centers for Medicare and Medicaid Services. (2020). *Outcome measures.* Author. https://www.cms.gov/Medicare/Quality-Initiatives-Patient-Assessment-Instruments/HospitalQualityInits/OutcomeMeasures

Chassin, M. R., & Loeb, J. M. (2011). The ongoing quality improvement journey: Next stop, high reliability. *Health Affairs, 30*(4), 559–568. https://doi.org/10.1377/hlthaff.2011.0076

Chin, M. H. (2014). How to achieve health equity. *New England Journal of Medicine, 371*(24), 2331–2332. https://doi.org/10.1056/NEJMe1412264

Donabedian, A. (1966). Evaluating the quality of medical care. *Milbank Memorial Fund Quarterly, 44*(Suppl. 3), 166–206.

Donabedian, A. (1980). *A guide to medical care administration: Medical care appraisal: Quality and utilization.* The American Public Health Association.

Donabedian, A. (1988a). The quality of care. How can it be assessed? *JAMA, 260*(12), 1743–1749. https://doi.org/10.1001/jama.260.12.1743

Donabedian A. (1988b). Quality assessment and assurance: Unity of purpose, diversity of means. *Inquiry, 25*(1), 173–192. https://www.jstor.org/stable/29771941

Donabedian, A. (2003). *An introduction to quality assurance in health care.* Oxford University Press.

Edwards, R. (2016). *Introduction to health outcomes.* Healthcare Financial Management Association (HFMA). https://www.hfma.org.uk/docs/default-source/our-networks/healthcare-costing-for-value-institute/institute-publications/introduction-to-health-outcomes

Greenberg, R. S. (2015). *Medical epidemiology, population health and effective health care* (5th ed.). McGraw Hill Education.

Health Quality Ontario. (2013). *Measurement for quality improvement.* Queen's Printer for Ontario. http://www.hqontario.ca/Portals/0/documents/qi/qi-measurement-primer-en.pdf

Hennekens, C. H., & Buring, J. E. (1987). *Epidemiology in medicine.* Little, Brown and Company.

Hostetter, M., & Klein, S. (2020). *Improve health care quality.* The Commonwealth Fund. https://www.commonwealthfund.org/publications/newsletter-article/using-patient-reported-outcomes-improve-health-care-quality>

Hughes, R. (Ed.). (2008). Patient safety and quality: An evidence-based handbook for nurses. Agency for Healthcare Research and Quality. https://www.ncbi.nlm.nih.gov/books/NBK2651/

Hussey, P. S., Wertheimer, S., & Mehrotra, A. (2013). The association between health care quality and cost: A systematic review. *Annals of Internal Medicine, 158*(1), 27–34. https://doi.org/10.7326/0003-4819-158-1-201301010-00006

Institute for Healthcare Improvement. (2020a). *Initiatives.* http://www.ihi.org/Engage/Initiatives/TripleAim/pages/default.aspx

Institute for Healthcare Improvement. (2020b). *Across the Chasm: Six aims for changing the health care system.* http://www.ihi.org/resources/Pages/ImprovementStories/AcrosstheChasmSixAimsforChangingtheHealthCareSystem.aspx

Institute of Medicine. (2000). *To err is human: Building a safer health system.* The National Academies Press. https://doi.org/10.17226/9728

Institute of Medicine. (2001). *Crossing the quality chasm: A new health system for the 21st century.* National Academies Press. http://www.nationalacademies.org/hmd/Reports/2001/Crossing-the-Quality-Chasm-A-New-Health-System-for-the-21st-Century.aspx

Institute of Medicine. (2015). *Vital signs: Core metrics for health and health care progress.* The National Academies Press. https://doi.org/10.17226/19402

Kendrach, M. G., Covington, T. R., McCarthy, M. W., & Harris, M. C. (1997). Calculating risks and number-needed-to-treat: A method of data interpretation. *Journal of Managed Care Pharmacy, 3*(2), 179–183. https://doi.org/10.18553/jmcp.1997.3.2.179

Kleinpell, R. M. (2013). Measuring outcomes in advanced practice nursing. In R. M. Kleinpell (Ed.), *Outcome assessment in advanced practice nursing* (3rd ed., pp. 1–43). Springer Publishing Co.

Langley, G. J., Moen, R. D., Nolan, K. M., Nolan, T. W., Norman, C. L., & Provost, L. P. (2009). *The improvement guide: A practical approach to enhancing organizational performance.* John Wiley & Sons.

Leapfrog Group. (2019). *Scoring methodology.* https://www.hospitalsafetygrade.org/media/file/HospitalSafetyGrade_ScoringMethodology_Spring2019_FINAL.pdf

Lee, T. H. (2010). Putting the value framework to work. *New England Journal of Medicine, 363*(26), 2481–2483. https://doi.org/10.1056/NEJMp1013111

Meyer G. S., Nelson E. C., Pryor, D. B., James, B., Swensen, S. J., Kaplan, G. S., Weissberg, J. I., Bisognano, M., Yates, G. R., & Hunt, G. C. (2012). More quality measures versus measuring what matters: A call for balance and parsimony. *BMJ Quality & Safety, 21*, 964–968. https://doi.org/10.1136/bmjqs-2012-001081

Mitchell, P. H. (2008). Defining patient safety and quality care. In R. G. Hughes (Ed.), *Patient safety and quality: An evidence-based handbook for nurses.* Agency for Healthcare Research and Quality. https://www.ncbi.nlm.nih.gov/books/NBK2681/

National Quality Forum. (2020a). *The ABCs of measurement.* http://www.qualityforum.org/Measuring_Performance/ABCs_of_Measurement.aspx

National Quality Forum. (2020b). *Improving healthcare quality.* https://www.qualityforum.org/Setting_Priorities/Improving_Healthcare_Quality.aspx

National Quality Forum. (2020c). *Measure endorsement.* http://www.qualityforum.org/Measuring_Performance/Consensus_Development_Process/CSAC_Decision.aspx

National Quality Measures Clearinghouse. (2015). *Tutorials on quality measures.* http://www.qualitymeasures.ahrq.gov/tutorial/

Pantaleon, L. (2019). Why measuring outcomes is important in health care. *Journal of Veterinary Internal Medicine, 33*(2), 356–362. https://doi.org/10.1111/jvim.15458

Porter, M. E. (2010a). What is value in health care? *New England Journal of Medicine (Appendix 1), 363*(26), 2477–2481. https://doi.org/10.1056/NEJMp1011024

Porter, M. E. (2010b). Measuring health outcomes: The outcomes hierarchy. *New England Journal of Medicine, 363*, 2477–2481. https://doi.org/10.1056/NEJMp1011024

Romano, P., Hussey, P., & Ritley, D. (2010). *Selecting quality and resource use measures: A decision guide for community quality collaboratives* (AHRQ Publication No. 09(10)-0073). http://www.ahrq.gov/professionals/quality-patient-safety/quality-resources/tools/perfmeasguide/index.html

Rondinelli, J., Zuniga, S., Kipnis, P., Kawar, L. N., Liu, V., & Escobar, G. J. (2018). Hospital-acquired pressure injury: Risk-adjusted comparisons in an integrated healthcare delivery system. *Nursing Research, 67*(1), 16–25. https://doi.org/10.1097/NNR.000000000000025

Sadeghi, S., Barzi, A., Mikhail, O., & Shabot, M. M. (2013). *Improving quality and strategy.* Jones & Bartlett Learning.

Scheinker, D., Ward, A., Shin, A. Y., Lee, G. M., Mathew, R., & Donnelly, L. F. (2020). Differences in central line–associated bloodstream infection rates based on the criteria used to count central line days. *JAMA, 323*(2), 183–185. https://doi.org/10.1001/jama.2019.18616

Scott, K. W., & Jha, A. K. (2014). Putting quality on the global health agenda. *New England Journal of Medicine, 371*(1), 3–5. https://doi.org/10.1056/NEJMp1402157

Scoville, R. (2015). *Advanced measurement techniques in improvement work.* Institute for healthcare Improvement (IHI). http://www.ihi.org/communities/blogs/_layouts/15/ihi/community/blog/itemview.aspx?List=7d1126ec-8f63-4a3b-9926-c44ea3036813&ID=119#:~:text=Outcomes%20measures%20provide%20feedback%20on,patient%2Dreported%20quality%20of%20life.&text=For%20example%2C%20length%20of%20stay%20or%20patient%20wait%20times

Stone, P. W., Glied, S. A., McNair, P. D., Matthes, N., Cohen, B., Landers, T. F., & Larson, E. L. (2010). CMS changes in reimbursement for HAIs: Setting a research agenda. *Medical Care, 48*(5), 433–439. https://doi.org/10.1097/MLR.0b013e3181d5fb3f

The Joint Commission. (2020). *Outcome and process performance measures.* https://www.jointcommission.org/-/media/tjc/documents/resources/health-services-research/clabsi-toolkit/clabsi_toolkit_tool_5-6_outcome_and_process_performance_measurespdf.pdf

Tinker, A. (2018). *The top seven healthcare outcome measures and three measurement essentials.* https://www.healthcatalyst.com/insights/top-7-healthcare-outcome-measures

Titler, M. G., Shever, L. L., Kanak, M. F., Picone, D. M., & Qin, R. (2011). Factors associated with falls during hospitalization in an older adult population. *Research and Theory for Nursing Practice, 25*(2), 127–148. https://doi.org/10.1891/1541-6577.25.2.127

Wakefield, M. K. (2008). The quality Chasm series: Implications for nursing. In R. G. Hughes (Ed.), *Patient safety and quality: An evidence-based handbook for nurses.* Agency for Healthcare Research and Quality. https://www.ncbi.nlm.nih.gov/books/NBK2677/

Weldring, T., & Smith, S. M. (2013). Patient-reported outcomes (PROs) and patient-reported outcome measures (PROMs). *Health Services Insights, 6,* 61–68. https://doi.org/10.4137/HSI.S11093

FIVE

FINANCIAL EVALUATION

Eileen R. Giardino and Angelo P. Giardino

> *. . . everything we discuss in reference to medicine, health care delivery or policy will merely be symptomatic of the overarching tension between our aspirations for health care and our resources to pay for them.*
> —C. Everett Koop
> *Surgeon General of the United States, 1981–1989*

GENERAL MANDATE TO UNDERSTAND ECONOMICS

Doctor of nursing practice (DNP)–prepared nurses are at the forefront of understanding and addressing the tensions between patient and community health care aspirations and the resources to pay for quality health care. DNP nurses are often accountable for determining the economic efficiency of health care interventions, programs to improve quality outcomes, and the health care delivery systems in which patient care and quality of care issues reside. *The Essentials of Doctoral Education for Advanced Nursing Practice,* published by the American Association of Colleges of Nursing (AACN, 2006), stated the ability to use principles of economics and finance to redesign care delivery strategies; evaluate the cost effectiveness of providing care; and evaluate quality improvement (QI) methodologies to promote safe, timely, effective, efficient, equitable, and patient-centered care competencies and skills of the DNP nurse. As DNP nurses develop and implement practice-level and systemwide initiatives that address care delivery, it is essential to know how to evaluate the economic impact of quality and safety initiatives within an organization (AACN, 2006). Quality principles underlie all aspects of health care, from the economics of relating reimbursement for patient care services, to achieving quality care measures, to understanding the relationship between the economics of developing QI initiatives to achieve better quality outcomes of care.

This chapter describes the concepts of economic evaluations used to appraise QI initiatives that DNP nurses implement in health care organizations. It describes the concepts needed to evaluate the economic impact and financial considerations of QI initiatives developed to improve the outcomes within a healthcare system. The chapter explores concepts of macroeconomics of the

U.S. health care system and how microeconomic principles relate to organizational and clinical unit finances, the reimbursement models that relate quality outcomes to providers' reimbursement for provision of care, the use of return on investment (ROI) calculation for developing QI initiatives, and the essential concepts and assumptions that support the economic evaluation as it relates to cost-effectiveness analysis (CEA), cost-utility analysis (CUA), and cost-benefit analysis (CBA).

IMPLICATIONS FOR THE DOCTOR OF NURSING PRACTICE

The 2001 Institute of Medicine (IOM) report, entitled *Crossing the Quality Chasm*, identified six areas for performance improvement within the U.S. health care system, namely safety, timeliness, effectiveness, efficiency, equity, and patient-centeredness (STEEEP) (IOM, 2001). In 2008, the Institute for Healthcare Improvement (IHI) framed the need for health care improvement in terms of a Triple Aim focused on "improving the individual experience of care; improving the health of populations; and reducing the per capita costs of care for populations" (Berwick et al., 2008, p. 760). In line with a call for the overall reform and improvement in health care delivery and outcomes, the value equation was introduced to address health outcomes per dollar spent, namely, the quality of the care being delivered divided by the lowest cost to deliver that care, representing the highest value: Value = Quality/Cost (Porter & Teisberg, 2006). *Crossing the Quality Chasm* identified the need for a redesign of the U.S. health care system and set in motion a framework for health care institutions to improve overall safety and quality of the care provided to individuals and populations (Fischer & Duncan, 2020).

The DNP nurse must understand principles of practice management that include strategies that balance cost and productivity with quality of care. The ability to improve practice outcomes and create sustainable change is achieved when financial and economic structures are in place to support change activities. The DNP nurse should be able to evaluate cost-effectiveness of care and apply economic principles to both evaluate care delivery and design effective strategies to improve care delivery (AACN, 2006). The ability to determine the costs of practice changes, and it is important to understand the economics to the organization when developing and implementing practice-level or systemwide initiatives to improve the quality of health care delivery. DNP nurses bring specialized knowledge to an interdisciplinary team and collaborate with other health professionals in issues that involve economic and budgetary components. A grounding in economic concepts and evaluation methods is necessary to lead discussions and develop programs that impact the health status of patients, the health care system, and health policies.

The AACN published the DNP Essentials that provided the educational framework for the preparation of nurses at the doctoral level (AACN, 2006). The update of *The Essentials: Core Competencies for Professional Nursing Education* (2021) continues to provide a structure for competencies that advanced practice nurses should know related to finance and nursing practice. Domain 5, Quality and Safety, notes that advanced-level education focuses on the DNP as an advocate for change related to financial policies that impact the relationship between quality care delivery and economics and the ability to develop a business plan for QI initiatives. Domain 7, Systems-Based Practice, states the importance of the DNP nurse having a knowledge of payment and financial models relative to reimbursement and health care costs as well as being able to apply strategies that improve cost-effectiveness and ROI for improvement initiatives (AACN, 2021).

MACROECONOMICS AND MICROECONOMICS

A Macroeconomic Perspective on Cost and Outcome

Macroeconomics is a branch of economics that studies the behavior and performance of the overall economy and how large-scale market systems behave in regard to aggregate changes in the economy, such as growth rate, inflation, unemployment, national economic planning, monetary policy, and gross domestic product (GDP). It examines how a country's policies and behaviors affect the economy and industries, rather than individuals or specific companies (Silver et al., 2020). Macroeconomics addresses questions such as "What should the rate of inflation be?" or "What stimulates economic growth?" Macroeconomics centers on industrial market performance and structure, whereas microeconomics focuses on market segments and individual firms or segments (Fetterolf & Shah, 2021).

The health care system in the United States is a multifaceted industry that employs approximately 16.2 million people, has over 6,100 hospitals and health systems in operation, staffs over 920,000 beds to provide care for over 36.3 million admissions, and had overall costs in excess of $3 trillion in 2018. Economists describe the dollars spent on health care in relative terms compared with other industries and as a percentage of the GDP. The GDP is a measure of total economic activity and the monetary value of all final goods and services produced within a country's borders in one year and serves as a way to understand a country's total output. In 2017, health care accounted for 16.9% of GDP (Tikkanen & Abrahms, 2020) and increased to 17.7% in 2018 (Centers for Medicare & Medicaid Services [CMS], 2020). Health care spending as a percentage of GDP and per capita spending in the United States have risen dramatically over the past several decades.

In 1970, U.S. health care spending was $75 billion, accounting for 7.2% of the GDP and representing an average of $356 per person as compared with $3.6 trillion in 2018 (17.7% GDP or $11,172 per capita; American Academy of Pediatrics, 2013; CMS, 2020). The CMS provides data related to the total health expenditure each year (federal data has a 2-year reporting lag; 2018 data are available in 2020). Exhibit 5.1 lists the total national health care expenditure for the United States in calendar year 2018 and breaks this expenditure down into two large components, consumption expenditures, namely, those costs attributed to providing care to patients, and investment, namely, those costs allocated to research efforts and to building and equipment projects. Exhibit 5.1 also displays a pie chart that shows that over 84% of the health care expenditures in the United States is spent on providing health care services to patients.

Exhibit 5.1
U.S. National Health Expenditure for Calendar Year 2018

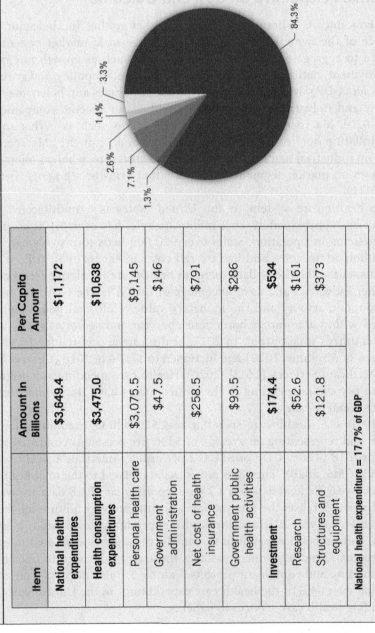

Item	Amount in Billions	Per Capita Amount
National health expenditures	**$3,649.4**	**$11,172**
Health consumption expenditures	**$3,475.0**	**$10,638**
Personal health care	$3,075.5	$9,145
Government administration	$47.5	$146
Net cost of health insurance	$258.5	$791
Government public health activities	$93.5	$286
Investment	**$174.4**	**$534**
Research	$52.6	$161
Structures and equipment	$121.8	$373

National health expenditure = 17.7% of GDP

Note: Numbers and percentages may not add to totals because of rounding. Dollar amounts shown are in current dollars.

Source: Centers for Medicare & Medicaid Services, Office of the Actuary, National Health Statistics Group; U.S. Department of Commerce, Bureau of Economic Analysis; & U.S. Bureau of the Census. https://www.cms.gov/Research-Statistics-Data-and-Systems/Statistics-Trends-and-Reports/NationalHealthExpendData/NHE-Fact-Sheet

In addition to the annual statistics, the CMS also provides economic forecast data that allow one to predict the dollar amounts of future expenditures. Table 5.1 demonstrates the anticipated growth of the national health expenditure in total dollar amount. The national health expenditure for the United States is projected to reach more than $5.5 trillion by calendar year 2026.

Health care is a worldwide industry in which health care systems are essential in supporting human healthcare economics and have major macroeconomic implications because of their effect on productivity, output, employment or labor, and research endeavors (Darvas et al., 2018). The Organization for Economic Co-operation and Development (OECD) provides data comparing the health care expenditures, workforce, and health status measures for different member countries. Exhibit 5.2 lists per capita health care spending for Australia, Canada, and several European countries as well as the number of physicians and nurses per 1,000 population.

TABLE 5.1   U.S. National Health Expenditure Projections

National Health Expenditure Projections					
	2018	**2020**	**2022**	**2024**	**2026**
Item	**Amount in Billions**				
National health expenditures	$3,649.4	$4,014.2	$4,456.00	$4,966.1	$5,549.5
Health consumption expenditures	$3,475.0	$3,832.6	$4,243.30	$4,731	$5,288.5
Personal health care	$3,075.5	$3,377.5	$3,765.5	$4,202.1	$4,703.0
Government administration	$47.5	$52.0	$58.4	$65.7	$74.3
Net cost of health insurance	$258.5	$295.2	$314.0	$350.0	$389.5
Government public health activities	$93.5	$98.9	$105.4	$112.8	$121.8
Investment	**$174.4**	**$190.7**	**$212.7**	**$235.5**	**$261.0**
Research	$52.6	$58.6	$66.4	$73.1	$80.6
Structures and equipment	$121.8	$132.0	$146.3	$162.3	$180.4

Note: Numbers may not add to totals because of rounding.

Source: Centers for Medicare & Medicaid Services, Office of the Actuary. https://www.cms.gov/Research-Statistics -Data-and-Systems/Statistics-Trends-and-Reports/NationalHealthExpendData/NHE-Fact-Sheet; Centers for Medicare & Medicaid Services. (2020). *NHE fact sheet.* https://www.cms.gov/Research-Statistics-Data-and-Systems/ Statistics-Trends-and-Reports/NationalHealthExpendData/NHE-Fact-Sheet

Exhibit 5.2

Comparative Health Care Spending of the United States and Other Countries

	Health Spending	Doctors	Nurses
	Per Capita (USD based on Purchasing Power Parities)	Practicing Physicians (per 1,000 Population)	Practicing Nurses (per 1,000 Population)
Australia	5,005	3.7	11.7
Canada	4,974	2.7	10.0
France	4,965	3.2	10.5
Germany	5,986	4.3	12.9
Sweden	5,447	4.1	10.9
United Kingdom	4,070	2.8	7.8
United States	10,586	2.6	11.7

Note: Data presented is from 2017.

Source: Organization for Economic Co-operation and Development. (2019). Health at a glance 2019: OECD indicators. Author. https://doi.org/10.1787/4dd50c09-en.

Health Spending Per capita

Australia	Canada	France	Germany	Sweden	United Kingdom	United States
$5,005	$4,974	$4,965	$5,986	$5,447	$4,070	$10,586

TABLE 5.2 Health Care–Related Measures

	Life Expectancy	Population Coverage	Infant Mortality
	Years of Life at Birth	Access to Care: Population Eligible for Core Services (% Population)	Deaths per 1,000 Live Births
Australia	82.6	100	3.3
Canada	82.0	100	4.5
France	82.6	99.9	3.8
Germany	81.1	100	2.8
Sweden	82.5	100	2.3
United Kingdom	81.3	100	2.8
United States	78.6	90.8	4.8

Note: Data presented is from 2017.

Source: Organization for Economic Co-operation and Development. (2019). *Health at a glance 2019: OECD indicators.* Author. https://doi.org/10.1787/4dd50c09-en.

While individual countries vary in their approach to health care delivery, per capita health spending in the United States is more than twice as much as it was in the European Union (Darvas et al., 2018). No matter what amount is spent, spending to improve the macroeconomic impacts should be efficient, achieve best practices, and decrease wasteful spending. Health care delivery systems influence overall macroeconomic outcomes (Darvas et al., 2018). However, a higher proportion of GDP spent on health care services does not translate into higher utilization because salaries, pharmaceuticals, and costs of care are much higher in the United States than in other countries (Mikulic, 2020). In addition, the United States spends significantly more on private health care services, as opposed to countries with universal health care or publicly funded health care systems. Additionally, with such a high per capita expenditure, one might expect the quality of health care to be higher than in countries where per capita spending is less, but that is not the case.

Uninsured Americans

A discussion of the U.S. health care system should include the plight of Americans without health insurance because this is a vexing characteristic of the U.S. approach to covering its population. Health care reform efforts in the latter part of the 2000s led to the passage of the Patient Protection and Affordable Care Act of 2010 (ACA), which was fully implemented in calendar year 2014. Table 5.2 presents statistics for the year 2017 that show that the United States has the lowest life expectancy, the lowest percentage of people with access to health care services, and the highest infant mortality rate as compared with other developed countries. Exhibit 5.3 lists the insurance coverage and level of those uninsured from 2012 through 2018 and displays the double-digit reduction in those uninsured in the years immediately

Exhibit 5.3

Insurance Coverage and Level of Those Uninsured From 2012 Through 2018

	2012	2013	2014	2015	2016	2017	2018
Enrollment							
				Amount in Millions			
Total private health insurance	191.1	191.0	194.7	200.3	201.8	202.1	200.5
Employer-sponsored private health insurance	169.5	169.2	169.8	172.2	173.1	175.6	175.2
Direct purchase	22.5	23.1	26.2	29.6	30.1	28.0	26.7
Marketplace	–	–	5.5	9.0	10.0	9.8	9.9
Medigap	9.8	10.3	10.6	11.6	12.1	11.9	11.8
Other direct purchase	12.7	12.8	10.1	9.0	8.0	6.4	5.0
Medicare	49.7	51.3	52.8	54.3	55.8	57.2	58.7
Medicaid	58.1	59.1	65.6	69.3	71.1	72.1	72.8
CHIP	5.8	6.0	5.9	6.0	6.5	6.9	7.1
Uninsured	44.7	44.1	35.5	29.5	28.7	29.7	30.7
Expenditures							
				Amount in Billions			
Total private health insurance	$922.0	$939.1	$994.1	$1,060.9	$1,119.9	$1,175.0	$1,243.0
Employer-sponsored private health insurance	$845.2	$856.2	$879.8	$925.1	$972.2	$1,018.7	$1,069.2
Direct purchase	$47.9	$52.7	$82.1	$102.3	$110.6	$116.9	$131.5
Marketplace	–	–	$23.8	$39.9	$47.2	$55.1	$70.5
Medigap	$24.8	$26.2	27.4	$29.8	$30.4	$31.8	$32.4
Other direct purchase	$23.1	$26.4	$30.9	$32.7	$33.1	$30.0	$28.6
Medicare	$568.5	$588.9	$618.5	$648.8	$676.8	$705.1	$750.2
Medicaid	$455.9	$445.2	$497.8	$542.6	$565.4	$580.1	$597.4
CHIP	$12.6	$13.5	$13.2	$14.7	$16.8	$18.1	$18.6

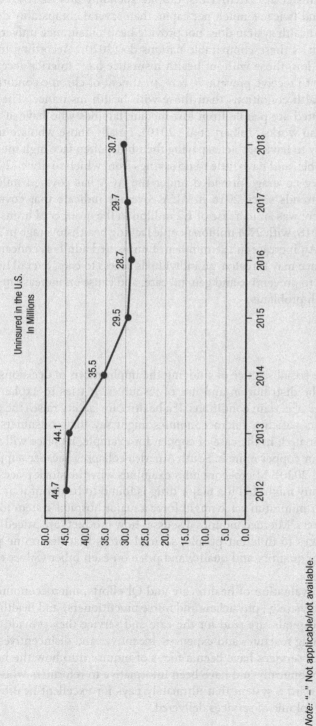

Uninsured in the U.S.
In Millions

44.7	44.1	35.5	29.5	28.7	29.7	30.7
2012	2013	2014	2015	2016	2017	2018

Note: "–" Not applicable/not available.

Source: Centers for Medicare Services, Office of the Actuary, National Health Statistics Group. https://www.cms.gov/Research-Statistics-Data-and-Systems/Statistics-Trends-and-Reports/NationalHe;athExpendData/NHE-Fact-Sheet; Centers for Medicare & Medicaid Services. (2020). *NHE fact sheet.* https://www.cms.gov/Research-Statistics-Data-and-Systems/Statistics-Trends-and-Reports/NationalHealthExpendData/NHE-Fact-Sheet

following the expansion of coverage that occurred after 2014 and the increasing number of uninsured from 2016 to 2018.

Estimates for the year 2020 indicate that approximately 12.5% of Americans were uninsured and that 43.4% of adults between the ages of 19 and 64 were inadequately insured (Collins et al., 2020).Thus, despite spending almost 18% of the GDP on health care, and twice as much per capita than several comparably developed nations, the U.S. health system does not provide health insurance universally to its entire population as these comparable nations do (2020). According to the Kaiser Family Foundation, those without health insurance have inferior access to care and are less likely to receive preventive care, treatment of chronic conditions, and care for major health conditions than those with health insurance. The vast majority of the uninsured are people from low-income families who have at least one family member who works (Tolbert et al., 2019). Finally, those who are uninsured are twice as likely to have problems paying their bills, often face high medical bills that are unaffordable, and have little to no savings from which to draw (2019).

Although insurance coverage provided under the ACA has covered millions of Americans, recent trends since 2016 in ACA coverage indicate that coverage gains have eroded. There was an increase of 1.2 million in the number of uninsured people from 2016 to 2018, with 27.4 million people lacking health coverage in 2018 (Tolbert et al., 2019). An increase in the number of uninsured adults is concerning because lack of insurance may threaten an individuals access to care, overall health and well-being, access to preventive and general care, and cause an increase in serious illnesses and health problems.

Microeconomics

Microeconomics is the social science of studying the implications of decisions and incentives regarding the distribution and use of resources. It tries to explain the outcomes of the change of certain conditions. If a health care facility raises the price of immunizations to its patients, microeconomics might say that consumers will decide not to get vaccinated. In the case of copper, for example, its price will most likely increase if a major copper mine in South America collapses because supply is restricted (Silver et al., 2020). Microeconomics examines why the stock prices of a pharmaceutical company might fall if a major drug is found to be harmful or ineffective or why a higher minimum wage might force a major hospital system to hire fewer health care workers. Microeconomics discusses how products are priced, why there are different prices to different people, societal forces that determine price levels, and the effect of quantity and quality and price on each other (Silver et al., 2020; Walsh, 2014).

As applied to the evaluation of health care and QI efforts, microeconomics is focused on how providers (e.g., physicians and nurse practitioners) and health care institutions such as hospitals, are paid for the care and service they provide. At a granular level, examining revenues and expenses, incentives and disincentives and managing utilization of services have been a focus of inquiry into how the health care system works economically and have been informative to reformers who seek to promote change toward a system that ultimately pays for excellent health outcomes rather than for volume of services delivered.

PAYMENT MODELS FOR U.S. HEALTH CARE SERVICES

Retrospective Payment

Over most of its history the payment model common in U.S. health care systems is a retrospective, fee-for-service (FFS) payment system. In an FFS payment model, health care professionals and/or health care facilities are compensated for the volume of covered services that were delivered and not necessarily for the quality and measured outcome for the care and services received (MacLeod, 2001). Within an FFS system, relatively complex coding systems are used that identify specific diagnoses being treated and specific procedures and services provided so that codes can be counted. These codes are then transmitted to the payer after the health care encounter with the patient, and payment is then transmitted back to the health care professional and/or facility. This process is retrospective because payment to the provider of services occurs after specific services are delivered.

The retrospective FFS payment model is routinely criticized since it has the potential to incent providers to overuse services since the more care or higher volume of care delivered likely leads to higher reimbursement for services. An example of overuse of services is the provider who routinely orders an extensive panel of commonly available laboratory tests on every patient admitted to the inpatient hospital unit rather than judiciously matching the laboratory tests ordered on admission with the specific characteristics of a given patient's clinical circumstances along with the differential diagnosis being considered for that admission.

Payment for Services and Quality Outcomes

As health care costs soared in the late 1990s and early 2000s, there were calls to address the retrospective, volume-based FFS system. The change was to transition from the FFS system toward a prospective fixed payment approach that would deemphasize the amount of service delivered in favor of a preset payment model that focuses on appropriate utilization of services and the achievement of quality targets. Generically referred to as a managed care approach, reimbursement is calculated as a capitated or per-member-per-month (PMPM) rate and combined with data systems and regular feedback to the providers in order to limit unnecessary utilization and to promote the adoption of standardized care pathways directed at achieving optimal outcomes, both clinical and financial (Kongstvedt, 2001). Because the prospective PMPM payments for individual patient care are fixed regardless of the volume of services provided, a health care professional or organization would likely lose money when they use more patient services than necessary to diagnose and treat a patient. The goal of the PMPM approach is to use only the necessary services to achieve the best outcomes for a patient's care. From the provider's perspective when receiving payment via a PMPM approach, there is a population-based ongoing reimbursement for the costs of the patient's care that is not dependent on what is or what is not ordered for that patient in a given time period. A well-managed prospective, capitated payment system (i.e., which provides an adequate PMPM) with quality monitoring should discourage overuse of services and lead to a health care delivery system that supports and encourages diagnostic and treatment services that are necessary and appropriate.

Value-Based Purchasing

The prospective managed care approach has evolved over several decades. Reformers now speak in terms of alternative payment models (APM) of reimbursement for patient care. APMs shift the volume of service, or the reimbursement approach that involves counting of codes submitted, to one that reimburses for the quality of the care delivered with the achievement of positive patient outcomes as the ultimate goal. APMs enthusiastically embrace the value equation: Value = Quality/Cost (Porter & Teisberg, 2006).

The CMS developed a four-category maturation framework that describes the shifting from the traditional FFS system toward value-based reimbursement. The categories are as follows:

1. FFS with no link to quality
2. FFS linked to quality
3. APMs built on a FFS architecture
4. Population-based payment that fully reflects payment for value

The type of payments described in Categories 2 through 4 are value-based purchasing payments, whereas Category 1 was the traditional payment model that did not require the provider to account for anything other than services provided. The models in Categories 2 through 4 involve a shift on the part of providers to be accountable for the quality and cost of care they provide as well as a shift in a practice to a population health management focus rather than a payment for specific services, as is the focus of Category 1. The significance of the relationship between payment models and quality care is that Catgories 2 through 4 focus on providing patient care that achieves quality outcomes that address outcome measures, whereas the FFS model (Category 1) was not connected at all to the quality of care that a patient received.

The Department of Health and Human Services, in partnership with private sector payers, wants to expand new health care payment models in order to reduce costs and improve the quality of health care delivered. Value-based purchasing involves paying for care provided that meets quality measures and is focused on better management of population health outcomes by providers and health care institutions rather than payment for specific services. The relationship between payment for services and provision of quality care is paramount, because the CMS only wants to reimburse provider services that achieve standard parameters for quality care (CMS, 2015).

The CMS recognizes the evolutionary process or reimbursement models and the many challenges health care professionals, health care facilities, and insurance payers face as they move through these stages toward a value-based payment model. The CMS wants to improve the way providers are paid and reward care coordination and value rather than care duplication of services and volume. Rewarding value of care addresses a reward to providing quality outcomes of care (CMS, 2015). However, the CMS is only one of many private and public payers. Health care providers have made operational changes in their approach to care as APMs and payment reforms have been adopted by a critical mass of payers. When providers encounter new payment strategies for one payer, but not others, the incentives to make fundamental change are weak. In fact, a provider that alters its system to improve quality outcomes to prevent admissions and meet quality measures may lose revenue from those payers that have continued FFS payments (CMS, 2015).

RETURN ON INVESTMENT

The ROI is an economic measure that indicates the degree of economic benefit derived in relation to the costs incurred to develop and implement the initiative (Agency for Healthcare Research and Quality [AHRQ], 2017; Brousselle et al., 2016). The ROI provides a determination of the net financial gains (or losses) after calculating the resources invested in a quality initiative and the amounts gained through either or both reduced costs and increased revenue that resulted from the initiative (AHRQ, 2015). An ROI can illustrate the time frame needed for the returns of the improvement initiative to offset the costs of the development implementation costs. Examples of public health messages related to ROI are (Brousselle et al., 2016):

- Every $1 spent on early childhood health and development saves up to $9 in future spending on health and social and justice services. ROI: 800%.
- Every $1 invested in tobacco prevention programs saves up to $20 in future health care costs. ROI: 1,900%.

An actual ROI can be determined after a quality initiative has been implemented to assess the overall value of the initiative and inform decisions on future improvement actions (AHRQ, 2017). In the planning stages of an initiative, the determination of the ROI can help planners estimate how the initiative will affect operating costs and revenue to optimize quality outcomes and financial performance. The ROI can be part of an informed decision-making process where examination of anticipated financial outcome data can help an organization prioritize resources for QI initiatives. A QI initiative in an organization should include the understanding of the initiative's ROI at various levels of operation.

Return on Investment and Quality Initiatives

The ROI is one aspect of the overall impact of a quality change initiative that should be considered when making the decision to invest in a quality initiative (Shah & Course, 2018). Although the main reason for a QI change initiative is to improve the experience of care delivery and care service and improve outcomes, the organization should consider the financial aspects of improved efficiency and productivity, reduced cost pressures/cost avoidance, and whether or not there are increased revenues that result.

The calculation of ROI requires the consideration of both costs and benefits to the organization. The many facets of a QI initiative make it challenging to demonstrate the specific cause and effects of the costs or the savings of the QI initiative and difficult to define the tangible ROI (Shah & Course, 2018). Developing a projected ROI is helpful in the planning stage of a QI initiative because it can estimate how implementing the change initiative will affect operating costs and provide data to then adjust the intervention in ways that optimize both financial performance and quality outcomes. In addition, planners can use an ROI to determine how long it will take for the initiative to offset up-front and ongoing implementation costs; that is, to break even (AHRQ, 2017). From the perspective of evaluating an implemented quality initiative, an ROI using the data from an actual quality initiative ROI can assess the value of that initiative to the organization and inform decisions on future improvement actions (2017).

Planners should consider the perspective of the economic evaluation when determining the ROI. The organizational costs of a QI initiative include the costs for the time invested by the improvement team, stakeholders and staff, as well as the training efforts needed to implement new change processes within the system. Consequently, accurately estimating the identifiable costs of an initiative may be challenging but is essential to the calculation; also, there may be hidden expenses that are either not understood or are so difficult to estimate that they may be excluded from the overall ROI calculations, and leaders must be cognizant that costs are likely to be underestimated, especially with complicated projects (Shah & Course, 2018).

Shah and Course (2018) developed a framework to evaluate ROI in QI initiatives that takes into account factors that lead to determining ROI. Their principles for calculating benefit and ROI from QI are determination of direct benefit of QI initiative outcomes to the customer, improvement of employees' work experience, improved productivity and efficiency, avoided costs, costs removed, and increase in business revenue (Shah & Course, 2018). The AHRQ provides a tool kit to estimate the ROI for an improvement initiative. The tool kit provides a step-by-step guide to calculate the ROI based on specified cost factors and complex determinants that reflect the project's implementation costs and the financial effects of improvement actions. Readers who want to use the AHRQ tool kit should go to the AHRQ website for a more robust description of the topics in the table and for the worksheets and descriptions that are useful to an evaluation team (AHRQ, 2017). Exhibit 5.4 provides a way to determine the calculation of an ROI.

Case Studies for Return on Investment

The following are two case studies that address the development and findings of an ROI. Case 1 describes the calculation of an ROI for a smaller scale QI initiative in a pediatric hospital, whereas Case 2 illustrates a larger scale, national quality initiative.

Case 1: Return on Investment Calculation for a Single Clinical Unit Quality Improvement Project

Context. An academic pediatric primary care practice serving patients and families from predominately underrepresented and underserved communities (e.g., more than 60% of those served spoke English as a second language). In 2015, the CMS began reimbursing for chronic case management (CCM) services that complied with regulatory standards and were appropriately documented and coded. This academic practice had been providing care coordination services for the children with special health care needs who were provided care in the practice. Thus, this opportunity to be reimbursed for CCM was seen as a potential opportunity to garner additional reimbursement for services that were already being delivered in this academic setting but that prior to 2015 had no billing mechanism (Hobson et al., 2018).

Project overview. Over approximately 15 months, the team undertook a QI project approach designed to refine clinic processes to ensure that appropriate patients who were to receive CCM services were properly enrolled, had documentation conducted in a compliant manner, created a registry of patients that could be monitored and used to provide operational and performance reports to ensure that CCM was occurring as planned, and, finally, developed care plans within the electronic medical record (EMR) that would allow for an automated billing process to be established.

Exhibit 5.4
Overview of AHRQ Tool Kit's Approach to ROI Calculation

Purpose	A ROI analysis is a way to calculate your net financial gains (or losses), taking into account all the resources invested and the amounts gained through increased revenue, reduced costs, or both.
Definition	ROI = Net financial returns from improvement actions/Financial investment in improvement actions Numerator and denominator of this ratio are defined as: ● *Net financial returns from improvement actions.* The financial gains from the implementation of the improvement actions, which are generated by net changes in quality, efficiency, and utilization of services or in payments for those services. ● *Financial investment in improvement actions.* The costs of developing and operating the improvement actions.

Step	Brief Description
Determine the basic ROI design	1. **Define the scope of services affected by the improvement actions.** 　—affecting one unit or department or broader, such as across all nursing units 2. **Define the timeline for implementation of improvement actions.** 　—the ROI analysis needs to capture when those actions change the hospital's operating procedures over time to estimate both the implementation costs and the financial effects of improvement actions. 3. **Define the comparison group.** 　—need to compare the hospital's finances under two conditions—with the improvement actions implemented and without them. Options include: 　　—comparison over time, with the "before" condition being the service processes before improvement actions, and the "after" condition the service processes after implementation. 　　—comparisons across units within the same institution. 　　—comparison across institutions. 　—be sure to choose comparison groups that have similar characteristics except that they did not implement the improvement actions. 4. **Capture complete information on financial contributors.** 　—identify and quantify as many of the financial contributors as possible for both the numerator and the denominator of the ROI formula. 　—planning phase ROI uses best estimates of improvement action costs and of the components of net returns. 　—postimplementation ROI uses actual data from financial system on those contributors.
Calculate return on investment	Develop estimates for both the numerator and the denominator of the ROI ratio: **ROI ratio numerator**: *Net returns from the improvement actions* **ROI ratio denominator**: *Implementation costs* (Tool kit includes worksheets to assist in these estimations)

(*continued*)

Exhibit 5.4

Overview of AHRQ Tool Kit's Approach to ROI Calculation (*continued*)

	1. **Considerations when estimating net return (ROI numerator)** —inherently complex estimation process —implementation of improvement actions may have many positive effects on patients' outcomes and health status, e.g., improvement actions might reduce hospital-associated infections, rates of pressure ulcers, or patient mortality, which do not have a direct monetary value but may affect revenues and expenses. —capture two types of financial effects: changes in the revenues and changes in operating costs. By reducing infection rates, a hospital could eliminate the costs it had been incurring to provide the extra care required to treat infections. It could also enhance or protect its revenues if insurers offered incentives for infection control or imposed penalties for occurrences of infections. —be mindful that the effects on revenues and effects on costs work in opposite directions; e.g., an increase in revenues is good, so a *higher revenue* due to improvement actions should be a *positive* number. On the other hand, a decrease in costs is good, so a *lower cost* due to improvement actions is good too. 2. **Consideration when estimating implementation costs (ROI denominator).** —the costs involved throughout the improvement process are included, e.g., planning and development of the initiative, training for staff, project start-up, ongoing operation, as well as monitoring and maintenance of the initiative. —cost categories include personnel, supplies, equipment, training, information systems, communication efforts, and external consultation. These costs may be incurred at different times during the improvement process but should be tallied and included in the calculation.
Interpret the ROI ratio obtained	Once calculated, the ROI ratio needs to be interpreted. 1. *ROI ≥1*: When an ROI is greater than or equal to 1, the returns generated by improvement actions are greater than or equal to the costs of development and implementation. In this case, ROI is considered to be *positive*. For example, an ROI of 1.8 indicates that for every $1 invested in the quality improvement program, $1.80 will be gained. 2. *ROI <1*: With an ROI of less than 1, the improvement actions yield a net loss from changes in quality and utilization. In this case, ROI is considered to be *negative*; e.g., an ROI of −1.5 indicates that for every $1 invested, $1.50 will be lost. An ROI of 0.8, on the other hand, indicates that for every $1 invested, 80 cents will be recouped. In other words, the entity loses 20 cents for every $1 it spends on the quality program.

AHRQ, Agency for Healthcare Research and Quality; ROI, return on investment.

Adapted from Agency for Healthcare Research and Quality. (2017). *Toolkit for using the AHRQ quality indicators.* https://www.ahrq.gov/patient-safety/settings/hospital/resource/qitool/index.html

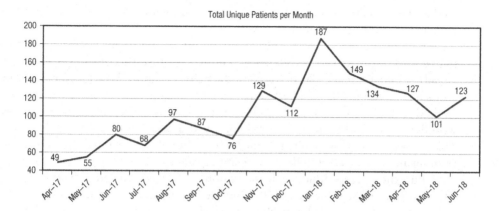

Figure 5.1 Unique patients enrolled in chronic case management service project.

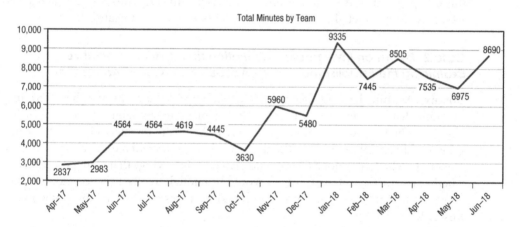

Figure 5.2 Total minutes spent by team on chronic case management activities.

Results. Between April 2017 through June 2018, 711 patients were enrolled in CCM (see Figure 5.1). Beginning in November 2017, the refinements in the EMR allowed for the initiative in the automated billing process resulting in better charge capture. Data tracking between April 2017 and June 2018 shows clinic billing for between approximately 2,500 and 9,000 minutes for CCM services (i.e., 42–150 hours). See Figure 5.2.

Of note, physicians billed for 10% of monthly CCM minutes (<1,000 minutes), nurses billed for 43% (between 2,500 and 3,000 minutes), and medical assistants billed for 47% (3,500–4,000 minutes). During the fiscal year running July 1, 2017, through June 30, 2018, $229,000 of charges were submitted, resulting in $70,000 of payments to the practice for CCM services that year.

ROI estimation. The net return (i.e., the numerator in the ROI ratio calculation; see Figure 5.2) for this CCM-related QI initiative included the $70,000 of payments for the majority of care coordination work that was already being done prior to the initiative but for which no reimbursement had been available until the CMS change in policy. In addition, a more formal enrollment process along with the operational and performance reporting that resulted allowed for more focused attention to be paid to the actual implementation of the care plans, which was viewed uniformly by clinicians as indicative of higher quality of care.

The implementation costs (i.e., the denominator) of this CCM-related QI initiative were estimated to be relatively minimal because this work was essentially already occurring. Time was invested in the planning around the EMR refinements, and some training was required to review the documentation standards required for both compliance with the CMS billing regulations and to understand the EMR workflow to correctly enroll patients for CCM as well as to correctly document. This, however, was viewed as part of the ongoing clinic operation, in which staff training and improvement efforts were anticipated.

Thus, the net return/net implementation cost was estimated to be positive and >1, which means that for each dollar invested, more than a dollar was returned to the practice. This, coupled with the perceived improved quality of care, resulted in the ROI being favorable. This initiative has since been disseminated to several other programs within the academic setting. As of June 2020, the total CCM payments to this complement of programs from April 1, 2017, through June 30, 2020, reached $258,000 (Hobson et al., 2018; Jason Fox, personal communication).

Case 2: Return on Investment Calculation for a National Initiative Examining the Establishment of an Accountable Care Organization

Context. Within the ACA, section 3022 established the Medicare Shared Savings program that was hinged on the establishment of accountable care organizations (ACOs), which were to coordinate the care of Medicare recipients in a manner that generated financial savings. At the time, ACOs were considered novel, and concern arose as to whether or not ACOs would generate the savings that were promised and whether the ACOs' potential upside would be enough to offset the formidable time, effort, and financial resources necessary to be invested at start-up (Haywood & Kosel, 2011).

Project overview. Using financial data from the CMS's evaluation of the Physician Group Practice Demonstration project, Haywood and Kosel (2011) constructed a financial model to estimate the average start-up cost per provider for an ACO as described in the Medicare Shared Savings section of the ACA. Using this estimate, they then projected the rate of return that would be necessary to offset this initial investment with a 3-, 5-, or 10-year time horizon. It should be noted that the ACA envisioned a 3-year time frame.

Results. Haywood and Kosel (2011) estimated that for an ACO composed of approximately 2,300 providers, the start-up cost would be $737 per provider. They determined what operating margin would be necessary for a 3-, 5-, and 10-year payback of that initial investment to get to breakeven. Figure 5.3 is the graphic from the journal article that reported this analysis.

For a 3-year payback, Haywood and Kosel (2011) projected that a 19.6% operating margin would be necessary. For a 5-year payback, a 12.7% margin would be necessary, and, finally, for a 10-year payback a 7.6% margin would suffice.

ROI estimation. Haywood and Kosel (2011) concluded that the 3-year 19.6% margin and the 5-year 12.7% margin would be unlikely, based on their analysis of the CMS Physician Group Practice Demonstration project data. The 10-year payback was the only scenario that appeared viable. In the authors' words:

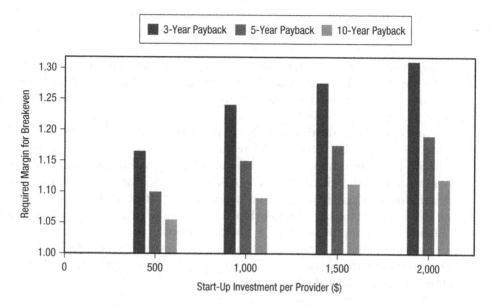

Figure 5.3 Projected operating margin for 3-, 5-, and 10-year payback.

Source: Data from Haywood, T. T., & Kosel, K. C. (2011). The ACO model–a three-year financial loss? *New England Journal of Medicine, 364*(14), e27. https://doi.org/10.1056/nejmp1100950

The high up-front investments make the model a poor fit for most physician group practices; the time frame in which one can expect a reasonable return on the initial investment is more than 5 years; and even the majority of large, experienced, integrated physician group practices could not recover their initial investment within the first 3 years. (Haywood & Kosel, 2011, p. e27)

Using the vocabulary of the AHRQ tool kit, the net return (i.e., the numerator in the ROI ratio calculation) for the ACO start-up in a 3- or 5-year time frame would be inadequate to offset the implementation costs (i.e., the denominator) for those time frames. The ROI ratio would be less than one in both time frames. For the 10-year time frame, the implementation costs may be offset by the net return in that longer time frame, and, therefore, the ROI ratio would be greater than one. This longer term payback situation still requires an optimistic view that the proposed ACO would be able to generate a 7.6% operating margin to recoup those start-up costs.

ECONOMIC EVALUATION

Basics of Economic Evaluation

An economic evaluation of an initiative to improve quality outcomes is an aspect of the domain of quality called efficiency, where the appropriate use of resources, both human and material, are optimally used to achieve a health care objective. Although finances are central to this evaluation, the efficiency domain occurs along a continuum from the fiscal elements of a clinical unit to the broader social measures of community well-being and patient individual and collective quality of life measures. By virtue of clinical training and doctoral education, the DNP nurse is ideally suited to being the team leader of quality and safety initiatives as well as to make sense of the financial and economic implications of improving outcomes and leading the team in implementing quality initiatives at all levels of the health care organization (AACN, 2006).

An economic evaluation is a type of evaluation research that focuses on clarifying the relationship between the required investment related to implementing a health care intervention and the amount of benefit achieved from the intervention. Criteria for conducting an economic evaluation include the identification or description of a problem within an organization that needs to be improved and the need to determine the relationship between the related consequences or actual outcomes of an improvement effort and the monetary cost of the efforts to achieve the outcomes, such as the resources and the time involved for the people needed to implement an initiative (Severens, 2003). Table 5.3 defines terms used when evaluating financial aspects of quality initiatives.

Economic Evaluation in Quality Improvement

When determining the economic investment involved in implementing one QI initiative over another, the comparison is between one or more QI strategies or between determining the cost of *doing nothing* or *usual health care* to a QI initiative. Also, the economic evaluation of an improvement initiative includes calculating the monetary cost or expense to the institution in dollars of the people and resources needed to implement the change initiative. Relating costs to the organization of the QI initiative to outcome(s) results in the efficiency or relative cost-effectiveness of a QI strategy is stated as a cost-effectiveness ratio. Economic evaluations of QI strategies are based on the comparison of alternative methods of introducing desirable changes (or doing nothing) in health care. A complete economic evaluation relates the costs incurred by people and resources to the (health) outcomes obtained (Severens, 2003).

Perspective in an Economic Evaluation

Before conducting an economic evaluation, one must first decide on the perspective of the analysis, because perspective is the point of view the organization or program developers adopt when deciding what types of costs and health benefits should be included in the economic evaluation. The viewpoint or perspective of the economic evaluation could be that of the health care system, society in general, the patient, the hospital, or clinic (Perspective, 2016).

The perspective reflects the scope of economic responsibility for costs and outcomes, and it establishes information that must be collected to determine the extent of cost of an initiative (Russell, 1996a, 1996b). For example, a practitioner who conducts an annual diabetes mellitus screening program for a local health clinic may want to determine the cost and outcomes of the intervention from the perspective of the clinic. Cost information would be limited to clinic expenses, and outcomes would be limited to the consequences of the program for the clinic population. On the other hand, a practitioner who conducted a state screening program

TABLE 5.3 Definitions of Economic Evaluations

Term	Definition	Units of Measurement
Cost-benefit analysis	A comparison evaluation of two or more interventions in which costs and end points are calculated in dollars	Monetary value (dollars), e.g., human capital, willingness to pay
Cost-effectiveness analysis	A comparison evaluation of two or more interventions in which costs are calculated in dollars and end points are calculated in health-related units	Life years gained
Cost-utility analysis	A comparison evaluation of two or more interventions in which costs are calculated in dollars and end points are calculated in quality of life units	Health years; e.g., QALYs, HYEs
Return on Investment	Degree of economic benefit derived in relation to costs incurred to develop and implement an initiative Identifies net financial gains (or losses) after calculating the resources invested in a quality initiative	Monetary value (dollars)
Cost (*of an initiative*)	Represents the amount of resources used to produce an item, service, or quality initiative	Monetary value (dollars)
Cost: ingredients approach	Components of the cost categories used determine the costs of an initiative and include personnel, supplies, equipment, and overhead expenses	Monetary value (dollars)
Incremental cost-effectiveness ratio	Represents the incremental cost and incremental outcome of an intervention when compared with one or more interventions.	
Incremental findings	The alteration in cost and outcome produced by the intervention of interest versus the alternative. This ratio represents the findings: $$\frac{\text{Cost of intervention A} - \text{Cost of intervention B}}{\text{Outcome of intervention A} - \text{Outcome of intervention B}}$$	
QALY	This is a year of life adjusted for its quality or its value. A year in perfect health is considered equal to 1.0 QALY. A measure used in cost-utility analyses	

HYE, healthy-years equivalent; QALY, quality-adjusted life year.

Source: Drummond, M. F., Sculpher, M. J., Torrance, G. W., O'Brien, B. J., & Stoddart, G. L. (2005). Methods for the economic evaluation of health care programmes. Oxford University Press; National Library of Medicine. (2016). *Health economics information resources: A self-study course: module 4. An introduction to the principles of critical appraisal of health economic evaluation studies.* Author. https://www.nlm.nih.gov/nichsr/edu/healthecon/04_he_06. html; Agency for Healthcare Research and Quality. (2017). *Toolkit for using the AHRQ quality indicators.* https:// www.ahrq.gov/patient-safety/settings/hospital/resource/qitool/index.html; Brousselle, A., Benmarhnia, T., & Benhadj, L. (2016). What are the benefits and risks of using return on investment to defend public health programs?. *Preventive Medicine Reports, 3,* 135–138. https://doi.org/10.1016/j.pmedr.2015.11.015; and Muennig, P. (2008). *Cost effectiveness analyses in health: A practical approach.* Jossey-Bass, a Wiley Imprint.

for lead poisoning in children would take a broader, state-level perspective. The collection of cost information would expand to include societal costs at the state level, which might consist of the cost of blood collection, testing the blood, following up abnormal blood tests, diagnosis, and treatment. Outcomes would expand to include the benefits and risks (if any) of the state screening program on the population of the state. If the perspective of an analysis is not specified, economists use the societal perspective as the default perspective.

Costs and Cost Data

Once the perspective of the economic evaluation is determined, the evaluator collects *cost* data to decide what costs for the improvement initiative should be described, measured, and valued. The *ingredients approach* is one method used to determine the costs of an initiative, in which the components of the cost categories include personnel, supplies and equipment, and overhead expenses (Drummond et al., 2005; Institute of Medicine & National Research Council, 2014; Olson & Bogard, 2014). The determination of specific costs relies on using competitive market prices or shadow prices based on current markets to determine the cost of the resources required for the QI initiative. Second, the specific ingredients or resources used to implement the intervention need to be described in terms of both quantity and quality, irrespective of how they are financed. Volunteers are not simply free because they are self-financed, because the market cost for that input would be paid if in another situation (Olson & Bogard, 2014). Cost-specific ingredients can be identified from documents, interviews, and observations of interventions conducted in the past.

The three primary categories for costs or resources are equipment or capital (machines), people and their time (personnel), and resources that need to be frequently replenished (materials and supplies; Center for Human Services, 2001). *Cost* represents the amount of resources used to produce an item or service and is usually lower than the amount presented as the charge for an item or unit of service. It is preferable to apply cost whenever possible because it more closely reflects actual resource usage.

All direct costs are generally included in a cost analysis. *Direct costs* may be described as the expenditures paid for health care. *Indirect costs* include productivity losses a patient and family may experience as a result of treatment, including days away from work and time traveled to and from a clinic or hospital (Luce et al., 1996; Muennig & Bounthavong, 2016; Sloan & Hsieh, 2017). They may also include other costs, such as the cost to the patient for hiring a caretaker after discharge. Indirect costs may be particularly important to collect when the evaluation takes a societal perspective. Describing, measuring, and valuing indirect costs can be difficult and problematic. If an evaluator decides that the inclusion of indirect costs is not feasible, the exclusion should be noted in the evaluation report.

Three types of comparative economic evaluations have been discussed in this chapter: CEA, CUA, and CBA, and an ROI, which is a way to determine the net financial gains or losses that occur with all resources invested along with the amounts gained through reduced costs, increased revenues, or both (AHRQ, 2017). Each type of economic evaluation represents a full analysis, in that the evaluator is describing, measuring, and valuing the costs and outcomes of two or more alternative interventions (Drummond et al., 2005).

Typically, the results of an economic analysis have been presented as a ratio, with cost in the numerator and outcome in the denominator. A project developer will want to know the cost and outcome of an intervention, as well as the incremental cost-effectiveness ratio (ICER), which represents the incremental cost and incremental outcome of an intervention when compared with one or more interventions. In this context, incremental findings refer to the alteration in cost and outcome produced by the intervention of interest versus the alternative (Drummond et al., 2005). The findings can be represented in the following ratio adapted from Muennig (2008):

$$\frac{\text{Cost of intervention A} - \text{Cost of intervention B}}{\text{Outcome of intervention A} - \text{Outcome of intervention B}}$$

The three types of economic evaluations, CBA, CEA, and CUA, are similar comparative evaluations, in that all measure costs the same way, but they measure and value outcomes differently. Each method provides a unique type of information that may be useful in helping to answer different questions. Occasionally, alternative interventions are evaluated using all three methods simultaneously.

Cost-Benefit Analysis

A CBA is a comparative evaluation of two or more interventions in which the costs and outcomes of each intervention are calculated in a monetary value (dollars) (Centers for Disease Control and Prevention [CDC], 2019). It is the best economic evaluation to address whether the benefits of an intervention exceed its costs. A CBA provides the net benefits (benefits minus costs) of an intervention, allows comparisons to be made across disease states, and provides an organization with information needed to determine whether an intervention is worth undertaking. A CBA evaluates/determines the costs of developing and implementing a change initiative and can identify the monetized value of health improvements such as medical costs averted or gained or productivity gains from the intervention (2019).

The true costs of a QI initiative include overt and covert costs that might occur in the development and implementation of the project. Costs incurred in the development and implementation of a quality initiative are determined by first identifying the criteria used to determine costs and then assessing the completeness of the costs incurred by covering the requirements needed to produce the project outcomes, the comparison of the costs to comparable prices in the local or national market (Olson & Bogard, 2014).

Quality Improvement Implications of a Cost-Benefit Analysis

The value of a CBA to QI planners is to identify the net benefit of the change initiative to the organization and compare the cost benefit in monetary terms of choosing one implementation strategy over another strategy or compared with keeping the system as it is currently (baseline). A CBA describes the costs of the components required to implement each alternative intervention and the benefits resulting from an intervention, such as medical costs averted, productivity gains, and the monetized value of health improvements (CDC, 2019). In QI initiatives, limitations of a CBA are that it can be challenging to identify the costs of various expenses in a CBA, and a CBA can only assess monetary benefits of a change initiative (Adhikari, 2018).

In an example of a CBA, Siddharthan et al. (2005) combined an observational study along with a CBA to determine the impact of a program designed to reduce the frequency and severity of staff injuries in the Department of Veterans Affairs (DVA) system. The 18-month study included 537 nursing personnel, and the perspective was the DVA hospital system. Costs included capital costs, training costs, and direct costs associated with the treatment of injured nursing personnel and work time lost because of the injuries. The program significantly reduced the annual injury rate from 24 per 100 workers to 16.9 per 100 workers. The program resulted in a $207,000 annualized net benefit stemming from a lower incidence and severity of injuries among nursing personnel. The authors noted that parts of the safety program had been integrated into national occupational health policy.

Cost-Effectiveness Analysis

Description of Cost-Effectiveness Analysis

A CEA examines the health outcomes in relation to the costs of one or more interventions by comparing Intervention A to the current situation or to Intervention B. A CEA does not place a monetary value on the cost of the initiative, as does the CBA, but makes a comparison by estimating the costs incurred to gain a unit of a health outcome as in a life year gained or a death prevented (CDC, 2019; Severens, 2003). It is useful when deciding to choose between alternative implementation initiatives that will achieve health care outcomes in a health care delivery system.

Examples of a unit of health outcomes or quantity of health benefits that might be considered in a CEA are the additional number of patients that might be treated in a primary care practice using Intervention A as opposed to Intervention B, or that the implementation of Intervention A would result in better outcomes for treating deep vein thrombosis (DVT) than if Intervention B was adapted and used in an emergency department setting.

The cost-effectiveness of a QI project is determined by a number of factors that come together to determine whether one initiative has an additional quantity of health benefits over a different initiative (Thompson et al., 2016). To calculate the cost-effectiveness of a QI intervention, a decision maker needs to know (a) the project costs, (b) the additional number of patients who will benefit from the project, and (c) the cost-effectiveness per patient of the quality initiative. It is important to consider the project's cost-effectiveness (PCE) prior to the project implementation to be a useful tool in prioritizing one initiative over the other (2016).

Because most decision makers have fixed resources, a CEA can help decision makers compare programs that produce different outcomes. For a particular level of health care resources, the goal is to choose from among all possible combinations of programs a set that maximizes the total health benefits produced. A CEA is a useful analysis to determine and understand the cost impact of different interventions or processes that lead to a similar or the same health outcome. It uses a common unit of measure that captures utility of outcomes (Thomas & Chalkidou, 2016). It is of value to know the cost of one health care intervention as compared with another. When an intervention that is more effective is more costly than the current intervention, the net costs are positive, and the results are presented as a cost-effectiveness ratio. When a more effective intervention costs less, the net costs are negative, and the results are considered to be a net cost savings (CDC, 2019).

Application to Quality Improvement Initiatives

A cost-effectiveness ratio of a QI strategy describes the relative cost-effectiveness or efficiency to outcome results (Severens, 2003). A CEA of a QI initiative may address outcomes such as the number of practices that received practice guidelines or the number of practices, departments, or professionals who, as a result of the quality initiative, now practice in accordance with a proposal care pathway or specific clinical guideline; or the number of patients who now receive treatment in accordance with the practice guideline, as compared with a different intervention strategy or program (2003).

CEAs are the type of analysis most frequently conducted in health care because they provide useful information to decision makers who must choose between two or more interventions or programs that have similar end points (Lämås et al., 2009). A disadvantage is that while CEAs provide information about the change in the quantity of patient health status, they do not address the value to the patient of having achieved the change (Torrance et al., 1996). Currently, more health economic analyses are including both cost-effectiveness (quantity) and cost-utility (quantity and quality) analyses.

The reason for doing a CEA either along with or instead of a CBA is grounded in what each of the analyses identifies. A CBA compares the cost of the intervention with the monetary benefit incurred and a net monetary benefit identified [Net benefit = Benefits − Costs] (Adhikari, 2018). The CBA compares "cost per consequence" of two or more interventions, where the consequences are measured by "natural" units such as life years gained or saved years of life and addresses nonmonetary outcomes achieved in a QI initiative (2018).

Cost-Utility Analysis

Definition of a Cost-Utility Analysis

A CUA is a type of effectiveness evaluation that compares the cost-effectiveness of one project with that of another project that has different effect measurements. The comparison is of the incremental cost of a program from a particular point of view with the incremental health improvement expressed in the unit of *improved general health* or quality-adjusted life years (QALYs; Rai & Goyal, 2018) and to determine cost in terms of a utility, which is, for example, the quantity and quality of life. Differing from a CBA, a CUA is used to compare two different drugs or procedures whose benefits may be different. A CUA relies on a general index that measures outcomes in terms of improved general health or gains in quality of life (e.g., QALYs), or gains in productive life years (e.g., DALYs or disability-adjusted life years). A CUA can compare two or more interventions in which costs are calculated in dollars and outcomes are calculated in quality of life units (QOLU), and the incremental cost of a program to the incremental health improvement expressed in the unit of QALYs (2018).

Application of a Cost-Utility Analysis

A CUA provides information to decision makers not only about the quantity of the outcome (e.g., years of life gained), but also about how individuals perceive the quality of the life years that were gained. CUA has been described as a type of CEA in which the health unit considers both quantity and quality (Elnitsky & Stone, 2005; Muennig & Bounthavong, 2016; Russell et al., 1996a). There are a number of measures that can be used in a CUA. These include QALYs, DALYs, years of healthy life (YHL), and healthy-years equivalent (HYE). The focus of this section is on QALYs because they are the most widely applicable and frequently used measure (Drummond et al., 2005; Russell et al., 1996a).

Use of Cost-Utility Analysis in Quality Improvement Initiatives

Using the CUA index allows decision makers for QI initiatives to compare the cost versus the benefit of two initiatives that produce the same to similar outcomes (The Quality Assurance [QA] Project, 2001). The CUA is of value in situations in which decisions are made to allocate limited funds among multiple programs (2001). One research study example of using a CUA was to determine whether the use of usual physical therapy versus an enhanced physical therapy program produced better QALYs results in patients with osteoarthritis of the knee (Kigozi et al., 2018).

SUMMARY

This chapter was designed to assist the DNP nurse in the evaluation of financial considerations of QI initiatives that improve processes of care and care outcomes in health care practices and institutions. It is challenging to evaluate the cost of a quality initiative in relation to what the initiative will achieve for the organization. It is important to define the relationship between the financial details of an improvement initiative and the overall value that improving quality outcomes brings to patient care because quality initiatives do not always tend to increase revenue within a health care organization. Although a CBA may identify the net benefit of the change initiative to the organization and compare the cost benefit in monetary terms of choosing one implementation strategy over another, the ROI may be a more useful process for the QI planner to estimate how a change initiative affects revenue and operating costs. An ROI can help planners adjust an initiative to optimize both quality and financial performance. The chapter also described financial aspects of providing care to patients and populations that effect quality outcomes because public and private payers expect health care providers to deliver care that achieves quality outcomes and payment is based on meeting outcome measures. The model of providing care that is linked to achieving outcomes is becoming the expectation rather than the norm. The DNP nurse is challenged to understand and apply meaningful financial evaluations to all aspects of health care.

REFERENCES

Adhikari, S. (2018). *21 differences between cost benefit analysis (CBA) and cost effectiveness analysis (CEA)*. https://www.publichealthnotes.com/21-differences-between-cost-benefit-analysis-cba-and -cost-effectiveness-analysis-cea/m

Agency for Healthcare Research and Quality. (2017). *Toolkit for using the AHRQ quality indicators.* https://www.ahrq.gov/patient-safety/settings/hospital/resource/qitool/index.html.

American Association of Colleges of Nursing. (2006). *The essentials of doctoral education for advanced nursing practice.* Author. https://www.duq.edu/assets/Documents/nursing/dnp/_PDF/DNPEssentials.pdf

American Association of Colleges of Nursing. (2021). *The essentials: Core competencies for professional nursing education.* Author. https://www.aacnnursing.org/Portals/42/AcademicNursing/pdf/Essentials-2021.pdf

Berwick, D. M., Nolan, T.W., & Whittington, J. (2008). The triple aim: Care, health, and cost. *Health Affairs, 27*(3), 759–769. https://doi.org/10.1377/hlthaff.27.3.759

Brousselle, A., Benmarhnia, T., & Benhadj, L. (2016). What are the benefits and risks of using return on investment to defend public health programs? *Preventive Medicine Reports, 3,* 135–138. https://doi.org/10.1016/j.pmedr.2015.11.015

Center for Human Services. (2001). *Concepts on cost and quality-core curriculum.* The Quality Assurance (QA) Project. U.S. Agency for International Development. http://www.qaproject.org/training/cq/ref.pdf

Centers for Medicare and Medicaid Services. (2015). Better care. Smarter spending. Healthier people: Paying providers for value, not volume. https://www.cms.gov/Newsroom/MediaReleaseDatabase/Fact-sheets/2015-Fact-sheets-items/2015-01-26-3.html

Centers for Disease Control and Prevention, Office of the Associate Director for Policy and Strategy. (2019). *Cost-benefit analysis (CBA).* https://www.cdc.gov/policy/polaris/economics/cost-benefit-analysis.html

Centers for Medicare and Medicaid Services. (2020). NHE fact sheet. https://www.cms.gov/Research-Statistics-Data-and-Systems/Statistics-Trends-and-Reports/NationalHealthExpendData/NHE-Fact-Sheet

Collins, S. R., Gunja, M. Z., & Aboulafia, G. N. (2020, August). *U.S. Health Insurance Coverage in 2020: A looming crisis in affordability—Findings from the commonwealth fund biennial health insurance survey.* Commonwealth Fund. https://doi.org/10.26099/6aj3-n655

Darvas, Z., Moës, N., Myachenkova, Y., & Pichler, D. (2018). *The macroeconomic implications of healthcare (No. 2018/11).* Bruegel Policy Contribution. https://www.econstor.eu/bitstream/10419/208018/1/1030935807.pdf

Drummond, M. F., Sculpher, M. J., Torrance, G. W., O'Brien, B. J., & Stoddart, G. L. (2005). Methods for the economic evaluation of health care programmes. Oxford University Press.

Elnitsky, C. A., & Stone, P. (2005). Patient preferences and cost-utility analysis. *Applied Nursing Research, 18*(2), 74–76. https://doi.org/10.1016/j.apnr.2005.02.005

Fetterolf, D., & Shah, R. K. (2021). Economics and finance in medical quality management. In A. P. Giardino, L. A. Riesenberg, & P. Varkey (Eds.), *Medical quality management* (3rd ed., pp. 197–244). Springer. https://doi.org/10.1007/978-3-030-48080-6

Fischer, H., & Duncan, S. (2020). The business case for quality improvement. *Journal of Perinatology, 40*(6), 972–979. https://doi.org/10.1038/s41372-020-0660-y

Haywood, T. T., & Kosel, K. C. (2011). The ACO model-a three-year financial loss? *New England Journal of Medicine, 364*(14), e27. https://doi.org/10.1056/nejmp1100950

Hobson, W. L., Hemond, J. A., Navar, E., Smith, L., Egusguiza, J., & Fox, J. (2018, December). *Improving coordination of care for children with special health care needs (CSHCN) by integrating chronic care management into a primary care practice.* National Forum on Quality Improvement in Health Care, IHI National Conference, Orlando, FL.

Institute of Medicine (US) Committee on Quality of Health Care in America. (2001). *Crossing the quality chasm: A new health system for the 21st century.* National Academies Press.

Institute of Medicine, & National Research Council. (2014). *Considerations in applying benefit-cost analysis to preventive interventions for children, youth, and families: Workshop summary.* The National Academies Press. https://doi.org/10.17226/18708

Kigozi, J., Jowett, S., Nicholls, E., Tooth, S., Hay, E. M., Foster, N. E., & BEEP Trial Team. (2018). Cost-utility analysis of interventions to improve effectiveness of exercise therapy for adults with knee osteoarthritis: The BEEP trial. *Rheumatology Advances in Practice, 2*(2), rky018. https://doi.org/10.1093/rap/rky018

Koop, C. E. (1989). Introductory remarks. In P. R. Magrab, & H. E. C. Millar (Eds.), *Surgeon general's conference. Growing up and getting medical care: Youth with special health care needs. Summary of conference proceedings* (pp. 3–5). Georgetown University, Child Development Center.

Kongstvedt, P. R. (Ed.). (2001). *The managed care handbook* (4th ed.). Aspen Publishers.

Lāmås, K., Willman, A., Lindholm, L., & Jacobsson, C. (2009). Economic evaluation of nursing practices: A review of literature. *International Nursing Review, 56*(1), 13–20. https://doi.org/10.1111/j.1466-7657.2008.00672.x

Luce, R. R., Manning, W. G., Siegel, J. E., & Lipscomb, J. (1996). Estimating costs in cost-effectiveness analysis. In M. Gold, J. Siegel, L. B. Russell, & M. C. Weinstein (Eds.), *Cost-effectiveness in health and medicine* (pp. 176–213). Oxford University Press.

MacLeod, G. K. (2001). An overview of managed health care. In P. R. Kongstvedt (Ed.), *The managed care handbook* (4th ed., pp. 3–16). Aspen Publishers.

Mikulic, M. (2020). *Percentage of GDP spent on health care in select countries 2018.* https://www.statista.com/statistics/268826/health-expenditure-as-gdp-percentage-in-oecd-countries/

Muennig, P. (2008). *Cost effectiveness analyses in health: A practical approach.* Jossey-Bass, a Wiley Imprint.

Muennig, P., & Bounthavong, M. (2016). *Cost-effectiveness analysis in health: A practical approach.* John Wiley & Sons.

Olson, S., & Bogard, K. (2014). *Considerations in applying benefit-cost analysis to preventive interventions for children, youth, and families: Workshop summary.* National Academies Press. https://www.ncbi.nlm.nih.gov/books/NBK219358/

Perspective [online]. (2016). *York; York health economics consortium.* https://yhec.co.uk/glossary/perspective/

Porter, M. E., & Teisberg, E. O. (2006). *Redefining health care: Creating value based competition on results.* Harvard Business School Press.

The Quality Assurance (QA) Project. (2001). *Cost and quality in healthcare.* U.S. Agency for International Development (USAID). http://www.qaproject.org/training/cq/ref.pdf

Rai, M., & Goyal, R. (2018). Pharmacoeconomics in healthcare. In *Pharmaceutical medicine and translational clinical research* (pp. 465–472). Academic Press.

Russell, L. B., Gold, M. R., Siegel, J. E., Daniels, N., & Weinstein, M. C. (1996a). The role of cost-effectiveness analysis in health and medicine. *Journal of American Medical Association, 276*(14), 1172–1180. https://doi.org/10.1001/jama.276.14.1172

Russell, L. B., Siegel, J. E., Daniels, N., Gold, M. R., Luce, B. R., & Mandelblatt, J. S. (1996b). Cost-effectiveness analysis as a guide to resource allocation in health: Roles and limitations. In M. Gold, J. Siegel, L. B. Russell, & M. C. Weinstein (Eds.), *Cost-effectiveness in health and medicine* (pp. 3–24). Oxford University Press.

Severens, J. L. (2003). Value for money of changing healthcare services? Economic evaluation of quality improvement. *Quality and Safety in Health Care, 12*(5), 366–371. https://doi.org/10.1136/qhc.12.5.366

Shah, A., & Course, S. (2018). Building the business case for quality improvement: A framework for evaluating return on investment. *Future Healthcare Journal, 5,* 132–137. https://doi.org/10.7861/futurehosp.5-2-132

Siddharthan, K., Nelson, A., Tiesman, H., & Chen, F. (2005). Cost effectiveness of a multifaceted program for safe patient handling. In K. Henriksen, J. B. Battles, E. S. Marks, & D. I. Lewin (Eds.), *Advances in patient safety: From research to implementation* (Vol. 3, Implementation Issues). Agency for Healthcare Research and Quality.

Silver, C., Chen, J., & Kagan, J. (2020). *Microeconomics vs. macroeconomics: An overview.* https://www.investopedia.com/ask/answers/difference-between-microeconomics-and-macroeconomics/

Sloan, F. A., & Hsieh, C.-R. (2017). *Health economics* (2nd ed). The MIT Press.

Thomas, R., & Chalkidou, K. (2016). Cost–effectiveness analysis. In J. Cylus, I. Papanicolas, & P. C. Smith (Eds.), *Health system efficiency: How to make measurement matter for policy and management.* European Observatory on Health Systems and Policies. Health Policy Series, 46. https://www.ncbi.nlm.nih.gov/books/NBK436886/

Thompson, C., Pulleyblank, R., Parrott, S., & Essex, H. (2016). The cost-effectiveness of quality improvement projects: A conceptual framework, checklist and online tool for considering the costs and consequences of implementation-based quality improvement. *Journal of Evaluation in Clinical Practice, 22*(1), 26–30. https://doi.org/10.1111/jep.12421

Tikkanen, R., & Abrams, M. K. (2020). *U.S. health care from a global perspective, 2019: Higher spending, worse outcomes?* Commonwealth Fund. https://doi.org/10.26099/7avy-fc29

Tolbert, J., Orgera, K., Singer, N., & Damico, A. (2019, December). *Key facts about the uninsured population*. The Henry J. Kaiser Family Foundation. https://www.kff.org/uninsured/issue-brief/key-facts-about-the-uninsured-population/#:~:text=In%202018%2C%2027.9%20million%20nonelderly,has%20grown%20by%201.2%20million.

Torrance, G. W., Siegel, J. E., & Luce, B. B. (1996). Framing and designing the cost-effectiveness analysis. In M. Gold, J. Siegel, L. B. Russell, & M. C. Weinstein (Eds.), *Cost-effectiveness in health and medicine* (pp. 54–81). Oxford University Press.

Walsh, K. (2014). Medical education: Microeconomics or macroeconomics? *The Pan African Medical Journal, 18*, 11. https://doi.org/10.11604/pamj.2014.18.11.4334

EVALUATION OF HEALTH CARE ORGANIZATIONAL IMPERATIVES

SIX

EVALUATION OF ORGANIZATIONS AND SYSTEMS

Nancy Manning Crider and Beth Ulrich

The hospital is altogether the most complex human organization ever devised.
—*Peter Drucker*

INTRODUCTION

Whether the goal is to assess an organization for benchmarking purposes, to select a new practice setting, or to better understand one's current organization in order to successfully lead organizational improvements, it is important for nurses to know how to assess and evaluate health care organizations and systems. Evaluation of an organization or a system requires a systematic review of key indicators, much like performing a systematic physical assessment of an individual patient. Like a patient, an organization has a structure (anatomy), ways of functioning that require all parts to work together for success (physiology), and the need for resources and support systems.

Organizations are social structures created by individuals to support collaboration and the pursuit of specific goals (Scott & Davis, 2015). They have defined objectives and, in order to provide and dispense products and services, must induce participants to provide services, garner resources from the environment, and work with their neighbors (Scott & Davis, 2015). Structure refers to the resources dedicated to provide patient care services. It is a key driver of organizational culture that influences institutional processes and ultimately determines clinical outcomes. Leadership skills, human resource management, nurse staffing, and the use of advanced practice registered nurses (APRNs) and other nurses with advanced degrees also influence the culture of the organization, practice models, and clinical outcomes (Glickman et al., 2007). Other factors including patient care technology, information management systems, and support services, as well as special designations provided by external organizations, reflect the comprehensiveness and quality of care delivered. Process addresses the organization's reputation and ability to sustain systems of care that are of the highest quality and that are recognized by peers through benchmarking databases. Outcome data on care effectiveness compare an institution's morbidity and mortality with comparable institutions and other threshold targets set by national organizations.

BOX 6.1 Key Components of Organization and System Evaluations

- History and overview
- Type of organization
- Sources of funding and revenue
- Size and scope of services
- Governance
- Mission, vision, and values
- Strategy, goals, and strategic culture
- Organizational structure
- Authority and decision-making
- Culture
- Patient safety
- Patient safety culture
- Work environment
- Reputation
- Quality and outcomes
- The role of nursing in the organization

This chapter provides a framework to assess health care organizations and health care systems using the concepts of structure, process, and outcome as developed by Avedis Donabedian (1978). Performing a comprehensive organizational assessment and evaluation requires knowledge of the structure and mission of the organization, understanding of how the organization functions in its current environment, knowledge of sources of relevant information, openness to see the organization as others see it (whether they are inside or outside the organization), and the ability to evaluate organizational performance in relation to other organizations (see Box 6.1).

HISTORY AND OVERVIEW OF THE ORGANIZATION

Similar to a physical assessment, the first step of an organizational assessment is to complete a history and overview of the organization or system. Widespread Internet access makes this fairly simple, as most health care organizations maintain websites to engage customers. The first question to ask is "When was the health care organization established and by whom?" Generally, hospitals were established to meet the health needs of the community or specific population (e.g., company employees, active military personnel, or patients with cancer). The organization may be privately owned by individuals or investors or publicly owned by a local, state, or federal agency. Many health care organizations were established by religious orders or have an affiliation with an established religious denomination (e.g., the Roman Catholic Church or a local Protestant or Jewish congregation). The ownership and purpose for establishing the organization strongly influence the current mission, vision, and values of the organization. Ownership and purpose also, at least partially, determine an organization's tax status. What are the defining moments in the organization's history?

TYPE OF ORGANIZATION

Not for Profit

The not-for-profit, for-profit, or governmental organization can offer information on the mission of the organization as well as on resources that may be available and restrictions that may apply to the use of "profit" or revenue over expenses. Key characteristics of a not-for-profit organization include the obligation to reinvest all profits back into the organization, required reporting of the community benefits offered by the organization, and an exemption from paying state and federal taxes on income and property (The Advisory Board Company, 2017). Tax-exempt organizations are also able to issue tax-exempt bonds that allow them to secure money at a lower interest rate and reduce their financing costs (Burns et al., 2012). Tax-exempt status also allows health care organizations to receive charitable donations that provide a tax subsidy to donors (Herring et al., 2018). While there is a lack of consensus on what constitutes a community benefit, such benefits including the provision of uncompensated care (e.g., cost of charity care, bad debt), Medicaid-covered services, and the provision of certain specialized services such as emergency care or labor and delivery have been identified as generally unprofitable (Congressional Budget Office, 2006). Other costs such as Medicare and Medicaid shortfalls, price discounts to private health insurance companies, and medical education costs have become more controversial (Herring et al., 2018) and raised the question of whether not-for-profit health care organizations provide enough community benefit to justify tax-exempt status (James, 2016). Subsequently, the passage of the Patient Protection and Affordable Care Act (ACA) of 2010 brought changes to the Internal Revenue Service (IRS) Tax Code that increased the financial reporting and transparency of not-for-profit hospitals. The ACA also included a requirement that mandated hospitals to conduct community health needs assessments and develop community health implementation plans every 3 years to address identified community priorities (James, 2016; Rozier, 2020). Key characteristics of a for-profit organization include the ability to distribute profits to its investors and to raise capital through investors and the obligation to pay income and property taxes (The Advisory Board Company, 2017). The third type of organization is governmental organizations, such as military, Department of Veterans Affairs, and county hospitals. According to the American Hospital Association (AHA), in 2018, there were nearly 5,200 nonfederal, short-term general, and other special hospitals in the United States: 2,937 not-for-profit hospitals; 1,296 for-profit hospitals; 965 state and local government hospitals; and more than 200 federal hospitals (AHA, 2018).

SOURCES OF FUNDING AND REVENUE

All organizations must have sources of funding and revenue to stay in business. Health care organizations are no different. Public hospitals and health care systems designed as safety net providers for the poor are, at least in part, funded by local, state, and/or federal tax dollars that must be approved by elected officials (e.g., city council, state legislature, or the U.S. Congress). Public hospital systems and private health care organizations may receive funds from publicly sponsored programs such as Medicare and Medicaid for services provided to patients. Operating revenue is also generated from fees for service or payments from private insurance companies or contractual agreements with major employers or managed care organizations. Payors may also negotiate with providers for bundled services or negotiate a risk-based per-member per-month contract to manage health care services. Revenue may also be generated from designated grants and cash payments.

Health care organizations frequently have a separate philanthropic organization to raise funds to provide services and support strategic initiatives and capital improvements. Many organizations also generate revenue through investments and other non-patient-care services.

Information on an organization's sources of funding and the percentage of revenue obtained from each source can contribute to the understanding of the organization's strategies and resources. Financial information about an organization can be found in the organization's annual report or in other public documents. Tax-exempt organizations file IRS Form 990, Schedule H, to provide federally mandated information about the organization's financial activities and community benefit requirements.

SIZE AND SCOPE OF SERVICES

The size and location of a health care organization will impact the type and scope of services that the organization provides as well as the available resources. What is the size of the organization (e.g., the number of beds, the number of patients cared for)? Is the organization located in an urban or a rural area? Is the organization a large health care system, a 600-bed urban tertiary care center, an acute care community hospital, or a primary care practice? What types of services are provided? Are specialty services available on site, or are patients referred to another provider? Does the organization provide pediatric and obstetrical care? Is the institution a teaching hospital? Are there academic or research affiliations? Is it a safety net hospital or regional trauma center? Is the organization an accountable care organization (ACO)? The organization's website and annual report are good sources for this type of general information.

The AHA annual survey is another source of information that describes the organizational structure and scope of hospitals and health systems. In 2018, more than 6,100 hospitals completed the self-reported survey that included detailed financials, bed size, and services offered (AHA, 2018). The survey also provides detailed staffing and physician data as part of the overall organizational structure. The AHA survey data, which have been collected since 1980, are used extensively for research and benchmarking purposes.

GOVERNANCE

Both for-profit and not-for-profit hospitals and health care systems are governed by a board of directors (BOD) or board of trustees (BOT). The BOD/BOT is responsible and accountable for the performance of the organization and has ultimate authority for the financial stability and quality of care provided by the institution. The BODs/BOTs comprise a specified number of members and include health care professionals and executives as well as business representatives and lay members from the community served by the organization. Not-for-profit BODs/BOTs for hospitals and health systems tend to be composed of local business leaders or individuals who have been heavily involved in raising money for the organization, while for-profit boards are often composed of a blend of investor representatives and community leaders (Cheney, 2019). When completing an organizational assessment, one should examine the composition of the board and determine whether all stakeholders, including nurses, are represented. Specifically, the evaluator should determine whether the chief nurse executive (CNE) of the organization or a nurse from the community is a member of the board.

MISSION, VISION, AND VALUES

The mission, vision, and values of an organization or a system flow from the original purpose for establishing the organization or system. While an organization's mission and vision should be aligned, they are not the same thing. Simply stated, the mission is the purpose or reason for which the organization exists. An organization's mission statements should be distinct, long enough to guide strategy, and short enough for staff members and the public to understand (Burns et al., 2012). The vision describes what the organization wants to achieve or looks like in the future. Vision statements should stretch and challenge an organization and resonate with those involved in the organization. The vision statement of an organization should reflect the feeling of pride in its members for being part of something much larger than themselves (2012).

The values of the organization determine how decisions are made. An organization's values are a visible guide for employees to follow and serve as an ethical compass for decision-making at all levels of the organization. Values should not be contingent upon circumstances. Rather, they should be constant and endure over time. While reviewing the values of the organization, it is important to consider not only the published values, but also what values are manifested in the actions of the organization.

STRATEGY, GOALS, AND STRATEGIC CULTURE

Strategy refers to the choices that the organization makes about who it will serve, where services will be provided, and how services will be delivered. Goals are specific outcome measures that are established to carry out the strategy and meet the mission and vision of the organization. Many organizations target specific segments (niches) of the health care market such as women and children, cancer care, orthopedics, cardiovascular surgery, and transplantation.

Miles and Snow (1978) described four types of organizational strategic cultures: prospectors, defenders, analyzers, and reactors. Prospector organizations are the most aggressive with their strategy. They tend to focus on creating innovative products and services and expanding services into new markets. They often create changes and uncertainty that require their competitors to respond. Defender organizations, on the other hand, prefer a rather narrow product line and maintain a secure and stable market. They focus more on internal efficiency and tend not to search for new opportunities. Analyzer organizations maintain a combination strategy and take less risk than prospectors, but are less committed to stability than defenders. Analyzers maintain a combination of established products and services and regularly update their business with new offerings that have been proven effective. Reactor organizations often lack focus and respond to external changes only when forced to. Some organizations demonstrate the characteristics of a mixed strategy by choosing to use different strategies in specific areas of the organization.

Strategies are also influenced by other variables. For example, not-for-profit organizations tend to have a more long-term view of the organization's viability, while for-profit organizations may focus more on short-term profitability (Cheney, 2019).

ORGANIZATIONAL STRUCTURE

The organizational structure formalizes the governance of an organization and provides rational direction to coordinate the activities required for an organization to survive and deal with the external environment. Box 6.2 identifies factors that influence the organizational structure.

Organizational structure may be conveyed by an organizational chart, which is a diagram that depicts how different parts of the health care organization/system relate to one another and who reports to whom. Organizational charts are typically shaped like a pyramid. A hierarchical organization has an organizational structure with many layers, where every entity in the organization, except the top one, is subordinate to another entity.

In recent years, some health care organizations have moved from the traditional hierarchal structure to a flatter, more horizontal structure with fewer layers in an effort to improve communication and respond more rapidly to consumer preferences and environmental changes. A flat organization has an organizational structure in which a number of middle-management levels have been eliminated. The result is an organizational structure with fewer layers that can foster communication by bringing top management in closer contact with the frontline employees and customers.

Organizational charts are useful in understanding the rational, formal nature of an organization. However, when doing an organizational evaluation, the evaluator should validate that the organizational chart is up-to-date and seek to understand

---

BOX 6.2   Factors that Influence Organizational Structure

The product;
The complexity and uncertainty of the work;
The environment in which the work is performed;
Skills and knowledge of the workers;
Characteristics of the objectives on which the work is performed;
Technical systems used to produce the work; and
Use of information technology in the production process

Source: Bolman, L. G., & Deal, T.E. (2013). *Reframing organizations: Artistry, choice, & leadership* (5th ed.). Jossey-Bass; Burns, L. R., Bradley, E. H., & Weiner, B. J. (2012). *Shortell and Kaluzny's: Health care management organization design and behavior* (6th ed.). Delmar; Scott, W. R., & Davis, G. F. (2015). *Organizations and organizing: Rational, natural and open systems perspectives.* Routledge.

the informal behavioral structures that impact employee performance and patient outcomes as well as the formal structure. The informal structure of the organization reflects the culture, norms, values, and social networks that exist within the organization.

AUTHORITY AND DECISION-MAKING

Rational–legal authority generally serves as the foundation of a permanent administrative structure. In a rational–legal organization, the position of authority is held because the leaders are either elected or hired (Scott & Davis, 2015). In the case of a health care organization, the final authority rests with the BOD/BOT members who hire the chief executive officer (CEO) to run the operations of the organization.

Decision-making within an organization may be centralized or decentralized depending on a number of factors such as organizational structure, leadership style of the executive team, and the culture of the system. In less hierarchal and bureaucratic organizations, decision-making may be delegated and shared among leaders and employees at various levels of the organization.

To evaluate the authority, decision-making, and leadership style of the organization, ask questions like the following: What is the leadership style of the executive team? Is there a shared/professional governance structure? How are nurses involved in decision-making? Is decision-making centralized, decentralized, or a combination?

ORGANIZATIONAL CULTURE

Organizational culture, as defined by Schein (2009), is a pattern of shared tacit assumptions that was learned by a group as it solved its problems of external adaptation and internal integration and that has worked well enough to be considered valid and, therefore, to be taught to new members as the correct way to perceive, think, and feel in relation to those problems (Schein, 2009). Culture is a set of shared goals, values, practices, and attitudes that characterize an organization or institution (Merriam-Webster, 2020). In reviewing the literature on definitions of culture, Groysberg et al. (2018) noted that common attributes of culture include a shared (group) phenomenon that is pervasive throughout the organization and enduring over the long term.

There are many cultures and subcultures within an organization, reflecting the written and unwritten "rules" of the organization, the norms, and what the acceptable behavior is. There is a culture of the organization as a whole, which may be influenced by such things as the organization's history, ownership, mission, values, and executive leadership. There are also subcultures in organizations within groups that are similar (e.g., nurses, physicians) and those who work together (e.g., patient care units, night shift).

In evaluating the culture or subculture of an organization, ask questions like the following: What is valued? What are the expectations of employees? What are the unwritten rules of the game? How do people relate to each other? Does the organizational culture support innovation or is it risk-averse?

PATIENT SAFETY CULTURE

Patient safety has been recognized as a core tenet of health care organizations since the days of Florence Nightingale. The first sentence of her book *Notes on Hospitals* says, "It may seem a strange principle to enunciate as the very first requirement in a hospital that it should do the sick no harm. It is quite necessary nevertheless to lay down such a principle" (Nightingale, 1863, p. iii). The release of the Institute of Medicine's (IOM, 2000) seminal report *To Err Is Human: Building a Safer Health System*, more than 20 years ago, focused the attention of health care professionals and the general public on the need to ensure patient safety; however, despite many efforts, preventable harm to patients remains an issue. In 2020, representatives from 27 organizations that comprise the National Steering Committee for Patient Safety (2020) collaborated in developing a plan "to achieve safer care and reduce harm to patients and those who care for them" (p. 6). Two questions asked by the Agency for Healthcare Research and Quality (AHRQ) in their hospital safety survey are good questions to use to initially evaluate patient safety issues in a health care organization: What overall rating would you give the organization on patient safety? What overall rating would you give the systems and processes the organization has in place to prevent, catch, and correct problems that have the potential to affect patients?

In 2009, a distinguished group of experts on patient safety found that despite all the programs and initiatives that had been implemented over the 10 years since the IOM's report entitled *Crossing the Quality Chasm* (IOM, 2001), little progress had been made in keeping patients safe. Their conclusion was that "Safety does not depend just on measurement, practices, and rules, nor does it depend on any specific improvement methods; it depends on achieving a culture of trust, reporting, transparency, and discipline" (Leape et al., 2009, p. 424). Since that time, the focus on patient safety culture has been shown in numerous studies to be related to a lower risk of adverse patient events and outcomes (including mortality).

Patient safety culture has been described as "the values shared among organization members about what is important, their beliefs about how things operate in the organization, and the interaction of these with work unit and organizational structures and systems, which together produce behavioral norms in the organization that promote safety" (Singer et al., 2009, p. 400). Three components of a safety culture are a just culture, a reporting culture, and a learning culture (Reason & Hobbs, 2003). In a just culture, there is trust; what is acceptable and what is not acceptable are clear; and fairness and accountability are consistent. In a culture that supports reporting, reporting errors and safety issues is the norm. Reporting is encouraged and facilitated, and the organization has a commitment to fix what has been found to be unsafe. A learning culture is a culture in which the organization learns from errors, near misses, and other safety issues. The three components are intertwined—without a just culture, employees are less likely to report errors and near misses; without reporting, opportunities to learn and improve are limited.

In 2004, the AHRQ identified the dimensions of a patient safety culture (with items for each dimension) and created survey instruments to measure those dimensions in various patient care settings. In 2019, the dimensions of patient safety culture for hospitals were updated (see Box 6.3; AHRQ, 2020). These dimensions can be used to evaluate the patient safety culture of an organization.

BOX 6.3   Agency for Healthcare Research and Quality Patient Safety Culture Dimensions—Hospitals

- Teamwork
- Staffing and workplace
- Organizational learning—continuous improvement
- Response to error
- Supervisor, manager, or clinical leader support for safety
- Communication about error
- Communication openness
- Reporting patient safety events
- Hospital management
- Handoffs and information exchange

Source: Agency for Healthcare Research and Quality. (2020). *Survey on patient safety culture (SOPS) hospital survey: SOPS hospital survey 2.0 – Hospital survey 2.0 items and composite measures.* AHRQ. https://www.ahrq.gov/sops/surveys/hospital/index.html

High-Reliability Organizations

One patient safety strategy is to create high-reliability organizations (HROs). HROs, according to Weick and Sutcliffe (2007), are organizations that "operate in an unforgiving environment rich with the potential for error, where the scale of consequences precludes learning by experimentation, and where complex processes are used to manage complex technology in order to avoid failure" (p. 164). They create a culture of persistent mindfulness that is founded on the belief that it is possible that any event is "known imperfectly and is capable of novelty" (Weick & Sutcliffe, 1999, p. 38), concentrating on prevention (anticipation) and resilience (containment; Sutcliffe, 2011). HROs focus on five processes: preoccupation with all failures (not just the big ones); reluctance to simplify interpretations (not stopping with the easy, first response); sensitivity to operations (maintain situational awareness for even small signals); deference to expertise (listening to the person who knows and understands the situation/event the best, regardless of their position in the organization); and a commitment to resilience (keep going in spite of the adversity, bounce back, and learn and grow from the experience; Weick & Sutcliffe, 2007). When evaluating an organization's patient safety culture, it is helpful to determine whether the organization has some or all of the elements of an HRO.

WORK ENVIRONMENT

Patient safety culture and healthy work environments share a number of similar components (e.g., communication, collaboration, engagement, staffing, decision-making), although the emphasis of the concept may be different. For example, when we talk about engagement in a healthy work environment, we are generally talking about the engagement of direct care staff into decision-making. When we talk about engagement in a patient safety culture, we are talking about the engagement of the patients and their families.

The environment in which people in health care organizations work impacts patient and employee outcomes. Poor work environments have been associated

---

BOX 6.4 Key Components of a Healthy and Positive Work Environment

Physical safety and mental safety;
Respect, communication, and collaboration;
Adequate staffing (the number of staff, competency of staff) to meet patient care needs;
Effective and authentic leadership;
Engagement and involvement of staff and, where applicable, patients and their families in decision-making;
A learning culture that supports professional development; and
Meaningful recognition.

Source: Institute of Medicine. (2004). *Keeping patients safe. Transforming the work environments of nurses.* The National Academies Press. http://www.iom.edu/Reports/2003/Keeping-Patients-Safe-Transforming-the-Work-Environment-of-Nurses.aspx; American Nurses Credentialing Center. (2020a). *ANCC's Magnet recognition program.* ANCC. https://www.nursing-world.org/organizational-programs/magnet/; Nursing Organizations Alliance. (2004). *Principles and elements of a healthful practice/work environment.* NOA. www.aone.org/resources/leadership%20tools/PDFs/PrinciplesandElementsHealthful WorkPractice.pdf; and American Association of Critical-Care Nurses. (2014). *AACN's healthy work environment initiative.* AACN. http://www.aacn.org/WD/HWE/Content/hwehome.content?menu=hwe

with negative outcomes for patients (e.g., lower quality of care, not prepared for discharge, falls, readmissions) and nurses (e.g., burnout, job dissatisfaction, turn-over; Aiken et al., 2011; Blake et al., 2013; IOM, 2004; Ulrich et al., 2019; Wei et al., 2018). There is also evidence that the quality of nurse work environments is significantly related to patient satisfaction, a key measure of Hospital Consumer Assessment of Healthcare Providers and System (HCAHPS; McHugh et al., 2011; McHugh & Chenjuan, 2013).

Components of healthy and positive work environments have been identi-fied by the IOM (2004), the Magnet® program (American Nurses Credentialing Center [ANCC], 2020a), the Nursing Organizations Alliance (2004), the Ameri-can Association of Critical-Care Nurses (AACN, 2014), and many others. Each component should be considered when evaluating the health of an organization's work environment. See Box 6.4 for key components of a healthy and positive work environment:

REPUTATION

Reputation reflects how the organization is viewed. For health care organizations, there are two main views of reputation—how the organization is viewed by the health care community (e.g., other health care organizations, health care profes-sionals) and how the organization is viewed by the lay community. Both views are important to the success of an organization and should be considered when evaluat-ing an organization.

A variety of external reference groups provide summary data related to excel-lence in clinical performance that can be used to compare an organization with other similar health care organizations. Examples of sources that one might review when assessing the reputation of a particular organization include hospital rankings by *U.S. News and World Report* and *Fortune*, as well as websites, patient portals, and social media sites.

U.S. News and World Report **Rankings**

In 1990, *U.S. News and World Report* introduced "Best Hospitals" as a resource to help individuals select those hospitals that might provide the best level of care for their specific medical issues and concerns (*U.S. News and World Report*, 2018). The annual *U.S. News and World Report* "Best Hospitals" list, prepared by the Research Triangle Institute International (2020), ranks hospitals in 16 specialties. Hospital rankings are primarily based on quality data as well as physician survey information. Metrics such as nurse staffing, use of technologies, and external recognition by organizations such as the ANCC (Magnet) are also factored into the hospital rankings (*U.S. News and World Report*, 2020). These hospital rankings provide information on specialty services as well as on reputation.

Fortune **100 Best Companies to Work For®**

On an annual basis, the Great Place to Work Institute (2020) publishes a list of the *Fortune* 100 Best Companies to Work For. In addition to other businesses, this list contains a list of and details on health care organizations that, via random employee survey, have indicated their work environment is one that reflects a partnership between the employer and employees and provides employees with unique and innovative programming reflective of common values.

Websites, Patient Portals, and Social Media

Social media sites such as Facebook, Twitter, and Yelp have become a popular means for the lay public to rate and comment on their experiences and interactions with health care organizations and other local businesses. Many organizations provide links to these social media sites from their home page. There are also sites in which employees provide information and opinions about their employing organization. Some organizations are utilizing 24/7 chatbots to engage both new and existing patients as well as potential employees.

Real-time text messaging and the use of telehealth technologies continue to gain popularity and have grown exponentially in response to many challenges related to the COVID-19 pandemic. Patient portals and the use of electronic health records have become ubiquitous in health care to communicate with both patients and staff members. Additionally, the Office of the National Coordinator for Health Information Technology implemented the Centers for Medicare & Medicaid Services (CMS) Interoperability and Patient Access final rule in 2020 that requires interoperability of electronic records and health care technology application programming interfaces to promote the exchange of information, facilitate remote patient monitoring, and support virtual patient visits (CMS, 2020a).

QUALITY AND OUTCOMES

Quality care, according to the IOM (2001), must be safe, effective, patient-centered, timely, efficient, and equitable. In the current age of transparency, there is no shortage of data for an objective review of an organization's performance. These reviews can be used to evaluate the quality and outcomes of an organization. In addition, accreditation and/or certification by organizations such as The Joint Commission (TJC, 2020b) or Det Norske Veritas Germanischer Lloyd Healthcare, Inc. (2020) are examples of ways an organization can be recognized for achieving standards.

According to The Commonwealth Fund, transparency and better public information on cost and quality are essential for three reasons: (a) to help providers improve by benchmarking their performance against others; (b) to encourage private insurers and public programs to reward quality and efficiency; and (c) to help patients make informed choices about their care (Collins & Davis, 2006). Transparency is also important to level the playing field through disclosure of accurate and comparable information on how all components of patient care are addressed. Accurate information is critical for the expected level of transparency related to health care.

Some of the outcomes and process measures collected in health care organizations are abstracted from databases that are used by payors, and many of these data are routinely published for review by both practitioners and the general public. Although, there are far more options for inpatient comparisons, data on the outpatient environment are improving. In recent years, a number of states have developed extensive data collection requirements and are publicly reporting clinical and quality outcomes. Payors, including the CMS, managed care, and fee-for-service organizations, also have additional reporting capabilities that are often utilized by employers to make choices for their employee health care needs. The CMS Hospital Compare website provides data for public review as does the Leapfrog Group. Examples of sources for quality and reputation data are shown in Box 6.5.

BOX 6.5 Examples of Sources for Quality Data

Hospital Compare
https://www.cms.gov/Medicare/Quality-Initiatives-Patient-Assessment-Instruments/Hospital
  -QualityInits/HospitalCompare

American Hospital Association
http://www.ahadataviewer.com/about/hospital-database/

***U.S. News and World Report* on Best Hospitals**
www.rti.org/besthospitals

***Fortune* 100 Best Companies to Work For**
http://www.greatplacetowork.com/best-companies/100-best-companies-to-work-for
http://archive.fortune.com/magazines/fortune/best-companies/2014/list/

ANCC Magnet®
https://www.nursingworld.org/organizational-programs/magnet/find-a-magnet-organization/
AACN Beacon Award for Excellence
https://www.aacn.org/nursing-excellence/beacon-awards

Leapfrog Group
http://www.leapfroggroup.org/

Healthgrades
http://www.healthgrades.com/business/services/

CORE MEASURE SETS

In 1998, TJC began the ORYX initiative to measure hospital quality. By 2001, TJC announced four initial core measures for hospitals, which included acute myocardial infarction, heart failure, pneumonia, and pregnancy. Beginning in 2002, TJC required hospitals to collect and report data on two of the four core measure sets. TJC released the quality outcome data to the public starting in 2004 (Chassin et al., 2010). Since 2004, TJC and the CMS have worked together to align these and other common measures and create one set of specifications and documentation with a common or an identical data dictionary, measurement information forms, and algorithms (TJC, 2020b). Common terminology and reporting methods minimize the time required for data collection and allow hospitals to focus efforts on the use of data to improve the health care delivery processes.

There are currently 14 core measure sets including acute myocardial infarction, children's asthma care, heart failure, hospital-based inpatient psychiatric services, substance use, tobacco treatment, hospital outpatient department measures, perinatal care, immunizations, pneumonia, stroke, venous thromboembolism, emergency department measures, and surgical care improvement project (TJC, 2020a). These measures are based on approved evidence-based guidelines adopted by TJC, the National Quality Forum (NQF), and the CMS. The success of core measures requires a multimodal approach with a major focus on a collaborative practice model, the nursing process, and an excellent technological support. The CMS (2016) reports data on the comparative effectiveness of health care organizations on core measures at its hospital compare website.

HOSPITAL-ACQUIRED CONDITIONS

Hospital-acquired conditions (HACs) are serious conditions that patients may acquire during an inpatient hospital stay (CMS, 2020b). Nurse leaders may wish to collect information on organizations similar to their organization to determine whether the organization being evaluated has a disproportionate share of poor outcomes such as HACs. Organizations that are outliers may have different processes from best practices or significant process failures.

HEALTH CARE-ASSOCIATED INFECTIONS

Health care-associated infections (HAIs) are infections caused by a wide variety of both common and unusual bacteria, fungi, and viruses that patients acquire during the course of receiving treatment for other conditions within a health care setting (Centers for Disease Control and Prevention [CDC], 2016). Medical advances have brought lifesaving care to patients, yet many of those advances come with a risk of HAIs. These infections can be debilitating and even deadly. Currently, the infections that are being publicly reported are bloodstream infections, urinary tract infections, and ventilator-associated pneumonias (CDC, 2014). These infections all carry a significant morbidity and mortality risk.

HOSPITAL VALUE-BASED PURCHASING

Value-based purchasing (VBP) is part of the CMS's long-standing effort to link Medicare's payment system to a value-based system to improve health care quality. Beginning in 2015, the program attaches VBP to the Medicare payment system including the quality of care provided in the inpatient hospital setting. Under the program, the CMS makes value-based incentive payments (or reduces expected payments) to acute care hospitals, based on either how the hospitals perform on certain quality measures or how much the hospitals' performance changes on certain quality measures from their performance during a baseline period (CMS, 2019). An example of a value-based incentive is 30-day readmissions. If a hospital's 30-day readmission rate is excessive, the hospital's payments from the CMS are reduced.

NURSING EXCELLENCE—MAGNET DESIGNATION AND BEACON AWARD FOR EXCELLENCE

Magnet designation and the AACN Beacon Award for Excellence are examples of programs that recognize excellence in nursing. Both have been associated with superior patient and nurse outcomes.

Magnet Designation

Of the 20 hospitals identified in *U.S. News and World Report* "Best Hospitals" in 2020–2021, all were Magnet-designated hospitals (ANCC, 2020b; *U.S. News and World Report*, 2020). Magnet criteria identify five domains and more than 60 sources of evidence that are essential for creating an environment in which nurses thrive and innovate (ANCC, 2020a). Leading these domains is transformational leadership, which addresses the quality of nursing leadership in an organization. A transformational nurse leader (i.e., CNE) is one who establishes a strategy that outlines the direction of nursing and effectively communicates the vision and the role of nursing in transforming health care processes in ways that can influence program innovation and quality outcomes for patients and families. Effective Magnet-designated organizations have nursing strategic plans that address the following elements: collaborative patient care delivery; workplace environment; community presence; evidence-based practice and research; innovation and technology; and financial stewardship (ANCC, 2020a).

Magnet designation and The Pathway to Excellence Program offered by the ANCC are indicators of a nursing enterprise that is focused on nurses, quality, service, and innovation in care. The initial designation is preceded by what has been referred to as the "Magnet Journey," which is when an organization engages in a rigorous self-assessment to determine whether it meets Magnet criteria and pursues the Magnet designation. For successful organizations, Magnet designation is awarded for a period of 4 years, and annual reports are submitted to demonstrate the sustainability of the Magnet culture and high-quality outcomes. A documentation system that tracks performance on nurse-sensitive indicators (i.e., pressure ulcers) with corrective action plans must be demonstrated for a 4-year period prior to every redesignation (ANCC, 2020a). The rigors of this process account for the fact that only about 7% of the nation's hospitals achieve Magnet designation (ANCC, 2020a).

American Association of Critical-Care Nurses Beacon Award for Excellence

In 2003, AACN established the Beacon Award to recognize excellence at the unit level (AACN, 2019). According to AACN (n.d.), the Beacon Award for Excellence "signifies a positive and supportive work environment with greater collaboration between colleagues and leaders, higher morale and lower turnover" and Beacon Award units "set the standard for excellence in patient care environments by collecting and using evidence-based information to improve patient outcomes, patient and staff satisfaction, and credibility with consumers" (p. 1). The Beacon Award designation process is based on meeting criteria in leadership structures and systems; appropriate staffing and staff engagement; effective communication, knowledge management, learning, and development; evidence-based practice and processes; and outcome measurement.

CONSUMER ASSESSMENT OF HEALTH CARE PROVIDERS AND SYSTEM

The HCAHPS survey is the first national, standardized, publicly reported survey of patients' perspectives on hospital care (CMS, 2020c). The HCAHPS is a survey instrument and data collection methodology for measuring patients' perceptions on their hospital experience. While many hospitals have collected information on patient satisfaction for their own internal use, until the HCAHPS, there was no national standard for collecting and publicly reporting information about patients' experience of care that allowed valid comparisons to be made across hospitals locally, regionally, and nationally. For many non-hospital health care entities (such as hemodialysis units, health plans, clinician and group practices, and surgical care centers), the Consumer Assessment of Healthcare Providers and Systems (CAHPS) surveys produce several measures of patient experience that include composite measures of two or more related survey items that reflect ratings of respondents on a 0 to 10 scale and single-item measures as well (AHRQ, 2015). Like the HCAHPS surveys, the CAHPS surveys ask consumers and patients to report on and evaluate their experiences with health care.

INFORMATION FROM OTHER ORGANIZATIONS

Press Ganey is an organization that has long been associated with the measurement of patient satisfaction/experience for health care organizations. In 2014, it acquired the National Database of Nursing Quality Indicators (NDNQI) from the American Nurses Association. The NDNQI is composed of nursing sensitive quality indicators that measure performance at the unit level (Press Ganey, 2020).

Private organizations such as Healthgrades (2020) and IBM Watson Health (n.d.) have developed proprietary methodologies to analyze public data sets to evaluate the quality of health care providers. Nurse leaders can gather the most recently published information on hospitals related to clinical quality outcomes for employers from these sources.

THE ROLE OF NURSING IN THE ORGANIZATION

The role of nursing in the organization is an important part of the organizational assessment. Questions that help to assess the role of the CNE within the organization are as follows: Where is the CNE positioned in an organizational structure in relation to other executives? Is nursing a part of critical committees and task forces? What is nursing's role in quality improvement? What leadership roles do nurses with advanced degrees hold in the organization? How does a new registered nurse (RN) or a nurse with an advanced degree move from a novice to an expert in this organization? How are APRNs and nurses with doctoral degrees integrated into the organization and what purposeful actions do they take to advance patient outcomes and use their knowledge and skills?

With the passage of the ACA in 2010, several new models of patient care delivery have emerged that are consistent with the holistic, patient-centered approach that is the backbone of professional nursing. The ACA addresses three emerging care delivery models: the ACO, the medical or health home, and the nurse-managed health center. RNs are fundamental to the success of all of these models. The elements of the holistic, patient-centered approach that are promoted and incentivized by the ACA include the family and community; prevention and wellness care; chronic disease management; care continuity; coordination and integration across settings and providers; patient education; and information management (ACA, 2010). Nurse practitioners and clinical nurse specialists provide significant organizational leadership within the ACO and health home models, which rely on an interdisciplinary, interprofessional team of providers comprised of medical specialists, nurses, pharmacists, nutritionists, dieticians, social workers, behavioral and mental health providers, and other licensed and unlicensed health care providers (American Nurses Association, 2010).

When assessing an organization, one should look for an organizational commitment to collaborative, interprofessional, and evidence-based practice that includes the development of specific goals that are measured and shared with both the individual and the organization. Nurses who are among the first APRNs or the first nurses with a doctorate (e.g., PhD, DNP) to be employed in a facility will have opportunities to educate administrators, employees, nurse leaders, executive colleagues, and collaborating physicians about their preparation, abilities, and scope of practice. Frequent communications and collaboration will offer the best opportunities for meeting expectations, achieving professional goals, and meeting organizational needs.

SUMMARY

Health care organizations and systems are complex structures that are frequently evaluated based on limited information and anecdotal data. This chapter provided nurse leaders with a systematic approach to complete a comprehensive organizational assessment. The approach is similar to a "head-to-toe" physical assessment of an individual patient and begins with a history and an overview of the institution, and it used the structure, process, and outcome measures in the assessment. The impact of the internal and external environment, leadership style and abilities, organizational culture, and the role of nursing in the enterprise are key factors that influence both clinical operations and patient care outcomes of an organization.

The evaluation methodology presented in this chapter provides an evaluation that can be used for a variety of purposes, for example, to select a new practice setting, to benchmark an organization among competitors, or to better understand one's current organization when planning and implementing a change in practice. Whatever the motivation, the consistent use of a systematic approach to organizational assessment will provide a better understanding of both the formal and informal structures of the health care organization or system being evaluated.

REFERENCES

The Advisory Board Company. (2017, August 17). *Daily briefing primer: What's the difference between for profit and not-for-profit hospitals?* Author. https://www.advisory.com/daily-briefing/resources /primers/whats-the-difference-between-for-profit-and-not-for-profit-hospitals

Agency for Healthcare Research and Quality. (2015). *CAPHS: Surveys and tools to advance patient-centered care.* Author. https://www.cahps.ahrq.gov/index.html

Agency for Healthcare Research and Quality. (2020). *Survey on patient safety culture (SOPS) hospital survey: SOPS hospital survey 2.0 – Hospital survey 2.0 items and composite measures.* Author. https:// www.ahrq.gov/sops/surveys/hospital/index.html

Aiken, L. H., Sloane, D. M., Clarke, S., Poghosyan, L., Cho, E., You, L., Finlayson, M., Kanai-Pak, M., & Aungsuroch, Y. (2011). Importance of work environments on hospital outcomes in nine countries. *International Journal of Quality in Health Care, 23*(4), 357–364. https://doi.org/10.1093/intqhc /mzr022

American Association of Critical-Care Nurses. (n.d.). *Beacon awards.* https://www.aacn.org /nursing-excellence/beacon-awards

American Association of Critical-Care Nurses. (2014). *AACN's healthy work environment initiative.* Author. http://www.aacn.org/WD/HWE/Content/hwehome.content?menu=hwe

American Association of Critical-Care Nurses. (2019). *The Beacon Award for Excellence handbook.* Author. http://mini.aacn.org/wd/beaconapps/content/beacon-program-overview.pcms?menu=beaconapps

American Hospital Association. (2018). *AHA annual survey database™ fiscal year 2018.* Author. https:// guide.prod.iam.aha.org/stats/total-us

American Nurses Association. (2010). New care delivery models in health system reform: Opportunities for nurses & their patients. Author. https://www.nursingworld.org/~4af0e8/globalassets/docs /ana/ethics/new-delivery-models---final---haney---6-9-10-1532.pdf

American Nurses Credentialing Center. (2020a). *ANCC's magnet recognition program.* Author. https:// www.nursingworld.org/organizational-programs/magnet/

American Nurses Credentialing Center. (2020b). *Find a magnet organization.* Author. https://www .nursingworld.org/organizational-programs/magnet/find-a-magnet-organization/

Blake, N., Leach, L. S., Robbins, W., Pike, N., & Needleman, J. (2013). Healthy work environments and staff nurse retention: The relationship between communication, collaboration, and leadership in the pediatric intensive care unit. *Nursing Administration Quarterly, 37*(4), 356–370. https://doi .org/10.1097/NAQ.0b013e3182a2fa4

Burns, L. R., Bradley, E. H., & Weiner, B. J. (2012). *Shortell and Kaluzny's: Health care management organization design and behavior* (6th ed.). Delmar.

Centers for Disease Control and Prevention. (2014). *Types of healthcare-associated infections.* Author. http://www.cdc.gov/HAI/infectionTypes.html

Centers for Disease Control and Prevention. (2016). *Healthcare-associated infections.* Author. https:// www.cdc.gov/hai/index.html

Centers for Medicare and Medicaid Services. (2020a). *CMS interoperability and patient access final rule.* Author. https://www.cms.gov/Regulations-and-Guidance/Guidance/Interoperability/index

Centers for Medicare and Medicaid Services. (2020b). *Hospital-acquired condition (HAC) reduction program.* Author. https://www.cms.gov/Medicare/Medicare-Fee-for-Service-Payment/Acute-InpatientPPS/HAC-Reduction-Program.html

Centers for Medicare and Medicaid Services. (2020c). *HCAHPS: Patients' perspectives of care survey.* Author. https://www.cms.gov/Medicare/Quality-Initiatives-Patient-Assessment-Instruments/ HospitalQualityInits/HospitalHCAHPS.html

Centers for Medicare and Medicaid Services. (2019). *Hospital value-based purchasing.* Author. https://www.cms.gov/Medicare/Quality-Initiatives-Patient-Assessment-Instruments/HospitalQualityInits/Hospital-Value-Based-Purchasing

Centers for Medicare and Medicaid Services. (2016). *Hospital compare.* Author. https://www.cms.gov/Medicare/Quality-Initiatives-Patient-Assessment-Instruments/HospitalQualityInits/HospitalCompare

Chassin, M. R., Loeb, J. M., Schmaltz, S. P., & Wachter, R. M. (2010). Accountability measures—Using measurement to promote quality improvement. *New England Journal of Medicine, 363*(7), 683–688. https://doi.org/10.1056/NEJMsb1002320

Cheney, C. (2019, September 3). 3 strategic differences between nonprofit and for-profit hospitals. Health Leaders. https://www.healthleadersmedia.com/clinical-care/3-strategic-differences-between-nonprofit-and-profit-hospitals

Collins, S. R., & Davis, K. (2006). *Transparency in health care: The time has come.* The Commonwealth Fund. http://www.commonwealthfund.org/publications/testimonies/2006/mar/transparency-in-health-care--the-time-has-come

Congressional Budget Office. The Congress of the United States. (2006). *Nonprofit hospitals and the provision of community benefits.* Author. https://www.cbo.gov/publication/18256

Det Norske Veritas Germanischer Lloyd Healthcare, Inc. (2020). *Hospital accreditation.* Author. http://dnvglhealthcare.com/accreditations/hospital-accreditation

Donabedian, A. (1978). The quality of medical care. *Science, 200*(4344), 856–864. https://doi.org/10.1126/science.417400

Glickman, S. W., Baggett, K. A., Krubert, C. G., Peterson, E. D., & Schulman, K. A. (2007). Promoting quality: The health-care organization from a management perspective. *International Journal for Quality in Health-Care, 19*(6), 341–348. https://doi.org/10.1093/intqhc/mzm047

Great Place to Work Institute. (2020). *Fortune 100 great places to work for.* Author. http://www.Groy.com/best-companies/100-best-companies-to-work-for

Groysberg, B., Lee, J., Price, J., & Cheng, J. Y. (2018). The leader's guide to corporate culture: How to manage the eight critical elements of organizational life. *Harvard Business Review, 96*(1), 44–52. https://hbr.org/2018/01/the-leaders-guide-to-corporate-culture

Healthgrades. (2020). *How America finds a doctor.* Healthgrades Operating Company, Inc. www.healthgrades.com/

Herring, B., Gaskin, D., Zare, H., & Anderson, G. (2018). Comparing the value of nonprofit hospitals' tax exemption to their community benefits. *Inquiry: The Journal of Health Care Organizations, Provision, and Financing, 55,* 1–11. https://doi.org/10.1177/0046958017751970

IBM Watson Health. (n.d.). *100 top hospitals.* Author. https://www.ibm.com/watson-health/services/100-top-hospitals

Institute of Medicine. (2000). *To err is human: Building a safer health system.* National Academies Press.

Institute of Medicine. (2001). *Crossing the quality chasm: A new health system for the 21st century.* National Academies Press. http://iom.edu/Reports/2001/Crossing-the-Quality-Chasm-A-New-Health-System-for-the-21st-Century.aspx

Institute of Medicine. (2004). *Keeping patients safe. Transforming the work environments of nurses.* The National Academies Press. http://www.iom.edu/Reports/2003/Keeping-Patients-Safe-Transforming-the-Work-Environment-of-Nurses.aspx

James, J. (2016, February 25). Nonprofit hospitals' community benefit requirements. *Health Affairs Health Policy Brief.* https://doi.org/10.1377/hpb20160225.954803

The Joint Commission. (2020a). *Core measure sets.* Author. http://www.jointcommission.org/core_measure_sets.aspx

The Joint Commission. (2020b). *What is accreditation?* Author. http://www.jointcommission.org/accreditation/accreditation_main.aspx

Leape, L., Berwick, D., Clancy, J., Conway, J., Gluck, P., Guest, J., Lawrence, D., Morath, J., O'Leary, D., O'Neilll, P., Pinakiewicz, D., & Isaac, T. for the Lucian Leape Institute at the National Patient Safety Foundation. (2009). Transforming healthcare: A safety imperative. *Quality and Safety in Health Care, 18,* 424–428. https://doi.org/10.1136/qshc.2009.036954

McHugh, M. D., & Ma, C. (2013). Hospital nursing and 30-day readmissions among Medicare patients with heart failure, acute myocardial infarction, and pneumonia. *Medical Care, 51*(1), 52–59. https://doi.org/10.1097/MLR.0b013e3182763284

McHugh, M. D., Kutney-Lee, A., Cimiotti, J. P., Sloane, D. M., & Aiken, L. H. (2011). Nurses' widespread job dissatisfaction, burnout, and frustration with health benefits signal problems for patient care. *Health Affairs, 30*(2), 202–210. https://doi.org/10.1377/hlthaff.2010.0100

Merriam-Webster. (2020). *Culture.* http://www.merriam-webster.com/dictionary/culture

Miles, R. E., & Snow, C. C. (1978). *Organizational strategy, structure, and process.* McGraw-Hill.

National Steering Committee for Patient Safety. (2020). *Safer together: A national action plan to advance patient safety.* Institute for Healthcare Improvement. www.ihi.org/SafetyActionPlan

Nightingale, F. (1863). *Notes on hospitals* (3rd ed.). Longman, Green, Longman, Roberts, and Green.

Nursing Organizations Alliance. (2004). *Principles & elements of a healthful practice/work environment.* Author. www.aone.org/resources/leadership%20tools/PDFs/PrinciplesandElementsHealthfulWork Practice.pdf

The Office of the National Coordinator for Health Information Technology. (2020). *Patient access to health records.* Author. https://www.healthit.gov/topic/patient-access-health-records/patient-access-health-records

Patient Protection and Affordable Care Act. (2010). P. L. 111-148. Sec. 3502. https://www.congress .gov/111/plaws/publ148/PLAW-111publ148.pdf

Press Ganey. (2020). *Insight and action that transform the care experience.* Author. https://www .pressganey.com/solutions

Research Triangle Institute International. (2020). *U.S. News & World Report's annual ranking of best hospitals.* Author. http://www.rti.org/BestHospitals

Reason, J., & Hobbs, A. (2003). Managing maintenance error. Ashgate.

Rozier, M. D. (2020). Nonprofit hospital community benefit in the U.S.: A scoping review from 2010 to 2019. *Frontiers in Public Health, 8,* 72. https://doi.org/10.3389/fpubh.2020.00072.

Schein, E. (2009). *The corporate culture survival guide.* Jossey Bass.

Scott, W. R., & Davis, G. F. (2015). *Organizations and organizing: Rational, natural and open systems perspectives.* Routledge.

Singer, S., Lin, S., Falwell, A., Gaba, D., & Baker, L. (2009). Relationship of safety climate and safety performance in hospitals. *Health Services Research, 44*(2), 399–421. https://doi .org/10.1111/j.1475-6773.2008.00918.x

Sutcliffe, K. M. (2011). High reliability organizations (HROs). *Best Practice & Research Clinical Anaesthesiology, 25*(2), 133–144. https://doi.org/10.1016/j.bpa.2011.03.001

Ulrich, B., Barden, C., Cassidy, L., & Varn-Davis, N. (2019). Critical care nurse work environments 2018: Findings and implications. *Critical Care Nurse, 39*(2), 67–84. https://doi.org/10.4037/ccn2019605

U.S. News and World Report LP. (2020). *2020–21 best hospitals honor roll and specialties rankings.* Author. https://health.usnews.com/health-care/best-hospitals/articles/best-hospitals-honor-roll-and-overview

U.S. News and World Report LP. (2018). *Celebrating 85 years: A timeline of events in the life of U.S. News & World Report, 1933–2018.* Author. https://www.usnews.com/info/articles/2018/06/11/celebrating-85-years

Wei, H., Sewell, K. A., Woody, G., & Rose, M. A. (2018). The state of the science of nurse work environments in the United States: A systematic review. *International Journal of Nursing Science, 5*(3), 287–300. https://doi.org/10.1016/j.ijnss.2018.04.010

Weick, K. E., & Sutcliffe, K. M. (2007). *Managing the unexpected: Resilient performance in an age of uncertainty* (2nd ed.). John Wiley & Sons, Inc.

Weick, K. E., Sutcliffe, K. M., & Obstfeld, D. (1999). Organizing for high reliability: Processes of collective mindfulness. In R. S. Sutton, & B. M. Shaw (Eds.), *Research in organizational behavior* (Vol. 1, pp. 81–123). Jai Press.

SEVEN

EVALUATION OF HEALTH CARE INFORMATION SYSTEMS AND PATIENT CARE TECHNOLOGY

Juliana J. Brixey and V. Gail Roberson Turner

> *Were there none who were discontented with what they have, the world*
> *would never reach anything better.*
> *—Florence Nightingale*

INTRODUCTION

This chapter discusses the role of the doctor of nursing practice (DNP)-prepared nurse in the assessment and evaluation of various types of technologies and information systems used by health care providers and patients. The purpose of this chapter is to equip the DNP nurse with increased knowledge of (a) the tenets of information technology (IT) evaluation and (b) effective partnerships and collaborations with informaticians and other members of the information systems team.

The first section addresses the framework of informatics and informaticians within the context of the clinical environment. It includes the following topics:

- Informatics and the role of the doctor of nursing informatician
- Collaborative relationship between the DNP nurse and informaticians
- National mandate for electronic health records (EHRs) and implications of reimbursement for eligible hospitals and providers
- The scope of the term *IT*

The second part of the chapter discusses the specific areas in which DNP nurses can make useful contributions to the assessment and evaluation of health care and ITs, including:

- Compare and contrast assessment and evaluation
- Unintended and unexpected consequences of the introduction of ITs
- IT as a communication tool and the emergence and implications of personal mobile devices in health care
- Patient portal and recommended evaluation criteria

● Recommended guidelines to support patients' searches for authentic health care information on the Internet
● Ergonomic and human factors evaluation of the work environment concerning ITs
● Evaluation of computerized patient care equipment

INFORMATICS AND DOCTOR OF NURSING INFORMATICIANS

Adding informatics to the discussion of assessment and evaluation of health ITs inserts a new and crucial domain of consideration. Nursing leadership organizations, such as the American Organization of Nurse Executives (AONE), have established baseline competencies for nurses in the executive and leadership roles, and research is emerging to define the nature and application of informatics competency for nurse leaders (Collins et al., 2015). The discussion begins by defining informatics, specifically nursing informatics (NI), and the relationship between DNP nurses and informatics practitioners. The American Nurses Association (ANA) states that the NI specialty integrates multiple analytical and information sciences with nursing science to define, communicate, and manage information and data in health care practice. NI practice seeks to improve the health of individuals and populations by identifying informatics-related issues in all domains of practice and then designing effective solutions using informatic technologies to improve the health and care of patients and families (ANA, 2015). A fundamental concept of the ANA's definition of the NI specialty is the inclusion and use of management and communication of data, information, knowledge, and wisdom to improve health. Informatics embraces IT in its multiple facets as a *tool* purposed to enhance information management and knowledge discovery. DNP informaticians are involved in research to determine best approaches to the development, implementation, and evaluation of informatics issues (2015) through the use of inquiry methods that evaluate information, knowledge, and data within data repositories (2015). The discovery of knowledge and understanding gleaned from the research findings will lead to models of health care delivery that are more effective, seamless, and transparent in the delivery of quality patient care and improvement of patient outcomes.

Preparation for informatics practice lacks standardization. Nurses may begin informatics practice through on-the-job training, completion of an informatics certificate program, and/or completion of a degree-granting program at the bachelor's, master's, or doctoral degree level. Degree domains include health informatics, health care informatics, clinical informatics, data science, NI, and similar informatics domains. The common thread among these entry-to-practice levels is the creation of tools that practitioners can use to promote patient safety, enhance the quality of care delivery, promote health maintenance and disease prevention, and improve outcomes for individuals and populations.

The ANA classifies nurses working in informatics based on interest, experience, and academic preparation as an informatics nurses (IN) and an informatics nurse specialist (INS). The IN is a registered nurse (RN) with experience and interest in the informatics field, while the INS RN is educated at the graduate level in an informatics-related field (ANA, 2015). Frequently, the role of the informatician focuses on the configuration and design of the clinical information system (CIS) in preparation for system implementation. Informaticians who have completed an undergraduate or a graduate program are prepared to embrace other vital dimensions that are fundamental to developing an information system that effectively supports critical thinking and decision-making. These dimensions include the following:

- The distinction between assessment and evaluation to help guide the DNP to assist in the selection and implementation of patient care technology software and hardware;
- Assessment of the sociotechnical (e.g., the convergence of people, relationships, systems, and organizational culture) facets of an IT implementation and the transformations that are deeply embedded in the implementation process;
- Awakening, promoting, and supporting innovative problem-solving, appropriately employing the tools of IT (Cassano, 2014);
- Assessment and evaluation in the design and management of the human–computer interface; that is, creating positive, intuitive, "error-free" experiences for practitioners as they use the technology;
- Assessment of current workflow, identifying opportunities for streamlining processes, for standardizing practice, and for the development of new workflows in the context of the IT system;
- Application of informatics science to align application design with the cognitive needs of practitioners;
- System assessment that ensures clinical staff are active, informed participants in evaluation and quality improvement decisions regarding IT systems (Jones et al., 2011);
- Establish, maintain, and update policies, processes, workflows, and/or technology designs that address EHR-related problems and issues (Jones et al., 2011);
- Strategic planning that anticipates and positions the organization for the cultural and practice transformation that is associated with the implementation of IT and information systems;
- System design that is aligned with the information management and knowledge management needs and characteristics of the organization (Greenes & Shortliffe, 2009; Jones et al., 2011; Koppel & Gordon, 2012; Koppel et al., 2008; McLane & Turley, 2011);
- The ongoing evaluation of health IT (HIT) projects; and
- Evaluation of the achievement of project goals and outcomes.

NATIONAL MANDATE FOR ELECTRONIC HEALTH RECORDS

The digital information age continues to influence the delivery of health care services. Health care adopted IT to support the financial imperatives of the organization in the 1970s. However, the complexities of patient care, the multiple environments in which health care is delivered, the diverse patient populations, and the variability of resources of the health care industry resulted in a much more tentative approach to embracing IT for documentation, display, and storage of clinical data. A few intrepid early adopters began the journey to digital CIS in the late 1960s, but the number of hospitals and health care systems using IT for clinical documentation increased very slowly over the next four decades.

The stimulus of the American Recovery and Reinvestment Act (ARRA) of 2009 provided incentives to health care organizations to implement EHRs. Between 2008 and 2013, 59% of the nation's hospitals adopted at least a basic EHR (e.g., patient demographics; problem lists; medication lists; discharge summaries; computerized provider order entry (CPOE) for medications; and lab, radiology, and diagnostic test results). While the rate of adoption is impressive, representing a fivefold increase between 2008 and 2013, it is interesting to note that adoption is highly variable across the individual states, ranging between 26% and 83% (Dustin et al., 2014). The adoption of EHR technology has been greater among urban hospitals. According to the National Institutes of Health National Cancer Institute (2020), nonfederal hospitals are nearing 100% adoption of EHRs. Nearly 80% of physician offices have adopted certified EHRs (Office of the National Coordinator for Health Information Technology [ONC], n.d.). The adoption of EHRs and IT in small and critical access hospitals lagged behind their urban counterparts due to capital and infrastructure challenges, as well as a limited access to a qualified workforce to support implementation (Adler-Milstein et al., 2014; Altarum Institute, 2011).

National health care policy, as established, provided direction to the Centers for Medicare & Medicaid Services (CMS) to responsively create meaningful use rules and criteria for eligible providers and eligible hospitals. The CMS also issued criteria for certification of EHRs, and eligible providers and eligible hospitals were required to report meaningful use of data from a certified EHR system by 2015 (HealthIT.gov, 2019; Obama, 2009). Due to the lack of meaningful use reporting functionality by several certified EHR systems, meaningful use reporting requirements were modified during the third quarter of 2014 (CMS, 2014; U.S. Government Publishing Office, 2015). Under the new rules, the timeline for Stage 2 reporting extended to 2016. In October 2015, the final rule was released with a focus on using certified electronic health record technology (CEHRT) to improve health outcomes (Stages of promoting interoperability programs, n.d.). Stage 3 was established in 2017 as a result of the 2015 final rule and focuses on using CEHRT to improve health outcomes. For 2015 and 2016, the CMS supported Modified Stage 2, and Modified Stage 3 was supported for 2017 and 2018 (Stages of promoting interoperability programs, n.d.). Modified Stage 2 requirements streamlined reporting requirements on redundant, duplicative, or topped out measures (Stages of promoting interoperability programs, n.d.)

The stages of meaningful use design were intended to assist eligible hospitals and eligible providers in moving beyond data capture and storage to the next level of improved quality of care for patient populations. The goal was to transform health care organizations into continual learning environments that iteratively improve outcomes and processes based on their performance as measured by the data. Table 7.1 provides a high-level summary of the purpose of each stage of meaningful use and the expected outcomes of each stage.

TABLE 7.1 Meaningful Use Stages

	Stage 1	Stage 2	Stage 3
Outcome	Data capture and sharing	Advanced clinical processes	Access to comprehensive patient data through patient-centered HIE
Criteria for success	Standardize electronic data capture	Increase the rigor of HIE	Continues to promote EHR interoperability
	Track key clinical conditions using EHR data	Increase requirements for e-prescribing and reporting of lab data	Providing more flexibility that simplifies the reporting requirements of the Medicare and Medicaid EHR Incentive Programs
	Improve care coordination processes	Electronic transmission of care summaries across multiple settings	Removal of topped out, redundant, and duplicative measures from reporting requirements
	Begin reporting of clinical quality measures and public health data	More patient-controlled data	Focused on only those measures that represent the most advanced use of the functions and standards supported by CEHRT
	Engage patients and families		Improve population health

CEHRT, certified electronic health record technology; EHR, electronic health record; HIE, health information exchange.

Source: HealthIT.gov. (2014). *Your mobile device and health information privacy and security.* https://www.healthit.gov/providers-professionals/your-mobile-device-and-health-information-privacy-and -security; Riesman (2017).

Beginning in 2015, Medicare payments to eligible providers and eligible hospitals that did not demonstrate meaningful use were reduced, and the level of reimbursement will continue to decline in the subsequent years. Recognizing the significant cost associated with the implementation of EHR systems, the CMS offered incentive payments to eligible providers and eligible hospitals, beginning in 2011 and running through 2015. Eligible providers and eligible hospitals that did not successfully demonstrate meaningful use by 2015 experienced payment adjustments to their Medicare reimbursement. These reimbursement changes created a compelling inducement to reluctant or uncertain health care organizations and eligible providers to embrace IT, specifically the EHR.

Since mid-2010, eligible providers and eligible hospitals accelerated plans for the implementation of an EHR, with an initial focus on achieving meaningful use. As of October 2018, more than 1,076,732 eligible providers and eligible hospitals have received payment for participating in the Medicare and Medicaid Promoting Interoperability (PI) Programs for a total of over $24.8 billion (CMS.gov, n.d.).

In 2018 and the entrance of Stage 3 meaningful use rules, the CMS decided to update the EHR Incentive Program with a name change to PI Program. The goal of the name change was to indicate a new focus on improving patients' access to their medical information and making program requirements less of a burden for eligible providers. The emphasis was to make it easier and less time-consuming for physicians to participate in incentive programs and give patients the power to control the usage of their health care data (2018 Updates to the EHR Incentive Program, 2018). Table 7.2 displays the stages of PI Programs since 2011.

The burden experienced by eligible providers varies as the measurements have changed over the years. An American Hospital Association (AHA) study found regulatory burden imposed by federal programs, including meaningful use costs health systems and postacute care providers close to $39 billion a year (Kate, 2017). Multiple resources are needed for the assessment and interpretation of the measures for the development of a plan to attest to the CMS requirements. According to ONC's final report in February 2020, there are multiple reported reasons that health care providers are feeling the increased burden. Some reasons that can present significant challenges for many health care organizations affecting program participation and accuracy of the data submitted include the following:

- Rapidly shifting certification requirements with short implementation timelines
- Frequent updates to certification of health IT

TABLE 7.2 Stages of Promoting Interoperability Programs

First Year Demonstrating Meaningful Use	Stage of Promoting Interoperability Programs								
	2011	2012	2013	2014	2015	2016	2017	2018	2019 and Future Years*
2011	Stage 1	Stage 1	Stage 1	Stage 1 or Stage 2	Modified Stage 2	Modified Stage 2	Modified Stage 2 or Stage 3	Modified Stage 2 or Stage 3	Stage 3
2012	N/A	Stage 1	Stage 1	Stage 1 or Stage 2	Modified Stage 2	Modified Stage 2	Modified Stage 2 or Stage 3	Modified Stage 2 or Stage 3	Stage 3
2013	N/A	N/A	Stage 1	Stage 1	Modified Stage 2	Modified Stage 2	Modified Stage 2 or Stage 3	Modified Stage 2 or Stage 3	Stage 3
2014	N/A	N/A	N/A	Stage 1	Modified Stage 2	Modified Stage 2	Modified Stage 2 or Stage 3	Modified Stage 2 or Stage 3	Stage 3
2015	N/A	N/A	N/A	N/A	Modified Stage 2	Modified Stage 2	Modified Stage 2 or Stage 3	Modified Stage 2 or Stage 3	Stage 3
2016	N/A	N/A	N/A	N/A	NA	Modified Stage 2	Modified Stage 2 or Stage 3	Modified Stage 2 or Stage 3	Stage 3
2017	N/A	N/A	N/A	N/A	NA	NA	Modified Stage 2 or Stage 3	Modified Stage 2 or Stage 3	Stage 3
2018	N/A	N/A	N/A	N/A	NA	NA	NA	Modified Stage 2 or Stage 3	Stage 3
2019 and Future Years	N/A	N/A	N/A	N/A	NA	NA	NA	NA	Stage 3

Adapted from *Stages of promoting interoperability programs: First year demonstrating meaningful use*. (n.d.). https://www.cms.gov/Regulations-and-Guidance/Legislation/EHRIncentivePrograms/Downloads/Stages _ofMeaningfulUseTable.pdf

- Regular program updates that require new quality measures or significant modification to existing measures
- Limited implementation timelines for certification and programmatic changes
- Access to quality and related data within certified health IT EHRs (ONC, 2020)

Leadership and Collaboration Opportunities for Doctor of Nursing Practice Nurses

DNP leaders and DNP informaticians have an opportunity to lead health care initiatives for their prospective organization by remaining current about (a) strategies to ease the burden of designing and implementing organizational specific tactics; (b) using strategies that focus on clinical documentation, health usability, and reporting requirements; and (c) public health reporting (ONC, 2020).

Collaboration between DNP nurses and nurse informaticians creates an ideal partnership for the effective use and design of a CIS. The nursing knowledge, clinical expertise, and experience of DNP nurses, in combination with the nursing knowledge, informatics knowledge, and CIS experience of nurse informaticians, merge to inform the design of a database that collects the information necessary to provide quality patient care. The synergy of clinical subject matter experts and informatics subject matter experts establishes a harmony of design and function. The DNP nurse's expert clinical knowledge and understanding of the data necessary to support clinical assessment, critical thinking, ongoing modification of the plan of care, and patient education are essential to the design of an effective CIS that will be useful and usable by practitioners. The nurse informatician carefully evaluates the knowledge and information needs as defined by the DNP nurse in the context of factors such as future workflow, data visualization, cognition, system navigation, information management, terminology and taxonomy, training, practitioner adoption of the system, and data analysis and reporting needs.

An exciting and a vital dimension of the design of an EHR information system is the duality of purpose. The primary focus of an EHR is the individual patient and the information that is necessary to provide effective and efficacious care. The second, yet compelling purpose of an EHR system is related to the data stored by the system, which can be used to evaluate practice, quality of care, outcomes, and many other dimensions for patient populations. Careful design of the system and thoughtful, intentional data input will create a database that can inform evidence-based practice and provide highly powered data regarding the quality of care and patient outcomes. While the quality of care for the individual who has presented for care is the primary focus of the moment, a system that is thoughtfully designed to support data input and data visualization by practitioners who understand and respect the importance and value of the prescribed data input has the potential to create a robust evidence-based database.

ASSESSMENT AND EVALUATION

The distinction between assessment and evaluation is fundamental to the correct use of the concepts in the discussion of health IT. Assessment and evaluation are used interchangeably in health care information systems and patient care technology. It is essential to know the specific context in which to choose the appropriate term. Table 7.3 provides a visual for the comparisons of assessment and evaluation.

TABLE 7.3 Types of Evaluation

Assessment	Evaluation
The need to collect and review data to improve a situation or performance	Define criteria and if goals or outcomes are established
Need to diagnose an issue or a problem to increase quality or productivity	Forms a conclusion on if desired goals or outcomes are obtained
Process-focused	Product-focused

Source: Centers for Disease Control.gov. (n.d.). *Types of evaluation.* https://www.cdc.gov/std/Program/pupestd/Types%20of%20Evaluation.pdf

Assessment determines whether deficiencies are present in a workflow or process and then describes those deficiencies. In information systems, an assessment is completed using workflow analysis. This method helps to determine the current state and assess the process that requires improvement once determined what needs improvement; goals are then related to how these goals are evaluated. Patient care technology requires continuous assessment to ensure that the latest and most efficient technology is in use.

Evaluation can be based on process measures or project outcomes. Process measures evaluate whether the parts or steps in the system are performing as planned and whether the efforts to improve the system are on track. Outcome measures determine the project's impacts on patients' health and stakeholders such as payers, employees, and the entire community (Institute for Healthcare Improvement [IHI], n.d.). Based on the project, it is determined which evaluation method is the most appropriate. Evaluation helps determine the value of the change and answer questions such as the following:

- Did the change add value and change the previous assessment?
- Was the change beneficial?
- Did the change add value to the process that needed adjustment?

The process of evaluation should underscore the significance of the project by using data analytics to ascertain whether established project goals are met or outcomes are achieved (Cusack et al., 2009).

Evaluation is further described as formative or summative. Both approaches examine intervention implementation, the barriers and facilitators to implementation, and the effects of the intervention on various outcomes. Formative evaluations engage stakeholders at the beginning and during the intervention development. The summative evaluation provides feedback to stakeholders at the end of program implementation. The benefit of formative evaluation is that stakeholders can identify when an intervention is not being delivered as planned or not having the intended effects so that the intervention can be modified in real time. Summative evaluation provides some challenges as there may be less than real-time discussions on progress, thus not providing timely information used to refine the intervention during implementation (Geonnotti et al., 2013).

Evaluation is an integral part of health IT to establish goals to improve clinical care, quality of care, and safety of patients. It is difficult to forecast a completed project's impact without evaluation. DNP-prepared leaders can ensure that evaluation is an important part of health IT to guarantee the achievement of the project's outcomes and goals. Evaluation provides the methods for DNP informaticians to systematically determine the achievement of project outcomes and goals. Lessons learned from evaluations help project team members and stakeholders involved in health IT implementation and adoption to improve upon and evolve into current practices (Agency for Healthcare Research and Quality [AHRQ], 2007).

UNEXPECTED AND UNINTENDED CONSEQUENCES

Unexpected and unintended consequences have been persistent topics of interest to NIs, patient safety experts, and health care professionals. For example, Merton attributes unintended consequences to ignorance, error, fixation with immediacy, basic values that entail or block action, and self-defeating prophecy (Merton, 1936). Furthermore, history has recorded many memorable quotations regarding unexpected and unintended consequences regarding technology. For example, Reilly's law and Murphy's law each point out that the unexpected and unintended consequences can and will occur (Oxford University Press, 2020; Reilly, 1931). Tenner comments that "Americans believe that things can be contrary by nature" (Tenner, 1997, p. 4) and "whenever we try to take advantage of some new technology, we may discover that it induces behavior which appears to cancel out the very reason for using it" (Tenner, 1997, p. 7). Therefore, from a historical perspective of "laws" regarding not only the perception, but also the actual performance of technology, it should not be astonishing that unexpected and unintended consequences should extend to EHRs and HIT.

Unexpected and unintended consequences in health care began to receive attention as the early adopters of HIT began to implement various patient care information systems (PCISs; Ash et al., 2004; Bloomrosen et al., 2011; Gruber et al., 2009; Campbell et al., 2006; Harrison et al., 2007; Jones et al., 2011; Middleton et al., 2013). Ash et al. noted that "PCISs might not be as successful in preventing errors as generally hoped, but could actually generate new errors" and "that PCIS applications seemed to foster errors rather than reduce their likelihood" (Ash et al., 2004, p. 105). The findings from their review of the literature and a series of qualitative studies identified that errors occurred in the process of data entry and retrieval as well as in the communication and coordination processes. Interest in unexpected and unintended consequences has continued with additional research studies and reports (Bloomrosen et al., 2011) with CPOE, clinician decision support (CDS), and bar code medication administration technology at the forefront of attention. In 2011, the RAND Corporation, under contract with the AHRQ, released the *Guide to Reducing Unintended Consequences of Electronic Health Records* (Jones et al., 2011). Clinicians should be well informed about the weaknesses as well as the benefits of technology (Kuperman & McGowan, 2013, p. 1666).

MOBILE TECHNOLOGY: BACKGROUND AND SIGNIFICANCE

Mobile wireless communication technology has become ubiquitous. Organizations have been challenged to keep pace with rapidly changing mobile technology and, before long, bring your own device (BYOD) surfaced.

BYOD in Health Care Organizations

Health care organizations are not exempt from the BYOD movement. Currently, 73% of hospitals permit some use of BYOD, and more than 50% have a specific BYOD policy (Spok, 2015). Clinicians are using their own devices, with physicians leading the charge. Approximately 96% of practicing physicians use personal smart devices for clinical communication (Spyglass Consulting Group, 2014a).

Furthermore, 67% of hospitals report that nurses use their own devices (Spyglass Consulting Group, 2014a); however, many hospitals prevent or discourage the use of smartphones, leaving nurses to use voice-only phones, multiple pagers, and/or wearable voice-activated two-way communication devices (Parker, 2014). A recent report indicates that physician use of BYOD continues to outnumber BYOD use by nurses (Spok, 2015). Although health care organizations have lagged in providing technologies to improve communication processes for nurses, more than 50% of hospitals in the survey were planning to acquire or consider smartphones within the upcoming 18 months, perhaps as early as late 2015 (Spyglass Consulting Group, 2014b). Spyglass conducted a similar study in 2016. The consultants commented that nurses have a need for expeditious communication as well as access to patient information at the point of care (Spyglass Consulting, 2016).

BYOD: Challenges and Management Recommendations

The term *BYOD* presents unique challenges to the health care organization. The IT department must maintain a secure network to protect the privacy and security of health and personal information. The IT department not only has to support the operating system for the health care organization, but also is charged with supporting additional operating systems such as iOS and Android. Furthermore, the use of the mobile device may not be exclusive to the owner. Family members and coworkers cannot and should not be excluded as possible users of the device.

Health care organizations need to consider infection control, as a mobile device may become a vector for the dissemination of disease. Microorganisms and fungi are known to survive on various surfaces, including plastics and fabrics. The microorganisms and fungi are easily transferred to other surfaces and objects, including by human hand contact (Sittig & Ash, 2011, pp. 203–210). In BYOD, the mobile device travels from one clinical setting to the next, most likely without disinfection. Employer-owned mobile devices are a similar source of disease dissemination and just as unlikely to be disinfected.

Employer policies regarding BYOD need to be carefully crafted to avoid standard of care issues. Some employees may be unwilling, financially or for other reasons, to use personal communication devices to support patient care communication activities. Employers need to ensure that these employees are provided with appropriate communication technology, so that patient care is not delayed or impeded due to ineffective or inefficient communication technology.

Data security and Health Insurance Portability and Accountability Act (HIPAA) compliance are significant concerns for health care organizations. HealthIT.gov (2014) offers tips to guide health care organizations as they decide if BYOD is the right solution for the organization. The organization must assess the risks, threats, and vulnerabilities and subsequently develop appropriate policies and procedures to protect health information. It is imperative to educate and train health care providers and professionals in strategies to protect the privacy and security of health information.

Health IT.gov (2013a, 2013b, 2014) offers recommendations to health care providers and professionals regarding BYOD in the clinical setting. Before using a personal device, a health care professional should consult with the IT department or privacy and security officers concerning the organization's BYOD policies and procedures. It is paramount that the device owner maintains physical control of the device at all times. Furthermore, the mobile device must be protected from breach and theft through encryption, security software, and user authentication, as well as securing and maintaining tracking software. It is obligatory that the most current security software and patches be installed upon release when personal devices are used in a clinical setting. All stored health information requires purging before discarding or reusing the mobile device.

THE PATIENT PORTAL

Meaningful Use Stage 2 mandated patient engagement through access to personal health information and bidirectional secure email communication with the health care team (CMS.gov, 2018). No longer would patients be blocked from personal health information. Access would occur electronically through the EHR patient portal. A patient portal is defined as "a secure online website that gives patients convenient, 24-hour access to personal health information from anywhere with an Internet connection" (HealthIT.gov, 2017, para. 1). The agency (HealthIT.gov, 2017) explains that typically the patient portal provides the patient with access to the following features: recent physician visits, discharge summaries, medications, immunizations, list of allergies, and laboratory results. Furthermore, some patient portals include additional features including secure messaging to a physician; request for prescription refills; scheduling of nonurgent appointments; checking benefits and coverage; updating contact information; ability to make payments; downloading and completing forms; and viewing educational materials.

Evaluation of the patient portal should be completed from the perspective of the end-user health care provider as well as the patient. Evaluation methods include both quantitative and qualitative methods. Cusack et al. (2009, pp. 4 and 5) prepared the *Health Information Technology Evaluation Toolkit* for the AHRQ. The toolkit recommends the following methods: clinical outcomes measures; clinical process measures; provider adoption and attitudes measures; patient adoption, knowledge, and attitudes measures; workflow impact measures; and financial impact measures. Other methods to consider include heuristic evaluation (Nielsen, 1998–2020); questionnaires; end-user think aloud (Lewis, 1982); cognitive walkthrough (Wharton et al., 1992); focus groups; and interviews.

WEARABLE TECHNOLOGY: ACTIVITY TRACKERS

Wearable technology, as activity trackers, continues to evolve. The price and features/functions of the technology vary. An *activity/fitness tracker* "is a type of electronic device that helps monitor some type of human activity, such as walking or running, sleep quality, or heart rate. An activity tracker can be a smartwatch, or device that syncs with a network or IT system to collect and store data. According to Vogels (2020), about one in five adults use a fitness tracker or smartwatch.

Furthermore, women, college graduates, and households earning more than $75,000/year are more likely to use the technology. Patients may present data from their fitness tracker to a health care professional during an office visit or submit to the EHR through the patient portal. It behooves the DNP nurse to develop familiarity with the various technologies.

The literature offers few suggestions regarding how to evaluate various entities. Xie et al. (2018) evaluated wearable technology for accuracy. Song and Stoylar (2019) suggested the following strategies to evaluate activity trackers: design and comfort, battery life, accuracy, and sensor and features. Additional research is needed to identify or develop methods to evaluate activity trackers.

GUIDING PATIENT DISCERNMENT OF HEALTH CARE INFORMATION ON THE INTERNET

As patients become increasingly adept in the use of IT and the Internet, the DNP nurse may notice a change in the questions patients ask and in the patients' knowledge about their health and self-care. They may also seek advice about the veracity of various websites. The DNP nurse must equip patients with information and tools that will guide their ability to make informed choices and feel confident that they can discern credible health care websites containing factual, accurate, and useful information.

The proliferation of health and health care information available on the Internet can be challenging to comprehend. To gain an appreciation of the pervasiveness of the Internet websites that address health or health issues, you need only "Google" the search term "health." A search conducted on April 19, 2020, disclosed eight billion five hundred million sites. The available information is overwhelming, and many patients need assistance to determine the validity of the information present on these websites.

A 2013 survey disclosed that 72% of the American population searched the Internet for health and health-related information in the previous year and that one in three Americans have used the web to determine the cause of the medical problems they or someone else was experiencing (Fox & Duggan, 2013). During the 2020 COVID-19 (SARS-CoV-2) pandemic, Anderson and Vogels (2020) reported that 70% of U.S. adults participating in a Pew Research Center survey acknowledged searching the Internet for information.

The authenticity of the information that patients find on the Internet is highly variable. Authenticity and accuracy concerns increase with the realization that the content of the Internet is not regulated. Consequently, health care information on the Internet should be carefully evaluated for accuracy and reliability before developing a level of confidence in the website content (Baildon & Baildon, 2012; Cornell University Library, 2020; Kent State University Libraries, 2020; Weber et al., 2010).

Two critical indicators of authenticity and accuracy of data on an Internet site are the source of the data and the date that the site was last updated. Interestingly, 75% of people who search for health information on the Internet do not check the data source (e.g., author, credentials, and affiliation) or the date when the website was last updated (Fox, 2006). Patients need to understand that virtually anyone can publish information on the Internet and that quality control is nominal at best

(Georgetown University Library, 2020). Consequently, health care professionals provide a critical service to their patients and the patients' family members by equipping them with criteria that empower them to cull their search results effectively.

Health care websites vary in quality and accuracy of the information, and patients seeking information are often vulnerable and not in the best position to discriminate among advice offered on health care websites. Researchers from the University of Florida (Weber et al., 2010) and Michigan State University (summarized in Table 7.4) provide guidelines to assist care providers and patients to more effectively evaluate website content on the Internet.

Proactive introduction of the subject of health care information available on the Internet and exploration of the patient's experiences when seeking such information on the Internet may assist the DNP nurse to determine the patient's readiness for education about the effective use of the Internet. Empowering patients with the knowledge of how to evaluate the information on the Internet provides the opportunity for patients to openly discuss information they may have discovered and may promote a greater sense of partnership and accountability for managing their health status. Once the DNP nurse understands the information and the sources that the patient is consulting, the DNP nurse can continue the patient's education by exploring when and where such new knowledge is complementary to the medical plan of care. Box 7.1 is a selected sample of current resources that can assist the DNP nurse to become more knowledgeable regarding the Internet evaluation.

GATOR WEBSITE ASSESSMENT CRITERIA

The acronym GATOR is used to identify key elements for the assessment of websites (Weber et al., 2010). *Genuineness* of information can be assessed by exploring the stated goals and purpose of the site. For example, the Internet addresses ending with ".com" are commercial websites that are usually selling a product or service; information provided by commercial websites should be independently verified with a credible resource. Care should also be taken to examine logos and website names, which may be ingeniously designed to resemble highly trusted and credible sites.

Accuracy of the information is a second consideration. Look for a date to determine the last time the website was updated, which is often at the bottom of the page. Also, look for indications of peer review. Consider seeking verification of information on other credible websites, mainly if the content is different from other credible sites.

Trustworthiness helps to ensure the veracity and reliability of the information. Check for references from credible sources, the credentials of site authors, and whether the authors are affiliated with established and respected organizations. The presence of contact information, such as telephone numbers and email addresses, is another indication of trustworthiness.

Origin or source of the site content is an additional indicator of trustworthiness. In most cases, authorship or sponsorship by a governmental (".gov" in the United States), an academic (".edu" in the United States), a research, or a health care organization lends some assurance that the content is trustworthy.

Readability is an indicator of how well the average consumer will be able to read and understand the website content. Patients need to recognize that some sites are designed for use by health care professionals, and therefore they should seek sites that are created and maintained for use by the lay information consumer.

TABLE 7.4 Telehealth Website Evaluation

Design	Links within the site or to other reference sources are recognizable and working. The site can be accessed from multiple browsers (e.g., Chrome, Bing, Internet Explorer, Firefox, and Safari).
Literacy	The site provides information that helps the user evaluate the credibility and trust-worthiness of the site.
Information	Readability is demonstrated through the limited use of jargon; tables and charts are clear and well-labeled; less common terminology is clearly explained.
Content	The site guides the readers' evaluation and understanding of the information presented, suggests questions they may direct to health care providers, directs users to other credible sources, and so on. Advertising, if present, should be clearly distinguished from the content of the site.

Source: Whitten, P., Holtz, B., Cornacchione, J., & Wirth, C. (2011). An evaluation of telehealth websites for design, literacy, information and content. *Journal of Telemedicine and Telecare, 17*, 31–35. https://doi .org/10.1258/jtt.2010.091208

BOX 7.1 Additional Health Website Evaluation Resources

- Health on the Net Foundation: *The HON Code of Conduct for Medical and Health Web Sites* (Health on the Internet Foundation, 2019)
- Medical Library Association: Find Good Health Information (Medical Library Association, 2020). http://www.mlanet.org/resources/userguide.html
- MedLine Plus: *Evaluating Internet Health Information: A Tutorial From the National Library of Medicine* (MedlinePlus, 2020)
- National Cancer Institute: *Using Trusted Resources* (NIH: National Cancer Institute, 2020)
- National Library of Medicine: *Guide to Finding Health Information* (National Library of Medicine, 2020)
- National Network of Libraries of Medicine (NN/LM): *Evaluating Health Websites* (National Network of Libraries of Medicine, n.d.)

HUMAN FACTORS AND ERGONOMICS

Human factors, or ergonomics, focus on the relationship of the worker with the work systems with which the worker interacts. In health care, human factors examine the systems that health care practitioners employ in the process of gathering data, assessing information related directly or indirectly to the care of the patient, and the actual delivery of care. Increasingly, technology is integral to the work processes of health care practitioners and, consequently, much of human factors research and engineering centers on patient safety and reduction of medical error.

Technology changes how individuals perform and complete their work, the task itself, and the workplace in general. Despite goals such as enhanced efficiency, improved quality, and reduced medical errors, the introduction of technology presents unique challenges that are not always immediately discernible by the health care practitioner (Carayon & Wood, 2010). Without careful attention to human factors, technologies intended to improve the quality of care can introduce new risks and negative consequences (Jones et al., 2011; Koppel & Gordon, 2012; Koppel et al., 2008; Norman, 1991; Patterson et al., 2006).

Ergonomics is an applied science that defines the physical, cognitive, and organization requirements of the work environment. Ergonomics is an important consideration when designing tools or configuring the spaces in which practitioners work; one crucial goal is to promote the effective and safe use of the tools (Harrison et al., 2007; Prensky, 2001). Ergonomics is an overarching principle embedded within informatics practice, is woven throughout each ANA NI practice standard, and recognizes the criticality of promoting a safe practice environment that minimizes the likelihood of injury (ANA, 2015). Incorporating ergonomic principles in the design of new environments or the retrofit of older work environments can reduce the risk of musculoskeletal injuries or other related injuries that often occur as the result of a poorly designed setting (Nielsen & Trinkoff, 2003).

An important ergonomic consideration is the computer workstation, which must be designed to enable the user to work with the computer without strain or risk of a temporary or permanent injury. The duration of sustained use of a computer workstation and the number of people who will use the workstation influence the necessary space modifications that will promote safe use. The design of workstations that are to be used by multiple individuals requires flexibility that enables each user to adjust the station to the best position for their physical and task needs.

Expert resources are available to guide objective purchase decisions for furniture and equipment, as well as to guide workstation design. The Occupational Safety and Health Administration (OSHA) offers evidence-based checklists for the evaluation of workstations and guidance for purchasing decisions. The consultative services of certified ergonomic professionals are also available as another expert consideration when planning computer workstations (Board of Certification in Professional Ergonomics, 2015). Given the personal anguish, lost productivity, and costs associated with ergonomic work-related injuries, some organizations choose to have a certified professional ergonomics engineer as a permanent part of the staff (OSHA, 2015a, 2015b, 2015c).

USABILITY AS AN EVALUATION TOOL

Usability is a dimension of the interface between people and technology. Zhang and Walji (2014) have addressed the concept of usability with the characteristic of how useful and safe it is to accomplish a desired task. The World Health Organization (WHO) articulates an essential nuance of usability in that good usability makes "it easier to do the work in the right way" (WHO, 2008).

User-friendly is a term often used to convey the concept of usability. However, user-friendly is a subjective descriptor and is absent of objective and measurable qualities or criteria. Zhang and Walji (2014, p. 29) at the University of Texas, School of Biomedical Informatics, developed TURF, a unified conceptual framework to quantify usability. TURF is an acronym for *Task, User, Representation,* and *Function* and is "a theory for describing, explaining, and predicting usability differences; an objective method for defining, evaluating, and measuring usability; a process for designing in good usability; and a potential principle for developing EHR usability guidelines and standards." Developers and clinicians can employ TURF as a framework for redesign or enhancement of an existing EHR system. Careful discernment of the TURF framework will equip the advanced practitioner to be a much more knowledgeable participant and consumer throughout IT acquisition and implementation.

Patient safety is a fundamental consideration when purchase decisions are made for equipment that will be used in the direct or indirect care of patients. A critical facet of equipment evaluation is the assessment of the usability of that equipment. Usability addresses the design of devices with attention to how the device will be used, how people may abuse the device, the types of errors people could make while using the device, and the outcomes people wish to achieve through the use of the device (Norman, 2002; Phansalkar et al., 2010; Zhang et al., 2003). Poor usability is a significant contributor to the unexpected and unintended consequences of IT.

An important means of evaluating the usability of equipment or software is to examine and observe how the system or equipment is used. A DNP nurse can apply some of the basic principles of usability that are embodied in a process called "heuristic testing," the principles of which are described in Table 7.5. These principles may prove useful in evaluating patient care technologies in DNP clinical practice. They are applicable when evaluating equipment, software, EHR designs, and other IT equipment. Heuristic evaluation principles are not difficult to apply and can support objective comparative information based on the usability characteristics of equipment, information systems, communication systems, as well as other systems.

Usability evaluation of patient care equipment is an essential measure in reducing risk, increasing safety, and minimizing human error in the delivery of patient care. Cost, return on investment, functionality, and compatibility with the current clinical environment are important considerations in the selection of patient care equipment from various vendor options. Equally important are the usability characteristics of each vendor's product. It is crucial to select equipment that is easy to use and that actively promotes the avoidance of error. The usability characteristics demonstrated by the equipment options under consideration for purchase should have at least equal weight with the other considerations in making the purchase decision. Zhang et al. (2003) suggested a rating scale to assist in assigning weights to the evaluation outcomes, which may be helpful when comparing the same equipment from different vendors.

A properly conducted heuristic evaluation is very unlikely to find no usability problems because the sophistication of human factors engineering has not attained that level of refinement to date. The primary intent of usability evaluation is to identify the product that is most appropriate for the target clinical environment. Additionally, usability evaluation will shed light on usability problems so that users can be informed of the risks and policies can be established to reduce and mitigate the identified risks.

SAFER GUIDES

The exploration of EHR assessment and evaluation would be remiss without an investigation of the Safety Assurance Factors for EHR Resilience (SAFER) guides. The guides are a collection of evidence-based tools to evaluate the safety and safe use of EHRs (AHA, 2020). Sittig et al. (2014) and Singh et al. (2013) published the guides for organizations and clinicians to complete a proactive self-assessment of an EHR. The guides can be used to detect particular areas of vulnerability in an EHR

TABLE 7.5 Usability Evaluation Using Heuristic Principles

Heuristic Principle	Example
1. Consistency and standards	Does the application use color consistently, and do the colors make sense? Are terms clear to the user, and are they used consistently? Are buttons consistently used for the same purpose? Is there consistency in the general layout between screens?
2. Visibility of the system state	Can the user tell when the system is working? Is the next action to be taken clear to the user?
3. Match between the system and the world	Does the use of the equipment match what the user would generally expect? Does pressing buttons or turning knobs result in expected outcomes? Does the user see what is expected?
4. Minimalist	Is the information present on the screen only what is needed to inform the user? Is superfluous information on the screen? Is there a logical and sequential level of detail and action?
5. Memory load is minimized	Does the system require the user to rely on memory to use the equipment, or is the user appropriately prompted? Are examples of data entry expectations offered (e.g., YYYY/MM/DD or YY/MM/DD)? Does the system progress through a logical hierarchy?
6. Feedback that is informative	Does the system offer immediate and understandable feedback to user actions, particularly incorrect actions? Is the feedback specific, providing clear direction regarding the next step to be taken?
7. Flexibility and efficiency	Does the system support shortcuts for the experienced user? Are the information needs of the novice distinguished from those of the expert?
8. Good error messages	When the user makes an error, does the system provide a meaningful and understandable feedback message, enabling the user to learn from the error? Does the system avoid the use of error "codes" (e.g., "Error 147")? Are error messages polite and helpful (e.g., "fatal error" and "illegal action")?
9. Preventing error	Is the system designed to help the user avoid mistakes? Does the system prevent egregious errors? Are audible or pop-up messages present when the user is about to perform an incorrect action?
10. Clear closure	Is it clear when a user is at the beginning, middle, or end of a task? Is it clear when a task, or required sequence of tasks, is completed?
11. Reversible actions	Does the system allow the user to recover from mistakes? Does the system prevent serious errors? Does the system allow the user to explore the system and back out without consequences?
12. User language	Does the system use language familiar to the user? Do the terms used by the system have a standard meaning?
13. User in control	Is the user in control of the system? Does the user, not the system, initiate action?
14. Help and documentation	Does the system provide context-sensitive help? Is the help embedded in the system? Is help available when needed?

Source: Graham, M. J., Kubose, T. K., Jordan, D., Zhang, J., Johnson, T. R., & Patel, V. L. (2004). Heuristic evaluation of infusion pumps: Implications for patient safety in intensive care units. *International Journal of Medical Informatics, 73*(11–12), 773–779. https://doi.org/10.1016/j.ijmedinf.2004.08.002; Nielsen, J. (1998–2020). *10 usability heuristics for user interface design.* http://www.nngroup.com/articles/ten-usability-heuristics/; Norman, D. A. (1991). Cognitive artifacts. In J. M. Carroll (Ed.), *Designing interaction: Psychology at the human-computer interface.* Cambridge University Press; Zhang, J., Johnson, T. R., Patel, V. L., Paige, D. L., & Kubose, T. (2003). Using usability heuristics to evaluate patient safety of medical devices. *Journal of Biomedical Informatics, 36*(1–2), 23–30. https://doi.org/10.1016/s1532-0464(03)00060-1; Zhang, J., & Walji, M. (2014). TURF unified framework of EHR usability. In J. Zhang & M. Walji (Eds.), *Better EHR: Usability, workflow and cognitive support in electronic health records.* UTHealth.

and develop strategies and culture change to reduce risks. The guides address the following nine areas: high-priority practices, organizational responsibilities, contingency planning, system configuration, system interfaces, patient identification, CPOE with decision support, test results reporting and follow-up, and clinician communication. The guides are available without charge from the ONC (HealthIT. gov, 2018) website and are organized by the following groups: foundational guides (high-priority practice and organizational responsibilities); infrastructure guides (contingency planning, system configuration, and system interfaces); and clinical process guides (patient identification, CPOE with decision support, test results reporting with follow-up, and clinician communication).

Each SAFER guide includes general instructions, an introduction, and a checklist. The checklist is organized by the recommended practice domain and the implementation status. The implementation status can be designated as fully implemented, partially implemented, or not implemented. In addition, the guide includes a team worksheet to document details of the self-assessment team. The practice worksheet is the last document in the guide to offer direction when implementing a specific recommended practice.

Clinicians should be engaged in identifying opportunities for increasing and maintaining the safety of the EHR. It is imperative to evaluate an EHR for safety. The SAFER guides provide systematic methods to complete an evaluation to support safe and effective clinical use.

SUMMARY

This discussion has established the role of an informatician and the criticality of developing and maintaining an ongoing partnership between nurse informaticians and DNP nurses. This partnership can provide significant guidance to IT project design and implementation. The scope and variety of IT and how deeply it is embedded in practice and in personal and professional lives are briefly addressed. The national mandate for EHRs was discussed along with why EHR selection and implementation are such a central focus at this time.

The DNP nurse is in an excellent position to influence nursing practice, technology implementation, and the integration of practice and technology. The DNP can influence and participate in BYOD/bring your own anything (BYOx) decisions by knowledgeably articulating the challenges and providing recommendations on the management of personal mobile devices. As a respected member of the health care team, the DNP nurse can identify the informatics competency needs of colleagues and staff and can influence the understanding of the power of this essential skill, advocating for resources that will support skill-building. The DNP nurse can empower patients to become more knowledgeable and involved in health maintenance, disease prevention, and management of chronic diseases through an understanding of the personal health record (PHR) and can identify the patients in their practice that would benefit from the PHR. Such understanding will inform the patient-teaching process and assist patients in discerning authentic, accurate information on the Internet.

The DNP nurse can be a powerful advocate for practice and patient safety through promoting and participating in usability evaluation as an integral part of the information system purchase decision. Also considered was the role of the DNP nurse in the influence of technology-driven patient care equipment purchase decisions through a constructive heuristic evaluation. The heuristic evaluation metrics presented can serve as important and objective criteria to evaluate patient care equipment. The design of computer workstations is vital to avoid or minimize user injury. We established underlying workflow design issues and, more importantly, directed readers to several evidence-based websites that described ergonomically appropriate computer design.

REFERENCES

2018 updates to the EHR incentive program. (2018, August 13). https://www.icanotes.com/2018/08/13/ehr-incentive-program-updates/

Activity/fitness tracker. (2020). Techopedia. https://www.techopedia.com/definition/32502/activity-tracker

Adler-Milstein, J., DesRoches, C. M., Furukawa, M. F., Worzala, C., Charles, D., Kralovec, P., Stalley, S., & Jha, A. K. (2014). More than half of US hospitals have at least a basic EHR, but stage 2 criteria remain challenging for most. *Health Affairs, 33,* 1664–1671. https://doi.org/10.1377/hlthaff.2014.0453

Agency for Healthcare Research and Quality (2007, October). *Health information technology evaluation toolkit.* https://www.healthit.gov/unintended-consequences/sites/default/files/pdf/ModuleIIpdf1.5.pdf

Altarum Institute. (2011). *Overcoming challenges to health IT adoption in small, rural hospitals.* t.ly/LOol

American Hospital Association. (2020). SAFER Guides. https://www.aha.org/guidesreports/2014-01-16-safer-guides.

American Nurses Association. (2015). *Nursing informatics: Scope & standards of practice* (2nd ed.). Author.

Anderson, M., & Vogels, E. A. (2020, March 31). *Americans turn to technology during COVID-19 outbreak, say an outage would be a problem.* t.ly/pIqu

Ash, J. S., Berg, M., & Coiera, E. (2004). Some unintended consequences of information technology in health care: The nature of patient care information system-related errors. *Journal of the American Medical Informatics Association, 11*(2), 104–112. https://doi.org/10.1197/jamia.M1471

Baildon, M., & Baildon, R. (2012). Evaluating online sources: Helping students determine trustworthiness, readability, and usefulness. *Social Studies and the Young Learner, 24*(4), 11–14. https://eric.ed.gov/?id=EJ1002590

Bloomrosen, M., Starren, J., Lorenzi, N. M., Ash, J. S., Patel, V. L., & Shortliffe, E. H. (2011). Anticipating and addressing the unintended consequences of health IT and policy: A report from the AMIA 2009 Health Policy Meeting. *Journal of the American Medical Informatics Association, 18*(82), e90. https://doi.org/10.1136/jamia.2010.007567

Board of Certification in Professional Ergonomics. (2015). http://www.bcpe.org

Campbell, E. M., Sittig, D. F., Ash, J. S., Guappone, K. P., & Dykstra, R. H. (2006). Types of unintended consequences related to computerized provider order entry. *Journal of the American Medical Informatics Association, 13*(5), 547–556. https://doi.org/10.1197/jamia.M2042

Carayon, P., & Wood, K. E. (2010). Patient safety: The role of human factors and systems engineering. *Studies Health Technology and Informatics, 153,* 23–46. http://www.ncbi.nlm.nih.gov/pmc/articles/PMC3057365/pdf/nihms274759.pdf

Cassano, C. (2014). *The right balance—Technology and patient care. Online Journal of Nursing Informatics, 18*(3). https://www.himss.org/resources/right-balance-technology-and-patient-care

Centers for Disease Control.gov. (n.d.). *Types of evaluation.* https://www.cdc.gov/std/Program/pupestd/Types%20of%20Evaluation.pdf

Centers for Medicare & Medicaid Services. (2014). *Medicare and medicaid programs; Modifications to the medicare and medicaid electronic health record (EHR) incentive program for 2014 and other changes to the EHR incentive program; and health information technology: Revisions to the certified EHR technology definition and EHR certification changes related to standards (45 CFR Part 170; 52910).* http://www.gpo.gov/fdsys/pkg/FR-2014-09-04/pdf/2014-21021.pdf

CMS.gov. (n.d.). Data and program reports. https://www.cms.gov/Regulations-and-Guidance/Legislation/EHRIncentivePrograms/Downloads/October2018_MedicareEHRIncentivePayments.pdf

CMS.gov. (2018). *Medicare promoting interoperability program stage 3 eligible hospitals, critical access hospitals, and dual-eligible hospitals attesting to CMS objectives and measures for 2018.* t.ly/j9QD

Collins, S., Kennedy, M. K., Phillips, A., & Yen, P. Y. (2015). *Nursing informatics competencies for nurse leaders/managers: A Delphi study.* Paper presented at the AONE 2015 Annual Conference, Phoenix, AZ. t.ly/VLWm

Cornell University Library. (2020, February 14). *Evaluating web pages: Questions to consider.* http://guides.library.cornell.edu/evaluating_Web_pages

Cusack, C. M., Byrne, C., Hook, J. M., McGowan, J., Poon, E. G., & Zafar, A. (2009). *Health information technology evaluation toolkit: 2009 Update.* Agency for Healthcare Research and Quality. t.ly/JPzL

Dustin, C., Gabriel, M., & Furukawa, M. F. (2014, May 14). *Adoption of electronic health record systems among U.S. non-federal acute care hospitals: 2008–2013.* http://www.healthit.gov/sites/default/files/oncdatabrief16.pdf

Fox, S. (2006). *Online health search 2006.* http://www.pewinternet.org/2006/10/29/online-health-search-2006/

Fox, S., & Duggan, M. (2013, January 13). *Health online 2013.* http://www.-pewinternet.org/files/old-media/Files/Reports/PIP_HealthOnline.pdf

Geonnotti, K., Peikes, D., Wang, W., & Smith, J. (2013, February). *Formative evaluation: Fostering real-time adaptations and refinements to improve the effectiveness of patient-centered medical home models.* Agency for Healthcare Research and Quality.

Georgetown University Library. (2020). *Evaluating internet resources.* t.ly/HTvf

Greenes, R. A., & Shortliffe, E. H. (2009). Informatics in biomedicine and health care. *Academic Medicine, 84*(7), 818–820. https://doi.org/10.1097/ACM.0b013e3181a81f94

Gruber, D., Cummings, G. G., Leblanc, L., & Smith, D. L. (2009). Factors influencing outcomes of clinical information systems implementation. *Computers Informatics Nursing, 27*(3), 151–163. https://doi.org/10.1097/NCN.0b013e31819f7c07

Harrison, M. I., Koppel, R., & Bar-Lev, S. (2007). Unintended consequences of information technologies in healthcare—An interactive sociotechnical analysis. *Journal of the American Medical Informatics Association, 14*(5), 542–549. https://doi.org/10.1197/jamia.M2384

Health on the Internet Foundation. (2019). *The HON code of conduct for medical and health web sites.* http://www.hon.ch/HONcode/Conduct.html

HealthIT.gov. (2013a). *How can you protect and secure health information when using a mobile device?* https://www.healthit.gov/providers-professionals/how-can-you-protect-and-secure-health-information-when-using-mobile-device

HealthIT.gov. (2013b). *You, your organization, and your mobile device.* http://www.healthit.gov/providers-professionals/you-your-organization-and-your-mobile-device

HealthIT.gov. (2014). *Your mobile device and health information privacy and security.* https://www.healthit.gov/providers-professionals/your-mobile-device-and-health-information-privacy-and-securityhttps://www.healthit.gov/providers-professionals/your-mobile-device-and-health-information-privacy-and-security

HealthIT.gov. (2017). *What is a patient portal?* https://www.healthit.gov/faq/what-patient-portal

HealthIT.gov. (2018). *SAFER guide.* https://www.healthit.gov/topic/safety/safer-guideshttps://doi.org/10.2147/AMEP.S63903

HealthIT.gov. (2019). *How to attain meaningful use.* http://www.healthit.gov/providers-professionals/how-attain-meaningful-use

Institute for Healthcare Improvement. (n.d.). Science of improvement: Establishing measures. t.ly/Ou8u

Jones, S. S., Koppel, R., Ridegely, M. S., Wu, S., Palen, T. E., & Harrison, M. I. (2011). *Guide to reducing unintended consequences of electronic health records.* AHRQ Publication No. 11-0105-EF. t.ly/JcQL

Kate, M. (2017, October 2). *Meaningful use, regulatory burden costing providers billions.* https://ehrintelligence.com/news/meaningful-use-regulatory-burdens-costing-providers-billions

Kent State University Libraries. (2020). *Criteria for evaluating web resources.* http://www.library.kent.edu/criteria-evaluating-web-resources

Koppel, R., & Gordon, S. (Eds.). (2012). *First, do less harm: Confronting the inconvenient problems of patient safety.* Cornell University Press.

Koppel, R., Wetterneck, T., Telles, J. L., & Karsh, B. T. (2008). Workarounds to barcode medication administration systems: Their occurrences, causes, and threats to patient safety. *Journal of the American Medical Association, 15*(4), 408–423. https://doi.org/10.1197/jamia.M2616

Kuperman, G., & McGowan, J. (2013). Potential unintended consequences of health information exchange. *Journal of General Internal Medicine, 28*(12), 1663–1666. https://doi.org/10.1007/s11606-012-2313-0

Lewis, C. (1982). *Using the "think aloud" method in cognitive interface design*. IBM.

McLane, S., & Turley, J. P. (2011). Informaticians: How they may benefit your healthcare organization. *Journal of Nursing Administration, 41*(1), 29–35. https://doi.org/10.1097/NNA.0b013e3181fc19d6

Medical Library Association. (2020). *Find good health information*. http://www.mlanet.org/resources/userguide.html

MedlinePlus. (2020, March 6). *Evaluating Internet health information: A tutorial from the National Library of Medicine*. http://www.nlm.nih.gov/medlineplus/webeval/webeval.html

Merton, R. K. (1936). The unanticipated consequences of purposive social action. *American Sociological Review, 1*(6), 894–904. https://doi.org/10.2307/2084615. http://www.d.umn.edu/cla/faculty/jhamlin/4111/Readings/MertonSocialAction.pdf

Middleton, B., Bloomrosen, M., Dente, M. A., Hashmat, B., Koppel, R., Overhage, J. M., Payne, T. H., Rosenbloom, S. T., Weaver, C., & Zhang, J. (2013). Enhancing patient safety and quality of care by improving the usability of electronic health record systems: Recommendations from AMIA. *Journal of the American Medical Informatics Association, 20*(e1), e2–e8. https://doi.org/10.1136/amiajnl-2012-001458

National Library of Medicine. (2020, March 9). *Guide to finding health information*. https://www.nlm.nih.gov/portals/public.html#find

National Network of Libraries of Medicine. (n.d.). Evaluating health websites. https://nnlm.gov/initiatives/topics/health-websites

Nielsen, J. (1998–2020). *10 usability heuristics for user interface design*. http://www.nngroup.com/articles/ten-usability-heuristics/

Nielsen, K., & Trinkoff, A. (2003). Applying ergonomics to nurse computer workstations: Review and recommendations. *CIN: Computers, Informatics, Nursing, 21*(3), 150–157. https://doi.org/10.1097/00024665-200305000-00012

NIH: National Cancer Institute. (2020, March 16). *Using trusted resources*. http://www.cancer.gov/about-cancer/managing-care/using-trusted-resources

Norman, D. A. (1991). Cognitive artifacts. In J. M. Carroll (Ed.), *Designing interaction: Psychology at the human-computer interface*. Cambridge University Press.

Norman, D. A. (2002). *The design of everyday things*. Basic Books.

Obama, B. (2009, February 9). *Obama's prime-time press briefing*. The New York Times. http://www.nytimes.com/2009/02/09/us/politics/09text-obama.html?_r=0

Occupational Safety & Health Administration. (2015a). *Computer workstation etools*. https://www.osha.gov/SLTC/etools/computerworkstations/

Occupational Safety & Health Administration. (2015b). *Computer workstation: Evaluation checklist*. https://www.osha.gov/SLTC/etools/computerworkstations/checklist_evaluation.html

Occupational Safety & Health Administration. (2015c). *Computer workstation: Purchase checklist*. https://www.osha.gov/SLTC/etools/computerworkstations/checklist_-purchasing_guide.html

Office of the National Coordinator for Health Information Technology. (n.d.). *2018 Report to Congress annual update on the nationwide system for the electronic use and exchange of health information*. https://www.healthit.gov/sites/default/files/page/2018-12/2018-HITECH-report-to-congress.pdf

Office of the National Coordinator for Health Information Technology. (2020, February). Strategy on reducing regulatory and administrative burden relating to the use of health IT and EHRs. https://www.healthit.gov/sites/default/files/page/2020-02/BurdenReport_0.pdf

Oxford University Press. (2020). *Murphy's law*. https://www.oxfordreference.com/view/10.1093/oi/authority.20110803100217459

Parker, C. D. (2014, November 20). *Evolution of revolution? Smartphone use in nursing practice*. http://www.americannursetoday.com/evolution-revolution-smartphone-use-nursing-practice/

Patterson, E. S., Rogers, M. L., Chapman, R. J., & Render, M. L. (2006). Compliance with intended use of bar code medication administration in acute and long-term care: An observational study. *Human Factors, 48*(1), 15–22. https://doi.org/10.1518/001872006776412234

Phansalkar, S., Edworthy, J., Hellier, E., Seger, D. L., Schedlbauer, A., Avery, A. J., & Bates, D. W. (2010). A review of human factors principles for the design and implementation of medication safety alerts in clinical information systems. *Journal of the American Medical Informatics Association, 17*(5), 493–501. https://doi.org/10.1136/jamia.2010.005264

Prensky, M. (2001). Digital natives, digital immigrants. *On the Horizon (Lincoln, NCB University Press), 9*(5), 1–6. https://doi.org/10.1108/10748120110424816

Reilly, W. J. (1931). *The law of retail gravitation*. Knickerbocker Press.

Reisman, M. (2017). EHRs: The challenge of making electronic data usable and interoperable. *Pharmacy & Therapeutics, 42*(9), 572–575.

Singh, H., Ash, J. S., & Sittig, D. F. (2013). Safety assurance factors for electronic health record resilience (SAFER): Study protocol. *BMC Medical Informatics and Decision Making, 13*(4). https://doi.org/10.1186/1472-6947-13-46

Sittig, D. F., & Ash, J. S. (Eds.). (2011). *Clinical information systems: Overcoming adverse consequences.* Jones and Bartlett Publishers.

Sittig, D. F., Ash, J. S., & Singh, H. (2014). The SAFER Guides: Empowering organizations to improve the safety and effectiveness of electronic health records. *The American Journal of Managed Care, 20*(5), 418–423. t.ly/YjVL

Song, V., & Stolyar, B. (2019, October 14). *How we test fitness trackers.* PC. https://www.pcmag.com/about/how-we-test-fitness-trackers

Spok. (2015). *BYOD trends in healthcare: An industry snapshot.* Retrieved http://cloud.spok.com/IB-AMER-BYOD-2015-Survey.pdf

Spyglass Consulting Group. (2014a). *Healthcare without bounds: Point of care communications for physicians 2014.* http://www.spyglass-consulting.com/Abstracts/Spyglass_PCOM_Physician2014_abstract.pdf

Spyglass Consulting Group. (2014b). *Healthcare without bounds: Point of care communications for nursing 2014.* http://spyglass-consulting.com/wp_PCOMM_Nursing_2014.html

Spyglass Consulting Group. (2016). *Healthcare without bounds: Point of care communications for nursing 2016.* http://www.spyglass-consulting.com/Abstracts/Spyglass_PCOM_Nursing2016_abstract.pdf

Stages of promoting interoperability programs: First year demonstrating meaningful use. (n.d.). https://www.cms.gov/Regulations-and-Guidance/Legislation/EHRIncentivePrograms/Downloads/Stages_ofMeaningfulUseTable.pdf

Tenner, E. (1997). *Why things bite back: Technology and the revenge of unintended consequences.* Vintage Books.

U.S. Government Publishing Office. (2015, September 9). *Health information technology standards, implementation specifications, and certification criteria and certification programs for health information technology.* Electronic code of federal regulations. http://www.ecfr.gov/cgi-bin/retrieveECFR?gp=&SID=c494467846b7f32b4bf2ee8526b425a3&r= PART&n=pt45.1.170

Vogels, E. A. (2020, January 9). *About one-in-five Americans use a smart watch or fitness tracker.* Fact Tank: News in the Numbers. https://www.pewresearch.org/fact-tank/2020/01/09/about-one-in-five-americans-use-a-smart-watch-or-fitness-tracker/

Weber, B. A., Derrico, D. J., Yoon, S. L., & Sherwill-Navarro, P. (2010). Educating patients to evaluate web-based health care information: The GATOR approach to healthy surfing. *Journal of Clinical Nursing, 19,* 1371–1377. https://doi.org/10.1111/j.1365-2702.2008.02762.x

Wharton, C., Bradford, J., Jefferies, R., Franzke, M. (1992). *Applying cognitive walkthroughs to more complex user interfaces: experiences, issues, and recommendations. CHI '92: Proceedings of the SIGCHI Conference on Human Factors in Computing Systems,* pp. 381–388. https://doi.org/10.1145/142750.142864

World Health Organization. (2008, June). *What is human factors and why is it important to patient safety?* http://www.who.int/patientsafety/education/curriculum/who_mc_topic-2.pdf

Xie, J., Wen, D., Liang, L., Jia, Y., Gao, L., & Lei, J. (2018). Evaluating the validity of current mainstream wearable devices in fitness tracking under various physical activities: Comparative study. *JMIR Mhealth Uhealth, 6*(4), e94. https://doi.org/10.2196/mhealth.9754

Zhang, J., Johnson, T. R., Patel, V. L., Paige, D. L., & Kubose, T. (2003). Using usability heuristics to evaluate patient safety of medical devices. *Journal of Biomedical Informatics, 36*(1–2), 23–30. https://doi.org/10.1016/s1532-0464(03)00060-1

Zhang, J., & Walji, M. (2014). TURF unified framework of EHR usability. In J. Zhang & M. Walji (Eds.), *Better EHR: Usability, workflow and cognitive support in electronic health records.* UTHealth.

EIGHT

PLANNING A PROGRAM OR PROJECT EVALUATION

Joanne V. Hickey

One of the great mistakes is to judge policies and programs by their intentions rather than their results.
—*Milton Friedman*

INTRODUCTION

The historical roots of systematic evaluation go back to the 17th century, whereas its contemporary interpretation coalesced in the 20th century (Alkin, 2004). Social science research methods for program evaluation evolved parallel to the growth and refinement of general evaluation research methods, which in turn followed ideological, political, and demographic trends (Rossi et al., 2014, p. 8). Following World War II, a number of major federal and privately funded programs in housing, hospital, and health care were launched, which naturally led to a need to judge the effectiveness and value of these programs. The methodologies, the information acquired through program evaluation, and the use of the acquired information for decision-making and action have developed to a point where evaluation is an intrinsic component of most programs. Most programs are well intended and are designed in what appears plausible and reasonable to address a problem. Unfortunately, good intentions and intuitive plausible interventions do not necessarily lead to better outcomes (Rossi et al., 2019, p. 4). Therefore, not only is evaluation critical, but it should also be conducted in a systematic science-based manner to support the reliability and validity of the results. Evidence-based practices and best practices are critical to sound evaluation.

Keep in mind the comparison of the terms *program* and *project* as they apply to evaluation. A *program* is a group of clear, related, complementary activities that are intended to achieve a desired outcome among the target group(s) (McGuire, 2016). Programs tend to be larger in scope and purpose. A *project* is a group of activities intended to achieve a specific goal, typically over a shorter period, and is more specific and narrower in focus and scope than a program (McGuire, 2016). Doctor of Nursing Practice (DNP) projects, and many unit-based projects, are focused on smaller, focused, and specific undertakings. Although project and program evaluations all follow basic principles and models for evaluation, *project* evaluations require much less detail and follow a simpler evaluation design. However, in reviewing the literature, the term *program evaluation* is used most frequently to refer to both program and project evaluations. In this chapter, both terms are used in ways that seem appropriate to the discussion.

DNP nurses are often enlisted to conduct program evaluations either as the leader or as a member of an evaluation team. The program evaluated may be small, such as for a DNP student project or comprehensive management of a heart failure patient population in a particular clinic, or large, such as a mental health care program offered by interprofessional teams at multiple facilities within a major health care system.

Program evaluation is an important competency for DNP nurses to develop so that they can influence health care delivery decision-making and enhance cost-effective high-quality outcomes for populations. Much has been written about program evaluation and many different views have been expressed. This chapter addresses the planning, design, implementation, and use of comprehensive program evaluation with the DNP evaluator in mind. It discusses the types of evaluations they will most likely conduct. The information is designed to be practical and useful. In this chapter, the term *evaluator* is used to refer to the person leading the evaluation. Also included are specific references made to DNP student projects and smaller unit-based or organizational projects for purposes of clarity.

EVALUATION RESEARCH VERSUS EVALUATION IN QUALITY IMPROVEMENT

What can often be confusing is the difference between an evaluation designed to be evaluation research and an evaluation designed to evaluate a project based on criteria designed to address a local problem. There is no uniformly accepted definition of what constitutes evaluation research. One basic definition is "the use of scientific methods to measure the implementation and outcomes of programs for decision-making purposes" (Rutman 1984, p. 10). This underscores the methods and intent of all evaluation. Evaluation research can also be described as a type of study that uses standard social research assessment and methodologies for evaluation of social programs (Powell, 2006).

This definition comes from the perspective of the social sciences and addresses the common components of evaluation. DNP students and graduates are not being prepared as social science researchers, but rather as health care professionals who must evaluate projects and smaller programs for it value to a specific setting and health care problem.

Whereas research is focused on generating new information that is generalizable, evaluation can also be focused on a project to determine its ability to influence change or quality improvement in a given setting and context. Evaluation, in this sense, is not designed for generalizability. The knowledge generated is used for decision-making to address a local problem within a specific context. This does not mean that this form of evaluation does not follow scientific methods or evaluation steps. By comparison, the differences between the two are difference in intent, the degree of rigor may be less stringent, and the scope of the evaluation is smaller. The DNP project and smaller unit-based or systems-based projects are more aligned with quality improvement science and its methods rather than evaluation research.

The following discussion provides an overview of some of the more frequently used research designs for program evaluation. An *experimental design* can establish causality, that is, a cause-and-effect relationship between the program and attainment of program objectives. This is possible because of three characteristics inherent in an experimental design: random assignment, control, and manipulation. Well-conducted experimental studies provide solid evidence that a program made a significant difference to a population. DNP nurses should keep in mind, however, that these studies have some drawbacks. They are conducted under ideal conditions with multiple controls to limit variations. They may be expensive and difficult to implement. They may also not be feasible because of ethical considerations. Health care studies that include experimental designs are frequently referred to as randomized controlled trials (RCTs).

A *quasi-experimental design* is less robust than an experimental design and cannot establish causality because it lacks one or more of the characteristics of an experimental design. Quasi-experimental studies are frequently used in health care evaluation because they are more feasible, less expensive, and usually easier to conduct in a real-world setting. A well-conducted quasi-experimental study will provide evidence that there is a significant association between a program and an outcome.

Observational designs are *nonexperimental* but may still offer important information if they are congruent with the purpose, perspective, and framework of the evaluation. Observational designs include descriptive studies, surveys, correlational studies, and case studies (LoBiondo-Wood & Haber, 2017).

DNP nurses may also want to consider using a *goal-based evaluation* (CDC, 2011). This design is constructed to measure the success of a program's goals as they were initially described by the program's developers. Closely related is the *objectives-oriented evaluation*, which is widely used in education (Fitzpatrick et al., 2004, p. 80). Both designs may incorporate evidence-based criteria, standards, and benchmarks into the development of program goals and objectives.

PROGRAM EVALUATION DEFINED

Program evaluation is a special subset of evaluation that utilizes the same general principles of evaluation but with a focus on programs. A *program* is "a set of resources and activities directed toward one or more common goals, typically under the direction of a single manager or management team. A program may consist of a limited set of activities in one agency or a complex set of activities implemented at many sites by two or more levels of an organization and by a set of public, nonprofit, and even private providers" (Wholey et al., 2010, p. 5). *Program evaluation* is the application of systematic methods to address questions about program operations and results. It may include ongoing monitoring of a program as well as a one-time study of program processes, outcomes, or program impact. It is the systematic assessment of the processes and outcomes of a program with the intent of furthering its development, improvement, and future. The approaches used for program evaluation are based on social science research methodologies and professional standards. The methods of program evaluation provide processes and tools that any evaluator can utilize to acquire valid, reliable, and credible data to address a variety of questions about the performance of programs (Wholey et al., 2010, p. 6).

Quality evaluations should provide useful information about program functioning that can contribute to program improvement (Kellogg, 2004). Program evaluation, just as any other evaluation, is designed to support decision-making and action about the program. Successful program planning and implementation require an evaluator who knows not only what the program expects to achieve, but also how it plans to achieve those outcomes. The evaluator must understand the principles on which a program is based (Weiss, 1998). Discussion about *how* and *why* a program is or is not successful requires credible evidence and attention to the means by which outcomes and impacts are produced. An evaluation serves two purposes. It elucidates how a program is working now and provides direction on how it can be improved in the future. The intent may be to help improve a program or to compare its value with other programs competing for resources. In some instances, it may be used to determine whether a program will continue or be terminated.

The evaluation of a program should gain knowledge about its effect and should help sponsors understand the relative contributions of its components. In general, program evaluation focuses not only on identifying the merits of the program, but also on deficiencies or areas for improvement to give stakeholders information that will help them make decisions regarding what to do next. To be most useful, program evaluation needs to equip stakeholders with knowledge of those program elements that are working well and those that are not. Program evaluation should facilitate stakeholders' search for appropriate actions for addressing problems and improving programs (Chen, 2005, p. 6).

Evaluation examines specific programs or interventions, proposed or in place, to measure their effectiveness in achieving agreed upon goals (e.g., does clinic's A treatment program reduce disease B deaths). Evaluators employ many of the same qualitative and quantitative methodologies used by researchers, and there is comparable rigor in evaluation. Evaluation is more client focused than research, and evaluators work closely with program staff and stakeholders to create and execute an evaluation plan that addresses the particular needs of the program. By its very nature, evaluation requires judgments to be made. Its purpose is to facilitate a program's development, implementation, and improvement by examining its processes and/or outcomes on the basis of some established criteria. According to a founding father of evaluation, the purpose of evaluation is not to prove but to improve (Stufflebeam et al., 1971).

Differentiation can also be made between evaluation and assessment, primarily regarding focus. Evaluation tends to examine a program's structure and process in relation to outcome and established criteria. Assessment is focused more on measuring the performance of component individuals or groups by appraising their skill levels on a variable of interest such as compliance with guidelines. In the next section, a discussion of types of program evaluation is provided that offers different perspectives for evaluation.

TYPES OF PROGRAM EVALUATION

Experts categorize types of evaluation in a variety of ways. Although terminology may differ, the fundamental concepts are similar, and much of the difference in terminology relates to the maturity of the program under scrutiny. Programs move through various stages of development. Program evaluation can address the performance of a program at any stage. The type of program evaluation conducted should align with the program's maturity (e.g., developmental, implementation, or completion), the purpose of conducting the evaluation, and the questions that it seeks to answer. The purpose of the evaluation points to the type of evaluation that is needed and helps the evaluator craft the appropriate design.

The following are common types of evaluation, as described by the Environmental Protection Agency (EPA). One may wonder how an evaluation model employed by such a huge agency, such as the EPA, is useful to the smaller scale projects that a DNP nurse might conduct. The answer is that the principles are similar regardless of whether one is conducting a large or small evaluation. Many other similar classifications are available from other organizations. Most evaluations may fall into more than one category, as noted in what follows (EPA, 2016). An evaluation may be focused on just one aspect of a program or may require investigation of all categories.

- *Design evaluation*—conducted early in the planning stages or implementation phase of a program to define the scope of a program or project and to identify appropriate goals and objectives. Design evaluations can also be used to pretest ideas and strategies.
- *Process evaluation*—examines whether a program or process is implemented as designed or operating as intended and identifies opportunities for improvement. Process evaluations often begin with an analysis of how a program currently operates. Process evaluations may also assess whether program activities and outputs conform to statutory and regulatory requirements, policies, program designs, customer expectations, and evidence-based practices.
- *Outcome evaluation*—examines the results of a program (intended or unintended) to determine the reasons for any differences between the outcomes and the program's stated goals and objectives. Outcome evaluations often examine program processes and activities to better understand how outcomes are achieved and how quality, efficiency, and productivity could be improved.
- *Impact evaluation*—a subset of an outcome evaluation is impact evaluation. It assesses the causal links between program activities and outcomes by comparing the observed outcomes with an estimate of what would have happened if the program had not existed.
- *Cost-effectiveness evaluation*—identifies program benefits, outputs, or outcomes and calculates the internal and external costs of the program.

Evaluations can also be classified as formative or summative (Chen, 2005, p. 47; Wholey et al., 2010, pp. 8–9), ongoing or stand-alone, objective observer or participatory, goal based or goal free, quantitative or qualitative, problem oriented or non–problem oriented. *Formative evaluation* is defined as an evaluation intended to furnish information for guiding program improvement that occurs during the conduct of the evaluation (Scriven, 1991). It is intended to monitor and evaluate the progress of the program and offers the opportunity to make changes in the program. *Summative evaluation* is defined as an evaluation conducted at the end of the evaluation to determine whether the expected outcomes have been achieved (1991). Often, both formative and summative evaluations are conducted. The value of the formative evaluation is that it allows the evaluator to examine how certain parts of the evaluation are proceeding so that a course correction can be made, as needed.

DOMAINS OF PROGRAM EVALUATION

Rossi et al. (2019) suggest that evaluation typically involves one or more of five program domains as a program matures through a sequence of developmental stages that include the need for the program, the design of the program, program implementation and services delivery, program impact or outcomes, and program efficiency and cost. Each domain will be briefly discussed from the perspective of relevance to nursing.

Need for the Program

A fundamental question to be answered in evaluating a program, either one being planned or one that exists, is the question "Is there a need for the program?" Begin by identifying the problem that is being addressed. The evidence to help identify the problem can come from a number of sources, such as interviews with stakeholders, organizational databases, national benchmarks/standards, and observation. Both quantitative and qualitative data are usually included.

Problem identification should be conducted systematically and with an openness of mind to follow the data. It takes an investment of time but is a critical step that cannot be overlooked or short-circuited. What may seem like the problem may only be a symptom of the underlying reality. Tools such as a root cause analysis, SWOT analysis, fishbone diagram, driver diagram, or brainstorming may help to clearly identify the problem causality. These tools and others are available through the Institute of Healthcare Improvement (IHI; http://www.ihi.org/). Unless the true problem and its cause are identified, it most likely will not be resolved.

Once the problem has been clearly and accurately identified, a needs assessment is conducted. A *needs assessment* is a type of evaluation that is conducted to determine the need for a program, the current methods for addressing that need, the existing gaps, and the proposed methods to alleviate the problem (Altschuld & Kumar, 2010; McGuire, 2016). The answers to a number of questions such as the following help to guide a needs assessment (Rutman, 1984; Watkins et al., 2012):

- What are the characteristics (e.g., signs, symptoms) and magnitude of the problem?
- What groups or entities (e.g., emergency department, discharge practices) are affected by the problem?
- What unmet needs or gaps are created by this problem? (gap analysis)
- What are the causes of this problem? (fishbone diagram)
- What solutions are proposed for the resolution of the problem by stakeholders?
- What kind of program is needed to solve the problem?
- What organizational, systems, or unit contextual characteristics are influencing the problem? (assessment of culture)

Design

Program design is a process of developing a program, including the plan of actions and activities that result in the expected outcomes. It is most often an iterative process, involving investigation, consultation, initial design, testing, and redesign (McGuire, 2016). The final design of the evaluation is based on a clear understanding of the program theory that guides selection of the design and its actions. *Program theory* is the knowledge about the problem, contributing factors, population, and clinical setting as well as the assumptions and expectations about how the program should work in order to achieve its expected outcomes (Rogers, 2020; Rossi et al., 2019, p. 19). Simply stated, *program theory* includes the assumptions, based on evidence, about why a program should result in the intended outcomes. It is created during the planning stage of a new program or revised during implementation when new information is acquired. The program theory can be developed by the program staff, an external evaluator, program designers, or collaboration with the community. For example, evaluators should keep in mind that an evaluation must be tailored to the political and organizational context of the program being examined.

Although programs vary in purpose and scope, the basic components of a program are essentially the same. All programs have objectives and a set of activities carried out by evaluator, staff, and participants that are intended to achieve those objectives. Programs operate within an organization and often within a broader system of similar programs (Bowen, 2012; McGuire, 2016).

Another term encountered in the evaluation literature is *theory of change,* which is described by McGuire (2016; design and methodology) as being the same as a program theory. The term is also often used interchangeably with the term *logic model* in the evaluation literature. In addition to describing the logic of a program, the theory of change should explain the underlying theory of why a program is expected to work (McGuire, 2016). The information included in the program theory can be in written format or diagrammed in a logic model that includes inputs, processes, outputs, outcomes, and impact. In short, the program theory is how you conceptualize the problem with all of its caveats and the interventions that you believe are needed to correct the problem.

In order to develop the program theory for the evaluation, an assessment is needed before a design can be developed to achieve the desired outcomes (Rogers, 2020). The following questions should help to guide that assessment:

- Are your assumptions and theory about the program and how it should work valid?
- Have you included all relevant information in developing the theory?
- What outcomes are you trying to achieve? Do they flow logically from the problem to the program theory, interventions, and outcomes?
- Have you targeted the appropriate population or entities for the interventions?
- What are the specific interventions that you plan to deliver, and are they appropriate and reasonable for the given setting?
- How is the program sequentially organized to achieve the outcomes? Are they realistic?
- Who will actually do the interventions, and is that adequate to implement the program?
- What resources are needed for the interventions, and are they reasonable?

The program design includes several elements that ground the conduct of the evaluation. These elements apply both to small and large programs that are undertaken. The first is the *need for the program* within the context of the given setting in which the program will be implemented. An example is the unmet needs of a population such as diabetics for comprehensive eye, kidney, and blood pressure management. Second, the *program objectives and outcomes* that the program is intended to accomplish must be clearly stated and measurable. An example of an expected outcome is that all patients seen in the diabetic clinic will have a yearly eye examination, assessment of kidney function, and blood pressure screening. Third, *program components,* which are the logically sequenced interconnected activities, are described in enough detail to guide the intervention processes. Fourth, the *cost/ budget/funding* of the program is addressed to determine the true cost, including "in kind" contributions. If the program cannot be supported within the current organizational structure, determine what funding opportunities might be available to support the program. Fifth, *responsibility for administering and leading the program* is clearly defined, including who is responsible and accountable for decision-making in the execution of the program (McGuire, 2016).

Implementation

Once a reasonable program theory designed to address the program intent has been developed, implementation is the next step. Although the designers may believe that their design is comprehensive and clearly articulated and written, it remains to be seen how workable the design plan is in achieving outcomes. During implementation, a number of pitfalls are common, such as design flaws that make execution impossible in the real world of practice, wrong personnel in place, poor management, political interference, or inadequate resources. The implementation can be evaluated from two perspectives of assessment of the program processes and ongoing program monitoring.

Assessment of program processes is addressed through process evaluation. *Process evaluation* is a method to monitor and document program implementation and determine how successfully the program followed the intended strategies and activities. It helps evaluators understand the relationship between specific program elements and program outcomes (Saunders et al., 2005). Process evaluation is a form of data gathering and measurement and constitutes one component of a comprehensive program evaluation plan

When developing a process evaluation plan, a number of important points should be considered, including (a) understanding the program and how it is intended to work; (b) defining the purposes of the process evaluation; and (c) considering program characteristics and context and how they may influence implementation (Saunders et al., 2005). A number of process evaluation models have been developed. One example is a six-step process evaluation model that includes the following: (a) describe the program; (b) describe complete and acceptable program delivery; (c) develop a potential list of questions; (d) determine implementation methods; (e) consider program resources, context, and characteristics; and (f) finalize the process evaluation plan (Saunders et al., 2005). Each step requires considerable detail and is best developed by a team of multidisciplinary stakeholders. Assessment of the implementation of a program also refers to fidelity. Implementation *fidelity* is "the degree to which programs are implemented as intended by the program developers" (Dusenbury et al., 2003). Failure to follow the intended implementation plan may lead to program goals and outcomes not being achieved. When the process evaluation is an ongoing component, it is referred to as *program monitoring* (Rossi et al., 2019, p. 21). Its area of interest is the ongoing performance of the program. Sample questions that might be of interest in implementation evaluation could include the following:

- Are the intended activities being delivered to the intended audience? If not, who is being missed?
- Are intended procedures, policies, and activities being followed as intended?
- Do the program activities place undue burden or distress on the recipient or deliverer?
- What kind of feedback is being received about the program? Is it being analyzed, and are changes being made as appropriate?
- Are the administrative, organizational, and personnel functions and responsibilities well managed?

A process evaluation can be conducted as a formative or summative evaluation; it is an iterative process that recognizes that there may be a need for change in implementation to achieve program goals based on collected data. Process evaluation generates data that can be used for both formative and summative purposes. Formative use of data involves using process evaluation data to fine-tune or tweak the program in order to keep the program on track (Devaney & Rossi, 1997; Helitzer et al., 2000; Viadro et al., 1997). Summative uses of process evaluation data involve making a judgment about the extent to which the intervention was implemented as planned and reached intended participants (Devaney & Rossi, 1997; Helitzer et al., 2000). Reports in the form of oral presentations, dashboards, charts, and other forms of communications are helpful in keeping all stakeholders informed and tracking progress. In summary, process evaluation systematically investigates how well a program is doing and helps evaluators determine why a program was successful or not.

Program Impact

Impact evaluation is an evaluation that makes a causal link between a program or intervention and a set of outcomes by answering the question: What is the impact (or causal effect) of a program on an outcome of interest (Gertler et al., 2016, p. 328)? It is an assessment of a program's effectiveness in achieving its ultimate goals and outcomes. Examples of evaluation questions that may be addressed in an impact evaluation could include the following (Rossi et al., 2019):

- Are the program objectives and outcomes being achieved?
- Are trends in data moving in the right direction?
- Is the program effective and having positive effects on the target recipients? What are those effects?
- Are there any unintended outcomes (both positive and negative) from the program, and what are they?
- Are the results of the dose of the intervention the same for all recipients, or are there differences? Why are there differences?
- Has the program addressed/alleviated the problem it was designed to correct?
- Has sufficient time passed to appreciate the full effect and value of the program? If not, how much more time is needed?

Impact evaluation is an attempt to understand the effect of the program, including unintended consequences (e.g., both positive and negative) at a given point in time. This evaluation must be free of bias and based on data driving the evaluation questions rather than the hopes and expected outcomes of the program designers. The information gained from an impact evaluation can influence ongoing support of the program and funding.

Cost Analysis and Efficiency Assessment

Cost-benefit analysis estimates the total expected benefits of a program and compares them with its total expected costs. It seeks to quantify all of the costs and benefits of a program in monetary terms and assesses whether benefits outweigh costs (Gertler et al., 2016, p. 326). Determining whether the benefits outweigh the costs examines comparative data of costs incurred without the program as compared with the costs related to program benefits. It requires analysis of cost and benefit not only for the present, but also for future milestones. The judgments made are often critical for the viability of the program for continuing, reducing, or eliminating funding. *Efficiency assessment* considers the relationship between a program's costs and its effectiveness. According to Rossi et al. (2019), efficiency assessment may take the form of either cost–benefit analysis or cost-effectiveness analysis. *Cost-effectiveness analysis* compares the relative cost of two or more programs or program alternatives in terms of reaching a common outcome, such as effectiveness in preventing pressure ulcers. Common questions that may guide this analysis might include:

- What are the actual total costs of operating the program, and who pays for these costs?
- Are resources used efficiently without waste or excess?
- Is the cost reasonable in comparison with the magnitude or monetary value of the benefits?
- Are other options available that provide equivalent benefits at less cost? If so, what are they?
- Is the program meeting a necessary societal need for a vulnerable or underserved population? If so, what is it?

Cost analysis and efficiency analysis are the practical questions important to decision and policy makers as programs vie for limited resources in a complex practice and health care delivery system.

PLANNING AN EVALUATION OF A PROGRAM OR PROJECT

In approaching the planning of a project or program evaluation, several modifying considerations of evaluation should be kept in mind. First, evaluation has two distinct yet closely related components that include a description of program performance and the standards or criteria for judging the performance of the program (Rossi et al., 2019, p. 29). As you consider the purpose and design of the evaluation, consider how you will evaluate performance and the criteria that you will use for that evaluation. What standards or criteria of performance are available? If these are available, who has published them and are they credible? The credibility of standards is often related to the best current evidence-based practices and best practices. Because of the nature of evaluation of specific questions, the evaluator may have to design performance standards that will be used to make judgments. These standards must be based on the best evidence and practices available. Think also about the practicality and availability of data that you will need to judge performance. Are these data easily available and accessible, and do these data clearly relate to performance criteria? Be focused on what data you need to collect.

A second consideration is how evaluation models compare with models for other purposes such as those related to middle range theories. Although most evaluation models are grounded in some theoretical frameworks, in practical terms, they tend to be less prescriptive, functioning often as a loose framework or structure for the evaluation. Evaluation models tend to guide thinking, but the evaluator must customize it to their needs. For example, a key component of the model is the purpose of the evaluation. Often, the model authors pose a number of general questions that relate to purpose. However, the evaluator must revise and customize these trigger questions so they apply to the specific evaluation planned. Sometimes these suggested questions are not applicable and thus should not be used.

Third, the size, scope, and details of an evaluation can vary. Recall the definition of a project as compared with a program, which is a much larger and detailed undertaking. Although project and program evaluations all follow basic principles and models for evaluation, project evaluations require much less detail and follow a simpler evaluation design.

Fourth, evaluation is not a linear process, in which one component is completed before the next is considered. Rather, there is a back and forth nature to the process; that is, as the planning proceeds, there is a need to return to previous developed components to make changes for clarity, flow, changing/modifying activities, and sequencing. It is the nature of the work.

Before one commits to conducting an evaluation, five basic questions should be answered (Wholey et al., 2010, pp. 7–8). First, can the results of the evaluation influence decisions about the program? Second, can the evaluation be conducted in time to be useful? Third, is the program/project significant enough to merit evaluation? Fourth, is the program/project performance viewed as problematic? Fifth, where is the program/project in its developmental life span? Rossi et al. (2019) suggests an additional question that addresses why the evaluation is being conducted. Reasons such as political pressure or a desire to eliminate the program may be the motivating factor for a stakeholder or decision makers to request an evaluation. This raises ethical concerns about the evaluation for the evaluator. The real reasons for the requested evaluation and whatever information is conveyed to the evaluator must be congruent. It will be up to the evaluator to determine the purity of motives for the evaluation.

An evaluation can answer many questions and assume many forms, not all of which are useful. Tailoring the evaluation to the needs of the stakeholders is perhaps the most important work of the evaluator. The evaluator collaborates with those requesting the evaluation and the recipients of the information to identify questions of value to the stakeholders that the evaluation needs to answer about the program/project. This is critical because if the evaluation does not address what is truly important to the stakeholders, it will have little or no value (Grembowski, 2001, p. 17).

There are many reasons to conduct a program evaluation and many types of programs previously discussed in the chapter. Frameworks, designs, and methods vary, and some are more congruent to one type of evaluation than another. As a result, the stages in program evaluation can be approached in a variety of ways; however, they generally fall into three categories: planning, implementation, and dissemination. The investment of time and energy in planning sets the course for the implementation and dissemination phase.

BASIC COMPONENTS OF PLANNING

Numerous models are available that outline the steps of planning. Although there are variations in labeling, all models address similar components to be included. Several interrelated components compose the evaluation plan process and can be classified as follows: (a) *purpose and scope*; (b) *design and methodology*; (c) *data collection, acquisition, and management*; (d) *data analysis and interpretation*; (e) *project management*; and (f) *dissemination*.

As noted previously, an evaluation is usually a collaborative process and brings together professionals with the expertise and interest required to evaluate a health care program. This is true of both large program and smaller project evaluations. For smaller project evaluations, the evaluator includes team members who represent the various stakeholders affected by the program/project and often represent various clinical areas and administrative personnel. However, you need a team, albeit small, to evaluate a project. Forming an effective team is often the key determinant of success regardless of the size of the program/project being evaluated. In Chapter 11, the different kinds of teams are discussed. Traditional teams are members who work together on a regular basis. However, in evaluation, members may come together periodically as needed. This is particularly true in the conduct of a DNP project. However, regardless of the type of team established, frequent and clear communications pathways must be maintained. An evaluation team that spends time to carefully plan and individualize the evaluation to the needs of stakeholders is more likely to conduct a meaningful evaluation. Each of the planning components is discussed in what follows.

Purpose and Scope

All members of the team should participate in determining and clarifying the purpose of the evaluation. The following are questions that can guide the discussion. Who requested the evaluation? Is the evaluation for internal and/or external use? Is the evaluation the result of an adverse event, or is it being made in response to an accrediting agency? What aspect of the program are we going to evaluate? What questions does the evaluation hope to answer? Who will use this evaluation? How will they use it? Why is the evaluation being conducted?

Perspective determines the scope and depth of an evaluation. Will the evaluation take the viewpoint of an organization (e.g., such as a hospital, clinic, continuous care, residential, community, or school of nursing), or will it take a more societal community approach (e.g., city, county, state, nation, or international)? The purpose and perspective will influence the design and methods. Perspective will also affect the design, required resources, cost, and the timeline for completion of the evaluation.

Design and Methodology

The decisions made about the purpose and perspective guide the selection of the design and methods (Wholey et al., 2010). *Design* refers to how the evaluation's questions, methods, and overall processes are constructed and organized. An organization with a clear focus helps those who will conduct the evaluation determine who will do what and what will be done with the findings. Furthermore, the process of creating and expressing a clear design will highlight ways that stakeholders can improve the evaluation and facilitate the use of the results. A series of questions such as those in the following list can help shape the design:

- For what purpose(s) is the evaluation being conducted; that is, what do you want to be able to decide as a result of the evaluation?
- Who is the intended audience (policy makers, chief nursing officers [CNO], chief executive officer, program directors, physicians, nurses)?
- What kinds of information are needed to make the decisions you need to make and/or to inform your intended audiences? With the varied intended audiences in mind, what kind of information does each group need to understand (its inputs, activities, and outputs): the product or program, strengths and weaknesses of the product or program, benefits to customers or clients (outcomes), or how the product or program failed and why?
- What are the sources from which the information should be collected (e.g., employees, providers, administrators, patients/clients, family members, program documentation, registries, and databases)?
- How can that information be collected efficiently (e.g., using questionnaires or interviews, examining documentation, observing patients or providers, focus groups)?
- What is the timeline (when is the information needed)?
- What resources are available to collect the information?

A model or framework can be used as part of the design process and provides a general roadmap for the evaluation; however, it must be congruent with its purpose and perspective. As part of the planning process, the team reviews models and frameworks to determine the best fit for evaluating the program under study. For example, the effectiveness–efficiency–equity framework (Aday et al., 2004) is frequently used for evaluating health policy but may not be appropriate for studying an educational program. The CIPP model context, input, process, and product, which is often applied in educational settings, would be a good choice in evaluating a service-learning program (Zhang et al., 2011). Logic models are generic and offer flexibility for matching with a number of both projects and program evaluation needs. The logic model is often used by DNP students to evaluate their DNP projects as well as for smaller unit-based projects.

Data Collection, Acquisition, and Management

After selecting and developing a design, the evaluation team may proceed to make decisions about required data, including data collection processes, data acquisition, and data management. These considerations are related to selected criteria and take the investment of considerable time to plan the details. Table 8.1 lists common

TABLE 8.1 Selected Categories of Data and Sources

Type of Data	Data Sources	Strengths	Limitations
Observation	Meetings and conferences Site visits	Allows for direct examination	Requires trained observer Complex and expensive
Surveys	Interviews Questionnaires Self-reports	Directly gathers data about client characteristics, satisfaction, and behavior	Cannot be certain client's statements are accurate May be complex and expensive
Discussion	Focus groups	Obtains a variety of opinions and suggestions	Requires a trained moderator May be difficult to interpret
Record review	Hospitals, clinics, meeting minutes, logs	Contains primary information Data have already been collected	Data may be missing or not pertinent May be difficult and expensive to access data
Vital statistics review	State health departments	Large available database with extensive health information	May not have needed data
Registries	CDC State and local public health departments Registries for selected diseases and programs	Contains epidemiological data about many diseases and conditions Data have already been collected	May not have needed data May be difficult to access data
Population data	U.S. Census Bureau	Large available database with extensive demographic information	May not have needed data
National data sets	CDC, Centers for Disease Control and Prevention.	Appropriate for evaluating large public health programs Data have already been collected	May not have needed data Complicated statistical analysis Often relies on individual self-reporting, which may not be accurate

Source: Adapted from Wholey, J. S., Hatry, H. P., & Newcomer, K. E. (Eds.). (2010). *Handbook of practical program evaluation* (3rd ed.). Jossey-Bass.

types of data and their sources along with the strengths and limitations of each type. The team should base their selection of data elements on the relevance of the program or project being evaluated, the reliability and validity of the data and method, the resources available to collect data, and the relevance of data to performance criteria/standards (CDC, 2011).

With the identification of data to be collected, the processes for data collection must be planned. Questions such as where the data will be found, in what format, and when they will be collected need to be addressed. The common sources of data found in Table 8.1 are helpful triggers to think about sources of data. Data can also be considered as primary or secondary data as well as quantitative or qualitative. *Primary data* are data collected from first-hand sources using methods such as surveys, interviews, or observations. Secondary data are data collected from the past by someone else and made available for others to use. Examples of secondary data are published reports, scientific literature, studies, surveys, and other methods that have been reported by others. Note that some types can be either primary or secondary depending on how they were collected. Although primary data are preferred over secondary data, sometimes primary data are not available or practical to access, so secondary data becomes the best option. *Quantitative data* come in the form of counts or numbers, whereas *qualitative data* are nonnumerical in nature and collected through selected methods of observations, one-to-one interviews, conducting focus groups, and similar methods. The type of data (e.g., quantitative or qualitative) collected for a particular evaluation depends on what questions the evaluator wishes to answer. Sometimes, both types of data are needed so that a mixed method is useful to provide the breadth and depth of information to answer the question adequately.

Data acquisition has to do with gaining possession of the desired data. This means that the evaluator needs to know what data are required, location/source of the data, the process for extracting the data, and its storage. Table 8.1 includes common sources and location of data. The data may be found in databases, websites, written documents, oral reports, and other sources. Data extraction depends on the kind of data, but most often it is extracted directly into a database established for the evaluation or through a process of extracting data from paper and other sources such as checklists and surveys into a temporary database that will then be entered into the overall evaluation database. Efficiency counts, in that elimination of steps before data are entered into the overall evaluation database will decrease data entry error. In order to ensure the fidelity of the data collection process, evaluators must be trained to ensure data collection processes are followed as intended. If possible, piloting the data collection–acquisition process answers practical questions and also helps the evaluators to feel comfortable. Checking for interrater reliability between data collectors further helps to identify questions or problems before beginning and during the evaluation so that corrections can be made immediately before data are lost. Finally, the timing of data collection is important, in that any interventions need time to have an effect. This decision is the responsibility of the evaluator, taking into consideration the intervention effect, environmental variations (e.g., weekend or holiday schedules or change in leadership that might influence availability of data or skew the data), or other contextual conditions not conducive to collecting credible data.

Data Analysis and Interpretation

Decisions about data analysis are largely based on the questions to be answered, the design, and the level of data collected (nominal, ordinal, interval, and ratio). Consultation with a statistician at the planning stage is recommended to ensure the data collected and the analysis plan are appropriate for the questions that you want the evaluation to answer. Program evaluation commonly uses descriptive, bivariable, or multivariable analysis or a combination of these, depending on the scope of the evaluation (Grembowski, 2001, pp. 246–252). Descriptive analysis produces measures of means, medians, frequencies, and percentages that are sufficient for many evaluations. Bivariable analysis constructs associations (or differences) between two items; for example, a handwashing program and nosocomial infections. Multivariable analysis employs more complex statistical techniques, such as multiple regressions, in order to determine the effect of a program, the direction of the effect, and how variables act separately and together. Once statistical analysis is completed, the evaluator and team need to interpret the findings in light of the questions that the project of program was to answer.

For DNP and smaller projects, the statistical analyses tend to be simpler, most often using descriptive and nonparametric statistics. The interpretation of the findings in light of the expected outcomes should be carefully considered by the evaluator and the team.

Project Management

Project management includes many activities designed to ensure the success of the project or program evaluation and it addresses a range of practical and administrative components for which the evaluator is responsible, such as personnel, resources, data management, timeline, and fidelity. A common thread for success in all aspects of project management is effective evaluator communications skills so that all participants understand the overall project, their responsibilities, and those of others. Communications are vital to the success of the evaluation and must be clear and transparent as well as updated periodically as the planning proceeds and changes over time.

The *personnel* for a large program evaluation brings special competencies required to execute specific roles such as data collector, content expert, or statistician. The number of personnel and needed roles will depend on the scope of the evaluation. For smaller projects such as DNP projects, there is the evaluator (e.g., DNP student) and other people who are loosely defined as team members and who participate to various degrees with the project planning. Regardless of the scope of the evaluation, the right people are needed with the right skills and competencies to plan the evaluation. Gathering the right people and establishing and executing an effective communication plan is the responsibility of the evaluator.

The *resources* needed for the conduct of any evaluation vary and, again, are based on the scope and available resources. It is the responsibility of the evaluator and team to identify the needed resources and communicate those needs to the sponsoring person/persons or organization sponsoring the evaluation. A budget is required and will include items such as personnel, equipment, and technology support. The cost and a rationale for each item are required. The budget for smaller projects, such as a DNP project, will be less extensive, but there are costs associated with even small projects. Those costs might include an estimate of the amount of staff time needed to attend an educational offering, printing of a questionnaire, technology support to design and launch a survey, and other items.

Data management consumes considerable time and focus on details in planning. Even before data are collected, the evaluator and team must consider what data are going to be collected so that it is quality as defined as valid and reliable are verified and also directly related to the focus of the evaluation. There must be a purpose in collecting specific data elements. Related considerations include securing permission for any copyrighted material such as instruments; permission to access any unit or organizational reports or databases; approval of processes for protection of human subjects for the organization's Institutional Review Board (IRB) if any human subjects data will be collected; and piloting of any evaluator-developed instruments or checklists to verify they are clear and appropriate for the data to be collected.

The downloading data into the established evaluation database may be necessary if data have not been directly entered into the final database. *Data storage* and accessibility to the data and evaluation materials must be clearly outlined. All evaluation data and related materials must be secured with password-protected access or storage in a locked drawer accessible to only key personnel such as the evaluator. If any identifiable data has been collected from subjects, which required IRB approval, a process for de-identification should be in place as required by the IRB. Although many evaluations do not require IRB approval, it is wise to check with the IRB whether there are any questions.

Planning an evaluation also includes time management requiring detailing all of the required activities in logical order, a responsible person, and the setting of a reasonable and realistic time frame for accomplishing these activities. Many tools are available to help organize these activities. One of them is a *Gantt chart*, which graphically shows activities or tasks (*y* axis) to be performed against time (*x* axis). It is a visual presentation of a project in which the activities are broken down, logically organized, and displayed on a chart for ease of understanding and communicating to others. Many examples of Gantt charts are available on the Internet. The Gantt chart can help to keep focused as well as provide a means for making changes in activities and timelines during the implementation phase. The responsibility for the overall management of the timeline falls to the evaluator as the leader and project manager.

Regardless of whether the evaluation is for a DNP project, smaller unit or organization-based project, or large program evaluation, all of the mentioned responsibilities for project management must be addressed. The difference between the larger program and smaller project evaluations are the complexity of the evaluation (i.e., scope) and the degree and depth of detail needed to properly execute it. In summary, the fuel for effective project management is open, clear, and transparent communications throughout the evaluation process, from inception, planning, implementation, and dissemination with all stakeholders to support the fidelity of evaluation.

Dissemination

No evaluation is complete until the results of the evaluation have been provided to the intended audience in a form that is meaningful and useful to the target audience. Many forms of dissemination can be used to report results, but the most common forms are a written report and an oral report. Both forms of communications will be briefly addressed in this section as methods of dissemination.

WRITTEN REPORTS

Multiple sources of models to write an effective evaluation report are available on the Internet and publications. Available resources can be overwhelming to both the novice and the experienced evaluator. In providing the reader with practical information, a few resources are cited as a beginning point. One excellent source, published by the CDC and National Center for Chronic Disease Preventions and Health Promotion (2013), is titled *Developing an Effective Evaluation Report*, which is available at the CDC website. (See pages 62–64 for sample outlines for writing an evaluation report.) These and other resources provide advice about writing an effective report. The intent of this section is to provide a generic outline of the content to be included in any evaluation report along with some suggestions to keep in mind when writing the report. The goal is to produce a well-organized and compelling evaluation report that convinces readers of the credibility of the findings, logical recommendations based on collected data and thoughtful analysis, and prompts for action based on the data and recommendations. The report must be practical and useful to the receiver.

Audience. Before putting fingers to the keyboard, think about the intended audience. The intended audience is whoever asked for the evaluation and what their reasons were for that request. Have a clear picture in your mind of these individuals or groups because this is whom you are addressing through the written word. Craft the report to the intended audience, providing the kind of information that they need and deliver it in a format that will be understandable and useful.

Message. Connecting with the intended audience and establishing and maintaining credibility are critical. The approach, style, and language must convey that you have a clear understanding of the questions that they wanted answered and that you have approached the evaluation in a respectful and unbiased manner. The evaluation report is not a term paper for a course. The report must be well written, concise, substantive, and conform to professional standards of a written report. Give the readers information that they do not already have, not a rehash of known facts. Considerable time is required to prepare a report for high impact and usability.

Format. The report must have the earmarks of a polished and professional product. Font type and font size should be easily readable. Trying to cram a lot of information into the report by using single spacing and a small font should be avoided. Formatting of the pages should include one-inch margins, page numbers, and clear headings. Consider the best way to present information. Judicious use of tables, graphs, and charts can be very effective in helping the reader to rapidly grasp the information. Paper quality and placing the report into a professional looking folder is expected if you are providing a hard copy. Be concise and clear. As a general guideline, the body of the report should be about 10 pages, with an executive summary of no more than two to three pages for the reader who just wants the big picture and key findings and recommendations.

Outline. As noted previously, multiple models are available to structure the report. Whatever form is chosen, it should follow a logical flow of information, taking the reader through the process followed in the conduct of the evaluation. Box 8.1 provides a basic outline for content to be included. Areas can be enhanced or deleted, as appropriate.

BOX 8.1   Components of a Written Evaluation Report

- Title page
- Executive summary
- Purposes and intended users
- Program description
- Evaluation focus and design
- Data sources and methods
- Results, interpretations, and conclusions
- Recommendations
- Appendix
- References

Components of the Written Report

The following provides a description of the components of the written report.

Title Page. Provide the title of the project and the date submitted center in the middle to upper third of the page. Do not include a page number on the title page.

Executive Summary. This is a very important component because some people may only read the executive summary. It should include the program description, evaluation questions or focus, design description, key findings, and recommendations. The executive summary should take no more than two to three pages.

Purposes and Intended Use. In this section, the purposes of the evaluation and the intended uses of the evaluation report are identified and described. In addition, the primary intended users and the evaluation stakeholder workgroup are identified. This section fosters transparency about the purposes of the evaluation, who is involved, and who will have access to the evaluation results.

Program/Project Description. A brief overview of the program/project, including background, program resources, program activities, stage of development, environmental context, statement of need, and any other key characteristics of the program that influence the evaluation are described (CDC & National Center for Chronic Disease Preventions and Health Promotion, 2013, p. 12). This description helps to focus the evaluation and leads to a common and shared understanding of the program as well as frames the evaluation questions and how they are prioritized. It is important to know the stage of development (e.g., planning, implementation, maintenance) of the program because programs are dynamic systems and change over time. The change in developmental stage will suggest different questions, priorities, and needs.

Evaluation Focus and Design. In this section, the focus of the evaluation is identified and clearly delineated. If there is more than one focus for the evaluation, the priorities assigned to each question by the evaluator should be based on stakeholder priorities and intended users of the evaluation. This is an important section because of the many areas that could be evaluated. Therefore, the specific focus must be identified so that an appropriate design can match the questions being addressed in the evaluation. The questions help to identify the data needed to answer the questions.

Data Sources and Methods. Several elements related to data and data collection processes are described in this section. With knowledge of the questions to be answered, the design of the evaluation process emerges with a clear notion of what data need to be collected. The evaluator must briefly describe the sources of the data, location of the data, and how they were collected. In addition, the rationale for selection of the data as well as data acquisition, management, analysis, and credibility of data sources are addressed to support reliability and validity.

Results, Interpretation, and Conclusions. This section discusses both processes and outcomes. The analytical processes are briefly described and interpreted in an understandable way for the intended audience. The results along with the interpretation are used to describe conclusions in relation to the questions that were the focus of the evaluation. Connecting the findings and interpretations with the questions being addressed is an important step that requires careful attention in the writing process. Conclusions must be justified. Guiding the reader from results to interpretations to conclusions in a logical format informs the reader of the process and supports transparency and credibility. As noted in the CDC and National Center for Chronic Disease Preventions and Health Promotion (2013) discussion of standards, the propriety standards play a role in guiding the evaluator's decisions in regard to how to analyze and interpret the data to ensure that all stakeholders' values are respected in the process of drawing conclusions.

Recommendations. The final narrative section of the report is recommendations. Based on the data collected, results, interpretation, and conclusions, what recommendations are offered in relation to the purpose and questions that were the focus of the evaluation? The recommendations should be clear directions with a timeline for action or the next steps to be taken. Take into consideration the resources needed to implement each recommendation. In presenting recommendations, give options with a brief analysis of consequences of action or no action.

Appendix. Place items into the appendix that provide more data and information addressed in the report. Tables, charts, and graphs may be included here or in the body of the report.

References. List the sources of information that were used in conducting the evaluation, including journal articles, external and internal reports, databases, websites, interviews, and other sources of information. The list of references helps to support transparency and credibility of the evaluation process.

In summary, a credible narrative report should be clear, concise, accurate, and logical and should provide answers to the questions important to the individual or group requesting the evaluation. It should follow best practices and standards of high quality (Sanders & The Joint Commission on Standards for Educational Evaluation, 1994). A compelling report is useful to build awareness, facilitate growth and program improvement, and inform decision-making of the stakeholders. The evaluation report is the property of the person or group sponsoring the evaluation and should be treated as confidential by the evaluator. Any requests from the outside for information about the report is directed to the sponsoring person or group.

ORAL REPORTS

In addition to a written evaluation report, an oral report may be requested as a means of communicating results. The oral presentation can take many forms and requires crafting for the particular audience, message to be delivered, and format. Audience, message, and format are intertwined and require careful consideration.

Audience. Knowing who the intended audience is serves a critical need in planning the oral presentation. There are often a variety of audiences, such as the C-suite, program directors or managers, program staff, and program recipients, all of whom will have different perspectives and information needs. The person or group who sponsored the evaluation should be consulted on who will be in the audience, when the presentation will take place, and what format will be used.

Message. The area of particular interest concerning the program evaluation for each group is often quite different. For example, members of the C-suite may have a particular interest of the program's market share, cost, profit margin, return on investment, and potential for growth. The program director or manager may be interested in the efficiency of delivery and program outcomes in relation to program objectives. The program staff may be interested in ongoing funding of the program, expansion, and increasing the number of personnel. Therefore, the message needs to be crafted to the needs and interests of the target group.

Format. The third intertwined consideration is the format or how the information is delivered. In addition to an oral presentation, PowerPoint slides, flip charts, handout material of PowerPoint slides, graphs, tables, executive summary, or other handout material may be used to augment the oral presentation. These are important decisions for the evaluator to make.

It is beyond the scope of this chapter to address the fine points of oral presentations, but suffice it to say it is a very important final step in coming to closure with the program/project evaluation.

IMPLEMENTING AN EVALUATION PLAN

Detailed and thoughtful planning greatly increase the potential for successful implementation of the evaluation. Surprises always crop up during an evaluation. Some are good, and some can drastically disrupt the procedure. Evaluators prefer a smooth and predictable experience; a way to accomplish this goal is by following a well-written management plan and carefully following the protocol. The management plan contains the study protocol, a timeline, a projected cost estimate, resources needed, and potential barriers. Evaluators should refer to the management plan frequently for guidance and direction as they move through the stages of the evaluation.

The management plan clearly establishes what will be done, when it will be done, and who is responsible for doing it. Each stage in the evaluation is linked to the person(s) responsible for the process. For example, one team member is accountable for supervising the ethical status of the study and seeking approval from the IRB, if approval is recommended. During data analysis, two members of the team may be responsible for assigning each variable a code name and value, checking the integrity of each value, and accurately entering data into a data set. Another member creates a data manual that contains management protocols (Grady et al., 2001, p. 247).

CASE STUDY

The following is intended to provide a brief overview of key elements of an evaluation to illustrate the operationalization of an evaluation project. The details of any project are specific to the particular evaluation.

A DNP graduate who is the director of cardiovascular clinical services at a major academic center is asked to evaluate the need for an outpatient cardiovascular program at one of the smaller community-based facilities of this large system. She begins with a clear understanding of the *purpose* of the evaluation and who is requesting the evaluation. A point person is identified as the person she can contact for any questions or if there is a need for assistance. A conversation also ensues in regard to what the deliverables will be at the conclusion of the project as well as the timeline and resources available to complete the project. It is agreed that an oral presentation to the leadership of both the academic medical center and the community facility will be provided in addition to a written report. The DNP nurse uses a planning, implementation, and dissemination format to conduct her evaluation.

Planning

She begins by identifying the stakeholders. These include the clinical facility (leadership, staff, resources, current cardiovascular services provided, etc.), the community it serves (demographics, socioeconomic profile, other cardiovascular services currently available in that community, etc.), and the relationship of this facility with the primary facility in the academic medical center. The point person is someone with whom to establish a working relationship because she will communicate the progress of the project and be available for assistance should any barriers be encountered. The next step in planning is to determine the subgoals of the project and what data are needed to answer the questions. Based on these considerations, the design for the evaluation can be determined. Data elements and data sources need to be identified, as well as how and by whom these data will be collected and stored. This step may include plans for interviews with stakeholders and key personnel, review of a variety of documents and databases, review of the literature and review of other data sources. Critical to any evaluation is a communication plan. This means that DNP nurses need to plan with whom communications are required, what messages need to be conveyed, and the related timeline. Many tools are available to assist the evaluator in conducting an evaluation, such as a logic model. The DNP nurse created a detailed logic model and used it not only for planning, but also to evaluate the success of the evaluation process based on identified outcomes (McLaughlin & Jordan, 1999). She also created a communication plan that included the person(s) with whom to communicate, as well as the key message and frequency of the communications. It is important to think through the project carefully in the planning phase to be efficient and effective in answering the questions posed by the evaluation purpose.

Implementation

Thoughtful and detailed planning leads to a smoother implementation. However, the DNP nurse recognized that she needed to conduct an ongoing environmental scan to assess progress in meeting milestones. Barriers were identified, and a new plan was devised to address them. For example, the CNO at the community facility was reluctant to give the DNP nurse access to the quality metrics for the facility. The DNP nurse was able to communicate with the point person for the evaluation, who discussed this matter with the CNO; the CNO now felt comfortable providing the information. The implementation of the evaluation plan continued. Frequent formative evaluations were conducted by the DNP nurse to assess progress as well as any need for change in the processes and activities. The DNP nurse spent time assessing the community needs for cardiovascular services; current available resources, including gaps; and the relationship of both clinical facilities. She determined that a business plan was needed to plan the outpatient program that could be used by the leadership for decision-making about creating this new service. A business plan is necessary when expenditure of capital funds is at stake. Preparing a business plan is beyond the scope of this case study, but many resources are available on the Internet and in the textbook for review. The DNP nurse might also work with the finance/business department to prepare a business plan.

Dissemination

A written report is prepared. (See the section on writing a report for models.) The DNP nurse completed the evaluation and met with the point person at the sponsoring facility to deliver the written report and the plan for an oral presentation. The DNP nurse verified who would be in attendance for the oral presentation so that she could tailor the presentation to the interests of the intended audience. She planned to keep it short, focused, and connected to the purpose of the evaluation. A few (6–8) slides were prepared to guide the discussion, and photocopies of the slides were distributed at the presentation.

Coming to Closure

The DNP nurse came to closure with the evaluation work by meeting with the point person, thanking that person for the opportunity to conduct this evaluation and for the point person's assistance. She returned any written or other materials that belonged to the facility. She kept in mind that this was confidential work and that she was therefore not at liberty to discuss the evaluation or disseminate any information about the project (in any form) without clear permission from the facility.

SUMMARY

Evaluation of programs and projects is a common and much needed focus in health care to evaluate value and relevance. Evaluation includes a description of program performance and the standards or criteria for judging the performance, both of which are interrelated and work in tandem. This chapter has described the differences and commonalities of program and project evaluation, although the literature lumps them together as program evaluation. Also addressed were the background of program evaluation, the special focus of program evaluation, the types of program evaluations, the domains of evaluation, and the planning of a program evaluation. Models and specific information related to evaluation were addressed, including the steps and components that guide the planning phase. Finally, a brief overview was provided on preparing both a written and an oral report of an evaluation for dissemination. DNP nurses are perfectly positioned and knowledgeable about the philosophy, frameworks, processes, and methods for conducting a credible and useful evaluation. It is clear from the evolving leadership positions of DNP graduates and the increasing requirement in health care for evaluation to determine the value of programs that DNP nurses will continue to be engaged as team members and leaders in the evaluation of programs and projects.

REFERENCES

Aday, L. A., Begley, C. E., Lairson, D. R., & Balkrishnan, R. (2004). *Evaluating the healthcare system* (3rd ed.). Health Administration Press.

Alkin, M. C. (Ed.). (2004). *Evaluation roots: Tracing theorists' views and influences.* Sage.

Altschuld, J. W., & Kumar, D. D. (2010). *Needs assessment: An overview.* Sage.

Bowen, S. (2012). A guide to evaluation in health research. Canadian Institute of Health Research. http://www.cihr-irsc.gc.ca/e/documents/kt_lm_guide_evhr-en.pdf

Centers for Disease Control and Prevention & National Center for Chronic Disease Preventions and Health Promotion. (2013). *Developing an effective evaluation report: Setting the course for effective program evaluation.* CDC.

Chen, H. T. (2005). *Practical program evaluation.* Sage.

Devaney, B., & Rossi, P. (1997). Thinking through evaluation design options. *Children and Youth Services Review, 19*(7), 587–606. https://doi.org/10.1016/S0190-7409(97)00047-9

Dusenbury, L., Brannigan, R., Falco, M., & Hansen, W. (2003). A review of research on fidelity of implementation: Implications for drug abuse prevention in school settings. *Health Education Research, 18*, 237–256. https://doi.org/10.1093/her/18.2.237

Environmental Protection Agency. (2016). *Evaluating EPA's programs.* www.epa.gov/evaluate/basicinfo/index.htm

Fitzpatrick, J. A., Sanders, J. R., & Worthen, B. R. (2004). *Program evaluation: Alternative approaches and practical guidelines* (3rd ed.). Pearson Education.

Grady, D., Newman, T. B., & Vittinghoff, E. (2001). Data management. In S. B. Hulley, S. R. Cummings, W. S. Browner, D. Grady, N. Hearst, & T. B. Newman (Eds.), *Designing clinical research* (2nd ed., pp. 247–257). Lippincott Williams & Wilkins.

Gertler, P. J., Martinez, S., Premand, P., Rawlings, L. B., & Vermeersch, M. J. (2016). Impact evaluation in practice (2nd ed.). International Bank for Reconstruction and Development/The World Bank.

Grembowski, D. (2001). *The practice of health program evaluation.* Sage.

Helitzer, D., Yoon, S., Wallerstein, N., & Garcia-Velarde, L. D. (2000). The role of process evaluation in the training of facilitators for an adolescent health education program. *Journal of School Health, 70*(4), 141–147. https://doi.org/10.1111/j.1746-1561.2000.tb06460.x

Institute of Healthcare Improvement. *Quality improvement essential toolkit.* http://www.ihi.org/resources/Pages/Tools/Quality-Improvement-Essentials-Toolkit.aspx

Kellogg, W. K. (2004). *Logic model development guide. W. K. Kellogg Foundation.*

LoBiondo-Wood, G., & Haber, J. (2017). *Nursing research: Methods and critical appraisal for evidence-based practice* (9th ed.). Mosby Elsevier.

McGuire, M. (2016). Program design & development resources. United Way of Toronto and York Region.

McLaughlin, J. A., & Jordan, G. B. (1999). Logic models: A tool for telling your program's performance story. *Evaluation and Program Planning, 22*(1), 65–72. https://doi.org/10.1016/S0149-7189(98)00042-1

Powell, R. R. (2006). Evaluation research: An overview. *Library Trends, 55*(1), 102–120. https://doi.org/10.1353/lib.2006.0050

Rogers, P. (2020). *Develop programme theory/theory of change.* Retrieved August 31, 2020, from https://www.betterevaluation.org/en/rainbow_framework/define/develop_programme_theory

Rossi, P. H., Lipsey, M. W., & Freeman, H. E. (2004). Evaluation: A systematic approach (7th ed.). Sage.

Rossi, P. H., Lipsey, M. W., & Henry, G. T. (2019). Evaluation: A systematic approach (8th ed.). Sage.

Rutman, L. (1984). Evaluation research methods: A basic guide. Sage.

Sanders, J. R., & The Joint Committee on Standards for Educational Evaluation. (1994). The program evaluation standards (2nd ed.). Sage.

Saunders, R. P., Evans, M. H., & Joshi, P. (2005). Developing a process-evaluation plan for assessing health promotion program implementation: A how to guide. *Health Promotion Practice, 6*(2), 134–147. https://doi.org/10.1177/1524839904273387

Scriven, M. (1991). Evaluation thesaurus (4th ed.). Sage.

Stufflebeam, D. L., Foley, W. J., Gephart, W. J., Guba, E. G., Hammond, R. L., Merriman, H. O., & Provus, M. M. (1971). *Educational evaluation and decision making.* Peacock.

Viadro, C., Earp, J. A. L., & Altpeter, M. (1997). Designing a process evaluation for a comprehensive breast cancer screening intervention: Challenges and opportunities. *Evaluation and Program Planning, 20*(3), 237–249. https://doi.org/10.1016/S0149-7189(97)00001-3

Watkins, R., Meiers, M. W., & Visser, Y. L. (2012). A guide to assessing needs: Essential tools for collecting information, making decisions, and achieving development results. World Bank.

Weiss, C. H. (1998). *Evaluations: Methods for studying programs and policies* (2nd ed.). Prentice Hall.

Wholey, J. S., Hatry, H. P., & Newcomer, K. E. (Eds.). (2010). *Handbook of practical program evaluation* (3rd ed.). Jossey-Bass.

Zhang, G., Zeller, N., Griffith, R., Metcalf, D., Williams, J., Shea, C., & Misulis, K. (2011). Using the context, input, process, and product evaluation model (CIPP) as a comprehensive framework to guide the planning, implementation, and assessment of service-learning programs. *Journal of Higher Education Outreach and Engagement, 15*(4), 57–84. http://openjournals.libs.uga.edu/index.php/jheoe/article/view/628

RECOMMENDED RESOURCES

There are countless resources available on the Internet to assist with program development and evaluation. Here are a few that may be helpful.

Centers for Disease Control and Prevention. (2012). *CDC approach to evaluation.* https://www.cdc.gov/eval/approach/index.htm

McGuire, M. (2016). *Program design & development resources.* United Way of Toronto and York Region. https://www.unitedwaygt.org/document.doc?id=538

McNamara, C. (n.d.). *Basic guide to program evaluation (including outcomes evaluation).* https://managementhelp.org/evaluation/program-evaluation-guide.htm

National Institutes of Health & National Cancer Institute. (n.d.). *Science at a glance: A guide for cancer control practitioners.* NIH Publication Number 19-CA-8055.

Savignac, J., & Dunbar, L. (2014). *Guide on the implementation of evidence-based programs: What do we know so far?* https://www.publicsafety.gc.ca/cnt/rsrcs/pblctns/gd-mplmnttn-vdnc-prgrms/index-en.aspx

University of Wisconsin-Madison. (n.d.). *Program development and evaluation (logic model templates).* https://fyi.extension.wisc.edu/programdevelopment/designing-programs/

NINE

EVALUATION IN QUALITY IMPROVEMENT

Eileen R. Giardino

The truth is rarely pure and never simple.
—Oscar Wilde

INTRODUCTION

Quality improvement (QI) in health care is a method of systematic and continuous actions, which cause measurable improvements in the health status of patient populations and health care services (Health Resources and Services Administration [HRSA], 2011a, 2011b). A QI initiative includes the assessment of what is currently happening within a given system regarding clinical outcomes and then determines systematic efforts to improve clinical and safety outcomes. The QI process uses science-based methodology to systematically approach the development and implementation of an innovative process to improve determined outcomes (Institute for Healthcare Improvement [IHI], 2020b; McCarthy, 2008).

An integral aspect of doctor of nursing practice (DNP) clinical practice is to be a leader in quality and safety initiatives. DNP nurses have the skills necessary to improve health care outcomes through translating research findings into practice (American Association of Colleges of Nursing [AACN], 2006). DNP graduates evaluate systems of care in health care organizations and then develop and implement QI initiatives that improve outcomes of care.

This chapter provides an overview of QI in health care and describes the intersection of the DNP nurse with QI and improvement initiatives. It also discusses essential components in the development and implementation of change initiatives and the role of the DNP nurse in the development, implementation, and evaluation of improvement initiatives within a health care system.

QUALITY IMPROVEMENT IN HEALTH CARE

Over 30 years ago, the Institute of Medicine (IOM) defined clinical QI as an interdisciplinary process designed to raise the standards for the delivery of preventive, diagnostic, therapeutic, and rehabilitative measures in order to maintain, restore, or improve health outcomes of individuals and populations (IOM, 1990). Since that

TABLE 9.1 Quality Improvement: Functions and Purpose

Function	Purpose
Monitor outcomes	Detect conformance with standards of care
Surveillance for negative outcomes	Detect predictable and unexpected outcomes (e.g., monitoring infection rates, surgical outcomes, examining sentinel events)
Performance reporting	Compare unit, group, or individual performance level to standardized performance measures
Measure patient-centered aspects of care	Measure outcomes to improve care

Source: From O'Kane, M. (2009). Do patients need to be protected from quality improvement? In B. Jennings, M. A. Baily, M. Bottrell, & J. Lynn (Eds.), *Health care quality improvement: Ethical and regulatory issues* (pp. 89–100). The Hastings Center; Healthhuman Resources and Services Administration. (2011b). *Quality improvement.* U.S. Department of Health and Human Services. https://www.hrsa.gov/sites/default/files/quality/toolbox/508pdfs/qualityimprovement.pdf.

time, the health care industry nationwide has seen the need to improve the safe delivery of health care through QI initiatives. It is not acceptable for clinicians and health care institutions to achieve outcomes that are below standard expectations and national-level benchmark.

QI is innovation and adaptation undertaken in a systematic, data-guided way (Baily et al., 2006). A quality initiative implements an evidence-based and best practices change protocol to achieve better outcomes than what the system was previously achieving (IOM, 1990). The Science of Improvement (SI) methodology uses principles of clinical science, psychology, systems theory, and statistical analysis to assess, monitor, and improve care outcomes (IHI, 2020b).

A QI initiative seeks to achieve higher levels of performance of clinical care and process outcomes to meet either internal or external benchmarks. A QI program includes clinically related activities within the organization designed to improve operations, finance, safety, and patient care (HRSA, 2011b). Table 9.1 shows activities that fall within the realm of QI and the purpose of each function (O'Kane, 2009).

To Err Is Human in Health Care

Quality is a direct link to an organization's care delivery systems and their ability to deliver service to patients and populations (HRSA, 2011b; Massoud, 2001). The U.S. health care system has trailed behind other industries in achieving safe and consistent outcomes for patient care and initiating safety efforts to prevent errors that result in morbidity and death (Schimpff, 2012). The airline industry is an exemplar of an industry that could not afford to allow tragic accidents to occur and since World War II has focused on providing safety systems. While the airline industry pioneered QI and safety initiatives to avoid preventable accidents (Reid et al., 2005; Shojania et al., 2001), the health care industry has not met the challenge of providing safe and quality care to the same degree as the airline industry.

The IOM report *To Err Is Human* revealed that the health care industry delivered inconsistent and unsafe care that harmed people (IOM, 2000), while *Crossing the Quality Chasm* (IOM, 2001) found that gaps in the quality of care delivered in institutions and health care systems nationwide were evidenced by suboptimal outcome measures along with breeches in patient safety measures. The identification of inconsistent and unsafe care practices in all health care delivery systems was widespread (Leape et al., 2009). Outcome studies across health care institutions identified widespread safety problems along with mediocre to poor patient care outcomes at all levels of health care delivery (IOM, 2001; Reid et al., 2005).

Errors and mistakes in health care that have resulted in harm or death range from giving the patient an incorrect medication dosage to performing the wrong surgery on the wrong body part. *To Err Is Human* revealed that between 44,000 and 98,000 Americans die each year as a result of medical errors (Botwinick et al., 2006; IOM, 2000). The report drew wide attention to overwhelming quality and safety problems in all areas of health care delivery, while a later study estimated the number of premature deaths associated with preventable harm to patients to be more than 400,000 per year (James, 2013). *To Err Is Human* recommended the need to improve the delivery of care to decrease medical errors, make health care outcomes more consistent across institutions, and decrease the rising cost of health care (IOM, 2000).

The delivery of health care has shifted from clinicians providing patient care they think is best based on their perceptions of quality care, to a system focused on delivering quality health science–based care designed to decrease preventable adverse events and premature deaths associated with preventable harm (Leape et al., 2009; U.S. Department of Health and Human Services [DHHS], 2000). The IOM report *Crossing the Quality Chasm* suggested the need for change in the delivery of health care and identified six aims that all health care organizations should achieve. Each aim describes a health care domain that addresses the quality, safety, and effectiveness of care from provider to patient (IOM, 2001; Slonim & Pollack, 2005). See Table 9.2 as a guide to the six aims of quality health care.

TABLE 9.2   The Six Aims of Quality Health Care

Aim	Description
Safe	Avoiding patient injury from care intended to help
Effective	Providing scientifically based services and refraining from services unlikely to benefit (avoiding underuse and overuse)
Patient-centered	Providing respectful and responsive patient care guided by patient values and focused on patient preferences, needs, and values
Timely	Reducing wait time and delays for patients and caregivers
Efficient	Avoiding waste of equipment, supplies, ideas, and energy
Equitable	Providing quality care to all that does not differ due to gender, ethnicity, geographic location, and socioeconomic status

Source: Adapted from Institute of Medicine. (2001). *Crossing the quality chasm: A new health system for the 21st century.* National Academies Press. https://doi.org/10.17226/10027.

Quality care focuses on providing the right care at the right time, every time, and ensures that fewer people are harmed or injured by incorrect procedures, incorrect medications, and incorrect treatment plans (Andel et al., 2012). It is less expensive, more efficient, and less wasteful to provide safe and effective health care than to provide care that engenders higher costs from errors and improper medical treatment plans. Therefore, it is incumbent that health care leaders and clinicians understand what quality care involves and how to develop protocols and programs that focus on quality of care and patient safety.

Cost of Preventable Harm

Since the IOM report, *To Err Is Human*, the U.S. health care system has not met the goal to decrease the rising costs of health care while improving patient outcomes and institutional safety and efficiency (IOM, 2000). The cost of errors or preventable harm that resulted in injury was estimated to be between $17 and $29 billion, with over 50% of these costs related to medical errors (Black et al., 2018). Medical errors are generally errors of omission and errors of commission. Omission errors occur when actions are not taken, while commission errors result from taking the wrong actions (Rodziewicz & Hipskind, 2020). A 2008 report showed that medical errors cost the $19.5 billion annually with approximately $17 billion associated directly with costs (Andel et al., 2012; Van Den Bos et al., 2011).

Past and current costs of preventable harm are an indication of inconsistency in the delivery of quality care in U.S. hospitals that results in high mortality rates, injuries that result in longer hospital stays, increased medical costs, and preventable disability (Brennan et al., 1991; Carter et al., 2014). It is difficult to quantify the costs of medical errors due to a lack of a standardized definition and nomenclature of what constitutes a medical error along with overlapping definitions that hinder the analysis and evaluation of medical error data (Rodziewicz & Hipskind, 2020).

THE ROLE OF THE DOCTOR OF NURSING PRACTICE NURSE IN QUALITY IMPROVEMENT

The IOM (2003) and the National Research Council of the National Academies (2005) stated that graduate nursing education should prepare nurses to lead patient safety and QI initiatives that improve health care outcomes (AACN, 2006). In keeping with the IOM recommendation, the DNP curriculum prepares graduates to appraise evidence through the evaluation of practice and create clinical strategies to improve health outcomes. The ability to translate evidence into practice through change initiatives is an important aspect of the DNP graduate's role as a leader and a clinician (Brown & Crabtree, 2013).

The DNP Essentials developed by the AACN outlines competencies that DNP graduates should achieve through program curricula and expectations and that DNP graduates have the ability to understand and apply change principles to improve health care outcomes (AACN, 2006). The 2006 DNP Essentials addressed what the DNP nurse should understand regarding quality issues and QI in the health care arena. Essential II: Organizational and Systems Leadership for Quality Improvement and Systems Thinking and Essential IV: Information Systems/Technology and Patient Care Technology for the Improvement and Transformation of Health Care state that the DNP graduate can assess and improve quality of care, identify improvement strategies needed to evaluate systems of care, and implement improvement initiatives (AACN, 2006; Vincent et al., 2010). The core essentials revised by the AACN (2021) continued to address the DNP nurse's role in QI in a number of ways. Domain 4: Scholarship for the Nursing Discipline states that there should be discernment for the appropriate application of QI initiatives, while Domain 5: Quality and Safety describes that quality and safety are core values of practice that are essential to the individual performance of clinicians and for system effectiveness. Furthermore, the DNP nurse has the expertise to advance QI practices (AACN, 2021).

Expertise in quality management and QI is clearly in the purview of the DNP nurse. The DNP nurse who practices at the highest leadership levels such as chief nursing officer, hospital administrator, chief executive officer (CEO), health information manager, and director of QI is positioned to analyze current systems of practice and lead QI initiatives (Melynk, 2013; Paplham & Austin-Ketch, 2015; Trautman et al., 2018). The DNP nurse practitioner and certified registered nurse anesthetist (CRNA) also assume leadership positions in the clinical areas of practice to improve patient care outcomes or process outcomes. The DNP nurse uses concepts of stakeholder engagement, project charters, logic models, driver diagrams, rapid cycle models, outcome measurement, and complex adaptive systems that are critical to the success of QI initiatives (Trautman et al., 2018).

Doctor of Nursing Practice Student Quality Improvement Projects

The focus of many DNP student projects is on small-scale QI and safety initiatives within health care clinical practices and organizations. The QI-focused DNP project enables students to learn how to evaluate the function of a current system of care and determine clinical and process-related outcomes that need improvement. Through the development and implementation of the DNP project, students learn to use QI assessment tools, identify processes in need of change, and develop a change plan designed to achieve desired outcomes. The implementation of the change initiative and ongoing evaluation of how well the change process is achieving desired outcomes give students the opportunity to develop expertise in developing and leading QI initiatives.

QUALITY IMPROVEMENT INITIATIVES AND RESEARCH STUDIES

Comparison of Quality Improvement Initiatives to Research Studies

QI activities intersect with human subjects research in that they are both systematic processes that provide significant contributions to the improvement of health care (Grady, 2015). However, there are distinctions between the purpose and scope of QI initiatives and research studies. A QI initiative is a systematic approach to improve health care outcomes and quality through adaptation in the processes of care systems and local innovations, while human subjects research is a systematic investigative process to develop or contribute to new knowledge that is generalizable to other populations about illness and health (Grady, 2007). The DHHS defines research as a systematic investigation designed to develop or contribute to generalizable knowledge (Office for Human Research Protections [OHRP], 2005; DHHS, 2020).

A QI initiative implements a best practice approach designed to improve post-implementation outcomes over current or baseline data within a specific setting. In contrast, the focus of a research study is on uncovering new knowledge that can be applied to the clinical setting. Research protocol may involve random assignment of subjects to compare the efficacy of outcomes of competing treatments (James, 2007) and may put subjects at risk by using unproven therapies for the purpose of generating new knowledge about efficacy and effectiveness of a treatment. Conversely, QI initiatives use evidence-based knowledge from research study findings or best practice protocols to improve care outcomes with a specific setting (McCarthy, 2008).

TABLE 9.3   Characteristics of Human Subjects Research and QI Initiatives

Characteristics	Human Subjects Research	QI
Purpose	Test hypothesis or establish clinical practice standards	System change to improve process, program, or system/establish best practices based on existing evidence (e.g., randomized controlled trials, observational studies, consensus expert opinion)
Starting point	Test hypothesis or answer a question	Identify need to improve performance or outcomes
Design	Follow a rigid protocol that remains unchanged throughout the research	Implementation protocol is adaptive, iterative, interactive, and modified, as needed
Benefits	Might or might not benefit current subjects; intended to benefit future patients	Directly benefits a process, system, or program; might or might not benefit patients
Risks	May put subjects at risk	Protocol does not cause risk to patients
Participant obligation	No obligation of individuals to participate	Responsibility to participate as component of care
Endpoint	Answer a research question	Improve a program, process, or system
Analysis	Statistically prove or disprove hypothesis	Compare program, process, or system to establish standards or baseline data
Adoption of results	Little urgency to disseminate results quickly	Results are already a part of local care delivery
Publication/ presentation	Investigator obliged to share results	QI practitioners share results of outcomes with systemic reporting insights

QI, quality improvement.

Source: Adapted from McCarthy, D. (2008). *Case study: Is it quality improvement or research? The experiences of Intermountain Healthcare and Children's Hospital Boston.* The Commonwealth Fund [On-line]. http://www.commonwealthfund.org/publications/newsletters/quality-matters/2008/july-august/case-study-is-it-quality-improvement-or-research-the-experiences-of-intermountain-healthcare; Marshfield Clinic, 2016.

QI methodology is not structured to compare and test two competing protocols, as might be done in a research study. Table 9.3 compares the characteristics of human subjects research and QI initiatives.

INSTITUTIONAL REVIEW BOARD OVERSIGHT OF QUALITY IMPROVEMENT INITIATIVES

The question arises as to whether QI initiatives fall within the continuum of research. Is a QI initiative a form of research and subject to the guidelines and obligations of research projects within an institution? Does a QI initiative need to seek Institutional Review Board (IRB) approval to protect the safety and rights of those individuals affected by the QI protocol? To answer these questions, it helps to compare the activities of QI initiatives to research studies that seek to describe, explain, predict, and control observed phenomena and, in turn, uncover new knowledge in health care.

The role of the IRB is to protect human subject participants' welfare and rights and ensure that ethical standards are followed throughout the study. An IRB reviews study protocol details, investigator brochures, and informed consent documents to make certain that all parts of the research protocol are in accordance with ethical standards to protect human subjects. After the IRB approves a research study protocol, it oversees the study from the start to the end to protect the rights of each participant in the research study (American Psychological Association, 2015; Food and Drug Administration, 2014). The Office for Human Research Protections (OHRP), supported by the DHHS, provides rules and regulations to protect the welfare, rights, and well-being of human subjects involved in research. They recognize that some QI initiatives may have a research-focused design that might require the protection of subjects in research (Marshfield Clinic, 2016; OHRP, 2005).

Institutional Review Board Review of Quality Improvement

A QI initiative does not usually require the same IRB oversight as a research study because the activities and protocols of most quality initiatives do not test new or untested interventions and are not considered as potentially harmful to human subjects (HHS). Regulations for the protection of human subjects in research do not apply to QI activities conducted by one or more institutions whose purposes are limited to (a) implementing a practice to improve the quality of patient care, and (b) collecting patient or provider data regarding the implementation of the practice for clinical, practical, or administrative purposes (OHRP, 2005). Because these activities are not defined as research under DHHS regulation Title 45 CFR 46.102, a QI initiative is not subject to IRB review and does not require informed consent of change initiative participants (OHRP, 2005).

The most consistent way to be certain that the QI initiative meets OHRP standards is to view every improvement project as being at risk for conflict of interest (James, 2007) and to submit the details of a QI initiative for IRB review. The review would identify whether there are any QI protocol details of concern (Holm et al., 2007).

Institutional Review Board Subcommittees Essential for Nonhuman Subject Research

Many institutions have instituted a subcommittee to fast-track nonhuman subject research (NHSR) proposals, of which QI initiatives are one example. For NHSR proposals, the IRB performs an expedited review in lieu of a full and more lengthy IRB review process required for human subjects research (Weiserbs et al., 2009). The expedited review is completed in accordance with the requirements set forth by the OHRP in Title 45 CFR 46 regulation (OHRP, 2005).

One academic medical center IRB access site provides an example of a typical submission process for a QI initiative. The website has a submission form for NHSR that instructs the submitter to select the category for QI described as "Collection of data with the sole purpose to conduct a quality improvement/quality assurance project for internal use only" (Rush University, 2020). The IRB reviews the project details, determines that the protocol does not describe research criteria, and reports back to the submitter in written format that the IRB does not need to oversee the project, or in this case, quality initiative. The notification states that if any changes to the project occur that might require review, contact the research affairs office to determine whether full IRB review is necessary (2020). The IRB statement regarding its decision of the status of the project is often necessary to use as documentation of the project's status for other institutions and when submitting a related paper for publication.

Doctor of Nursing Practice Projects and Institutional Review Board Review

The determination of the IRB regarding the status of the project is important in moving forward with implementing the QI initiative. In the university setting where students conduct a DNP project, the nursing program and its academic institution require IRB review of the DNP project and ruled that the project is not human subjects research and does not require IRB oversight. Health care institutions such as hospitals and outpatient clinics require IRB review of a QI initiative with the resultant documentation letter.

Guidelines for Quality Initiatives Requiring Institutional Review Board Review

There are some QI initiatives with components that overlap with human subjects research studies and have potential for ethical or safety risks. Such initiatives may require a formal IRB review (Holm et al., 2007; National Ethics Committee of the Veterans Health Administration, 2002; Weiserbs et al., 2009). When overlap exists, the IRB completes a full review of the project to determine whether the federal regulations that protect research participants apply (Children's Hospital of Philadelphia, 2020). Table 9.4 describes the characteristics of QI initiatives that may require a full IRB review.

TABLE 9.4 Characteristics of QI Initiatives That May Require Full IRB Review

Component of QI Initiative	Reason for IRB Review
Testing of untested intervention	• Involves human subjects or their identifiable data • Intends to test a new, modified, or previously untested intervention, service, or program to determine whether it is effective and can be used locally or elsewhere
Part of a research study	• QI project is a component of larger already-determined research study
Expanding results to a research study	• Original QI project did not meet definition of research, but its results are interesting, and a decision is made to expand findings into a research project
Change initiative includes specific research details	• Novel treatments • Involvement of researchers • Delayed feedback of monitoring • Findings to develop generalizable knowledge • Involves external funding (S28, S34)
Use of standard research design methodology, such as randomization	• Patients randomized into different groups to enhance confidence in differences that might be obscured by nonrandom selection
Uses protocol with rigid goal, methodology, population, time period, etc.	• QI initiative makes frequent adjustments in the measurement, intervention, and possibly goal over time as experience accumulates
Funding from outside organization	• Third-party payor gives clinical reimbursement incentives, or internal clinical/operations funds versus research funds • Organization with interest in project results • A manufacturer with interest in outcome relevant to its products • Nonprofit foundation that typically funds research • Internal research accounts
Identifies possible risks from the intervention to participants that are greater than minimal	Randomly assign patients to different QI interventions to determine which evidence-based care is the most effective (distinguished from nonrandomized pilot test comparing the experience of different organizational subunits)

IRB, Institutional Review Board; QI, quality improvement.

Source: Adapted from Children's Hospital of Philadelphia. (2020). *Quality improvement vs research.* https://irb .research.chop.edu/quality-improvement-vs-research; Baily, M. A., Bottrell, M. M., Lynn, J., & Jennings, B. (2006). Special report: The ethics of using QI methods to improve health care quality and safety. *Hastings Center Report, 36*(4), S1–S40. https://doi.org/10.1353/hcr.2006.0054; Scheller, L. A. (2016). *Program evaluation, including quality assurance and quality improvement: Determining the need for IRB review document.* https://www.marshfieldresearch.org/Media/Default/ORIP/Documents/Program%20Evaluation.pdf; and James, B. C. (2007). Quality-improvement policy at Intermountain Healthcare. In B. Jennings, M. A. Baily, M. Bottrell, & J. Lynn (Eds.), *Health care quality improvement: Ethical and regulatory issues* (pp. 169–176). The Hastings Center.

METHODOLOGY FOR QUALITY IMPROVEMENT

The Science of Improvement

The SI is an applied science that guides QI initiatives through a systematic plan that uses evaluation tools, improvement methods, and rapid cycle testing to achieve improved outcomes (IHI, 2020b). The methodology combines academia with health service delivery using scientific methods and principles that benefit patients, populations, and health systems to improve quality, safety, and care efficiency (Marshall & Mountford, 2013).

The IHI has been instrumental in developing and refining the SI methodology used to improve safety and quality in health care (IHI, 2020b). The SI approach applies the IHI Model for Improvement to systematically test change processes designed to improve specific outcomes. A hallmark of the SI method is to implement the iterative process of rapid style tests of change to produce improvements and achieve the desired aim of the change initiative (IHI, 2020b).

The SI approach to a QI initiative includes these steps:

1. Identify a clear aim for improvement.
2. Define a measurement plan to achieve the project aim.
3. Implement small tests of changes that will lead to improvement in a short time period.
4. Refine the small change tests to achieve outcomes.
5. Broaden the testing process and scale-up of the changes.
6. Determine the best path for improvement that emerges from prior tests of change.
7. Implement changes in a sustainable way.

The Quality Improvement Team

The QI team is a group of individuals within an organization charged to carry out the change efforts for a QI initiative. The collective wisdom of a QI team adds to the identification of the problem and development of solutions to improve current outcomes in the system or organization. Since successful change efforts are collaborative and require interdisciplinary and multidepartmental support, the ideal QI team includes members who represent all areas that are affected by the proposed improvement, as well as patient representatives when appropriate (Knox & Brach, 2013).

An improvement effort needs the support and input of people within the system who want a change to take place. The QI team is formed with members who represent the organizational entities needed to effect change and improve outcomes, and it includes key players from departments and professions in the organization that are affected by the changes. The team members include key players who have organizational expertise in the areas of system leadership and clinical and technical expertise (IHI, 2020f). Team members who bring their area of expertise to the planning and implementation process ensure that there is the right balance of leadership, management, and power for the quality initiative to succeed (Silver et al., 2016b).

The success of a QI initiative is dependent upon a person with executive authority to say that changes that affect departments and personnel can take place (IHI, 2020f). The executive sponsor, also known as the project sponsor, is a person who has organizational authority and connections to senior management who make decisions regarding change strategies that have financial, structural, and personnel implications (IHI, 2020f). Take the example of a change initiative to decrease the 30-day readmission rate from an inpatient stroke center. If the implementation plan

TABLE 9.5 Characteristics of QI Team Members

Executive Sponsor	<ul><li>Has organizational power to secure resources and remove barriers</li><li>Authority to provide liaison with other areas of organization</li><li>Link to senior management and strategic aims of the organization</li><li>Reviews team's progress on a regular basis</li></ul>
Team Leader	<ul><li>Driver of QI projects</li><li>Responsible for day-to-day management of the QI project</li><li>Ensures tests are implemented</li><li>Oversees data collection</li><li>Understands system details and effects of making change(s) in the system</li><li>Works effectively with project champion(s)</li></ul>
Clinical/System Leader	<ul><li>Authority in organization to test and implement a change</li><li>Able to deal with issues that arise</li><li>Understands clinical implications of proposed changes and consequences of change in a broader system</li></ul>
Technical Experts	<ul><li>Are part of the system in which changes need to take place</li><li>Expert on improvement methods</li><li>Help team determine outcome measures and measurement tools</li><li>Understand specific components of the quality of care issue</li></ul>

QI, quality improvement.

Source: Adapted from Institute for Healthcare Improvement. (2020f). *Science of improvement: Forming the team.* http://www.ihi.org/resources/Pages/HowtoImprove/ScienceofImprovementFormingtheTeam.aspx; Silver, S. A., Harel, Z., McQuillan, R., Weizman, A. V., Thomas, A., Chertow, G. M., Nesrallah, G., Bell, C.M., & Chan, C. T. (2016b). How to begin a quality improvement project. *Clinical Journal of the American Society of Nephrology, 11*(5), 893–900. https://doi.org/10.2215/CJN.11491015.

requires the hiring of a part-time registered nurse to call patients after they have been discharged to home, it takes a person with executive authority to authorize the hiring of a nurse to make postdischarge phone calls. The QI team members may not have the authority to make those financial and personnel-related decisions.

A well-structured team has a leader who oversees every detail of the initiative from the start to the end and is responsible for the day-to-day management of the QI project (IHI, 2020f; Knox & Brach, 2013; Silver et al., 2016b). The leader guides team members individually and collectively to evaluate the current system, to assess performance data and outcomes, to identify relevant research findings and best practices, to determine the development and implement of a change plan, and to evaluate how well the change process is achieving project aims. Table 9.5 identifies the characteristics of team members (IHI, 2020f). See Chapter 11 for more information about interprofessional teams.

Contextual Factors in Quality Improvement Initiatives

A successful QI initiative involves a multidisciplinary approach of staff and clinicians who work in teams to develop and implement a change process that will improve patient and system outcomes. Contextual factors influence the success of quality initiatives and affect how people work together to achieve shared goals of a change initiative. In organizations, contextual factors reflect a particular context, characteristics unique to a particular group, community, society, and individual.

The success of a QI initiative can vary depending on contextual factors at the individual, organizational, or teamwork levels (Shea et al., 2018).

There is growing consensus in health care, which suggests that the context or the contextual factors of a quality initiative may be a reason that a successful change initiative in one setting may fail in another (McDonald, 2013). Kaplan looked at variations in the outcomes of QI initiatives and saw that the success that QI projects achieved varied greatly even in environments that supported change initiatives. Some QI teams struggled more than others and could not make desired improvements (Robert Wood Johnson Foundation, 2012). The Model for Understanding Success in Quality (MUSIQ) was developed as a framework for understanding contextual factors in QI. MUSIQ describes 25 contextual factors within a health care system that might influence the success of QI efforts. The contextual factors with the greatest total effects on QI success are as follows (2012):

- QI team characteristics (leadership, skills, and decision-making processes)
- The QI capability and motivation of the microsystem (i.e., the unit/department/office)

Contextual factors are important to the success of quality initiatives, and it is important to address contextual factors systematically. A successful QI initiative "takes a village" to develop and implement. If there is no QI team to address the change, or the team does not work together to achieve desired goals, then the improvement efforts to achieve desired outcomes will struggle and most likely fail. Along with that, there have to be motivated people at all levels of the organization and within the QI team to buy into the change idea and support each other when the inherent challenges within a system occur during the change initiative.

Contextual factors should be taken into consideration even before a QI team is developed, and those factors can be used to inform the design of the change initiative. Implementation strategies that address contextual factors promote cross-understanding of QI among team members and promote effective collaboration and, ultimately, effective implementation of QI programs (Shea et al., 2018).

Aim and SMART Aim Statements

A QI project has a clearly defined aim statement that reflects the desired performance that the organization wants to achieve and an ultimate goal as well as incremental goals that gauge the short-term progress of the intervention plan. The ultimate goal should reflect the gap between the current state of the situation and the desired outcomes to be achieved (Edgman-Levitan et al., 2020). A SMART aim is an explicit statement that describes what the QI initiative is expected to achieve (IHI, 2020g). The acronym "SMART" refers to specific, measurable, applicable, realistic, and timely. The SMART aim statement identifies the improvement goals in time-specific, quantitative, and measurable terms with identification of the specific population that is affected by the change and time-specific. The organization and QI team need to agree upon the SMART aim statement to guide the change process and determine the resources and people necessary to accomplish the aim (IHI, 2020g).

Quality Improvement Tools for Evaluating Organizational Systems

An essential component of a QI initiative is to evaluate an organizational system to identify and clarify the reasons as to why clinical outcomes are not up to a desired or required level. The purpose of the evaluation is to identify the problem, understand the problem and its causes, identify system factors that contribute to the problem, and determine strengths and weaknesses of the processes that lead to the problem. The system evaluation should include input from key players involved with the situation as to what changes might improve processes that lead to desired clinical outcomes.

There are helpful tools that assist in evaluating the system in QI initiatives. The use of assessment tools assists in identifying and understanding dynamics at play that cause poor outcomes. This section describes a number of system assessment tools useful in managing performance improvement (IHI, 2020a).

Cause and Effect Diagram

The cause and effect diagram, known also as a "fishbone" or Ishikawa diagram, is a valuable organizational tool that provides a visual conveyance of process variations and consequences of a specific problem (Agency for Healthcare Research and Quality [AHRQ], 2018). The fishbone diagram visually displays potential root causes of a problem into category areas of people/staff; environment; materials; methods; equipment/supplies; and rules, policies, and procedures (2018). Through questioning and brainstorming sessions with key players in the system, improvement teams identify steps, inadequacies, and problem areas within the diagram categories that lead to the overall problem and need improvement (IHI, 2020a).

The fishbone diagram displays the problem at the head of the fish or end of the diagram. Realities in the system that can be contributing causes to the problem are listed within specific cause categories on the smaller "bones" of the diagram (IHI, 2020a). The improvement team questions personnel who have first-hand knowledge of the processes and systems involved in the problem or event to be investigated. Figure 9.1 shows a fishbone diagram developed from a patient satisfaction survey with descriptors in each category that could play a part in patient dissatisfaction.

Key Driver Diagram

A key driver diagram is an assessment tool developed by improvement team members which visually displays what issues "drive" or contribute to the achievement of a desired outcome or improvement aim. The content of the diagram helps an improvement team to understand key components that contribute to the problem and what is needed to organize improvement strategies and achieve desired goals. There are different renditions to the structure of key driver diagrams as evidenced by key driver diagrams that include secondary drivers, while the Agency for Healthcare Research and Quality (AHRQ) model (see Figure 9.2) does not include secondary drivers (AHRQ, 2019; IHI, 2020a).

The structure and content of the driver diagram communicate relationships between the overall aim or goal of the improvement initiative and identify key drivers that contribute directly to achieving the aim and secondary drivers or change strategies that relate to the primary drivers (AHRQ, 2019; IHI, 2020a). Key drivers

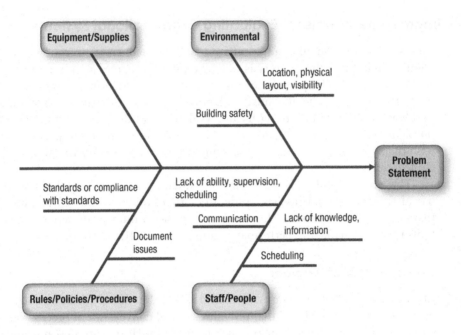

Figure 9.1 Example of fishbone diagram.

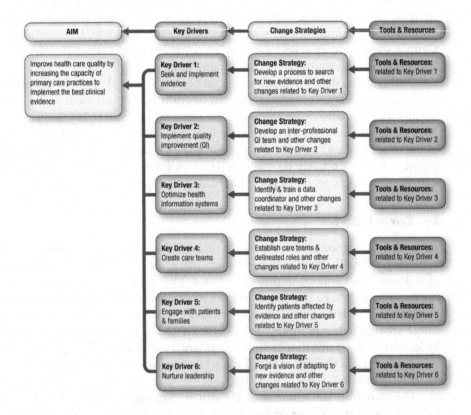

Figure 9.2 Key driver diagram.

Source: From Agency for Healthcare Research and Quality. (2019). *The EvidenceNOW key driver diagram.* Author. https://www.ahrq.gov/evidencenow/tools/keydrivers/index.htm.

are important influencers on the aim, as they state an act or a process that needs to be done to reach the aim, while secondary drivers are specific change ideas. There is an established way to measure each driver (IHI, 2020a).

Process Mapping

Process mapping breaks down events or processes, such as workflow, into individual steps that enable evaluation of how the steps in the processes can be made more efficient (DeGirolamo et al., 2018). A process map or flowchart visually identifies the steps, pathways, and transitions in a process that lead to an outcome and shows where improvement in a clinical system is needed or required to achieve an improved outcome (IHI, 2020c). The map shows the complexity of steps, people, and transitions that must occur to achieve a given outcome. It is a simple way to evaluate the journey of a process through the organization to identify areas for change that could occur to strengthen or streamline the details and achieve more effective outcomes and goals.

The example of a process map depicting the transfer of a patient from the emergency department (ED) to an inpatient unit can show why the transfer can take longer than desired. The method shows the steps between the ED and inpatient unit and identifies areas of delay and bottlenecks that occur between hospital departments such as housekeeping, patient care units (ED and admitting unit), and staff (housekeepers, nurses, physicians, aides).

In a quality initiative, a process map is developed for both the current process and the new, revised process intended to change and improve the process. Comparing the current process with the new process shows how the change addresses inefficiencies in the current process and how the new process is designed to achieve improved processes.

Surveys and Questionnaires

Surveys and questionnaires completed by key players and stakeholders in the system who interact with the system can provide information about attitudes, behaviors, or characteristics of individuals and groups. Respondents can identify strengths and weaknesses of current processes and barriers to change and suggest potential solutions to identified problems (Victorian Quality Council, 2008).

Key Informant Interviews

Key informant interviews are an evaluation strategy to gather in-depth information from well-informed people in the system. The evaluation of stakeholder perspectives, views, insights, and recommendations through focus groups and key informant interviews guides the development and implementation of QI initiatives (Victorian Quality Council, 2008). The input of knowledgeable people within an organization can help to diagnose problems and understand the views and experiences of people who are directly involved with the problematic outcomes.

SWOT Analysis

A SWOT analysis is a tool used to identify strengths, weaknesses, opportunities, and threats that exist within the system in which the identified problem lies. The SWOT analysis assesses the strengths and weaknesses of internal and external factors that lead to problematic outcomes, as well as current and future potentials within the system that can be used to develop a strategy to achieve improved system outcomes. To complete the SWOT analysis, the evaluator gathers information about the details of the system and talks with key players to describe each strength, weakness, opportunity, and threat to the system (Blayney, 2008).

DEVELOPMENT OF THE IMPLEMENTATION PLAN IN QUALITY IMPROVEMENT INITIATIVES

A Theory for Change

Change concepts are useful in the development of more specific ideas for changes as they stimulate creative and critical thinking, which lead to imaginative and specific improvement ideas (Langley et al., 2009). A change concept is a general idea with proven merit and sound scientific or logical foundation that can stimulate specific ideas for changes that lead to improvement (Plsek, 1999).

A specific and an actionable idea for changing a process is a change idea. The idea that change is needed within a system or an organization comes from a number of creative and practical sources: creative thinking, observation and critical evaluation of current processes, insight from a different situation, and hunches or intuition. A more evidence-based is scientific literature and the expert opinion of others (Plsek, 1999), while a practical source may be from seeing that other organizations recognized a problem and an improvement on a specific issue. People who work in health care settings experience processes that are cumbersome and time-consuming. Clinicians see that approaches to care are ineffective and outcomes of care and treatment are variable.

Framework for Change

The process of translating research findings into clinical practice in QI initiatives should be based on a model or strategy for implementing research evidence into practice. The framework should consider theoretical approaches to understanding behavior change, as implementing change into a system is challenging due to the structure of organizations and the complex nature for humans that make change practice from what is familiar to what is new and different. A QI team approach that addresses specific barriers to change is more likely to lead to sustained and effective changes in practice. Conversely, a passive dissemination plan that does not address inherent challenges in a complex system might prove to be ineffective (Grol & Grimshaw, 1999).

Grol and Grimshaw (1999) described a five-phase framework for QI initiatives that guides the change initiative. The five phases are the following: the development of a concrete proposal for change; analysis of the target setting and group to identify obstacles to change; linking interventions to needs, facilitators, and obstacles to change; development of an implementation plan; and monitoring progress with implementation (Grol & Grimshaw, 1999, p. 503). Another framework is the IHI

Model for Improvement used to first identify what needs to be changed within the system and then focuses on the changes that will result in improvement (IHI, 2020e) (see section on Model for Improvement). The IHI framework supports developing an implementation plan that is then tested using small tests of change that are adapted to the specific initiative and environment. A change plan that works in one clinical unit or organization may not work in another environment (IHI, 2020e; Langley et al., 2009; Silver et al., 2016b).

The details of a change protocol or implementation plan are based on the collective information that is derived from evaluation data from within the system and the input of QI team members. The QI team determines the most appropriate interventions and steps to address the identified problem and achieve the desired aim and outcomes of the QI initiative (see Quality Improvement Team section). The implementation strategy involves comparing the benefits of alternative interventions and selecting the most appropriate interventions for the situation. The steps or interventions of the implementation plan emerge from a combination of research findings, expert opinion, stakeholder input, personal experience, evidence-based practice, best practices, and even intuitions as to what might work to improve outcomes (HRSA, 2011a, 2011b). Information derived from system evaluation tools such as process maps and fishbone diagrams is also used to develop a change process (Victorian Quality Council, 2008).

THE EVALUATION OF QUALITY IMPROVEMENT AND PATIENT SAFETY INITIATIVES

The evaluation of a QI initiative to determine the extent to which the implementation plan and strategies are working to achieve the aims of the project is an ongoing process. A well-organized QI initiative clearly outlines implementation strategies, evaluation tools, and statistical measures to determine whether the desired outcomes of the initiative were achieved (Hopkins Medicine, 2015; Mittman & Salen-Schatz, 2012). A weak QI initiative results from poor conceptualization of evaluation methods that failed to determine whether the implementation strategies achieved the project's desired outcomes.

The Plan–Do–Study–Act Cycle: Evaluation and Change

The implementation process of the SI methodology is the Plan–Do–Study–Act (PDSA) cycle. PDSA cycles provide a systematic approach to the iterative process and action-oriented hallmark of QI initiatives and are an integral part of the evaluation process where small tests of change lead to the desired aim (IHI, 2020b). Change starts by planning the steps needed to achieve the aim of the project, trying the implementation steps, observing and evaluating the outcomes that the plan achieves, and acting on what is learned.

PDSA cycles are a blueprint for project managers to gain practical knowledge of the effects of the QI protocol and evaluate and revise the plan in an immediate and a sequential process. The iterative nature of an improvement protocol results from implementing small tests of change and rapid-cycle testing that allow for refinements of or modifications to the implementation plan through each cycle (Langley et al., 2009; Scoville & Little, 2014).

The Plan (P) is the test of change, change interventions, or observations and details to collect data. The Do (D) is the implementation of the action plan and carrying out the test of change, including data collection on the plan. Study (S) is observing the Do and learning from the consequences. At this point, the plan is evaluated and modifications are made that can better achieve the aim of the project. The Act (A) step is an iterative process where changes in or modifications to the plan are implemented before repeating the next PDSA cycle. Project planners make modifications to the plan based on what was learned in the Study step and go through the cycle again with a different plan. If the plan was successful, project planners incorporate wider changes from what was learned from the prior cycle (American Society for Quality [ASQ], 2009).

The length of a PDSA cycle varies with each iteration of change. A cycle could last from one day to weeks, depending on how well the processes and implementation steps are working to achieve the project aims. The evaluation of the implementation plan in relation to the outcomes achieved is at the center of PDSA cycles. The Study (S) part of the PDSA cycle is where the team evaluates how well the processes of the implementation plan are working to reach the project outcomes.

The study process identifies problems or strengths in the plan and determines what needs to be modified or changed in order to achieve the overall outcome of the project (IHI, 2020b). Each new or revised change plan is immediately under scrutiny to determine how effective the change is in achieving the aim or desired outcome. If the change process is working as evidenced by data tracking toward the project goals, the implementation steps may stay in place. If a part of the implementation plan is cumbersome, and comparison of the data with the aim predictions is not in line, then modifications to the implementation plan should be made (IHI, 2020d; Silver et al., 2016b).

Data in Quality Improvement Initiatives

Data drive QI initiatives from the problem identification through the analysis of how well change processes have improved outcomes, while playing an essential role in monitoring the performance of interventions and drawing conclusions as to how well the change initiative is achieving project goals (Langley et al., 2009). Data analysis describes the effectiveness of current system functioning, tracks how well the change processes are trending toward the desired outcomes, and enables the comparison of current or prechange outcomes with desired outcomes of the change initiative. Data measurement identifies problems with processes, systems, and care outcomes that need improvement and shows whether improvement processes are achieving the desired effects (HRSA, 2011a).

There is a clear role for the use of data in each phase of a QI initiative. Table 9.6 describes five activity phases of the QI cycle and how data relate to each phase of the change initiative. Data are the information that identifies the problem, describes whether improvement processes are achieving project aims, and shows the measure to which change interventions helped achieve project goals.

TABLE 9.6   Data in the Development and Evaluation of QI Initiatives

QI Project Phase	Data
1. Project definition phase	● Identifies current outcomes as problem areas that do not meet desired standards of process or care ● Baseline data that show why current outcomes are not sufficient
2. Diagnosis phase—[What can we improve?]	● Analyzed to evaluate existing processes within interest area and diagnose potential quality problems and/or opportunities for improvement
3. Intervention phase—[How can we achieve improvement?]	● Identified to determine performance measures ● Used to monitor improvement progress
4. Impact measurement phase—[Have we achieved improvement?]	● Analysis identifies the impact of interventions on performance measures
5. Sustainability phase—[Have we sustained improvement?]	● Analyzed to monitor desired outcome[s] ● Identifies whether interventions are sufficient to maintain achievement of outcomes ● Shows whether change processes are integrated into health care delivery

QI, quality improvement.

Source: Adapted from Victorian Quality Council. (2008). *A guide to using data for health care quality improvement.* Victorian Government Department of Human Services. https://aci.health.nsw.gov.au/__data/assets/pdf _file/0006/273336/vqc-guide-to-using-data.pdf.

Data in Improvement Initiatives

Improvement initiatives often start with a question or a problem that is data related, such as:

● Why are patient satisfaction scores low for the spinal surgery practice?
● How can the ED improve the average wait time to see the health care provider?

Data identify the extent of problems in the system, such as the length of wait times in EDs or low patient satisfaction scores for hospital stays. It identifies the extent of a problem and provides information that describes current or baseline performance and performance gaps as compared to standardized databases or the norm of other organizations. Data "pushes" improvement by identifying problems and "pulls" improvement by identifying opportunities that can improve quality outcomes in a system (Victorian Quality Council, 2008). Qualitative data as gathered through interviews, observations, and questionnaires help a system understand the needs of the organization, opinions of stakeholders, and what can or should be done to improve the organization (Langley et al., 2009).

Data Measures

The second question of the IHI Model for Improvement is "How will we know that change is an improvement?" This question addresses the need to identify data analytic measures that will show whether the change processes have achieved an improvement toward the desired outcomes (IHI, 2020e). Data are used to set measurable targets that are linked clearly to the aims, objectives, and outcomes of an improvement initiative.

Measuring outcomes during a change initiative is an ongoing process to determine how well the change strategies are trending toward the goal. Collecting both quantitative and qualitative data is essential to identifying or evaluating the effectiveness of change strategies in achieving a project's aim.

Table 9.7 defines the three types of measures used in QI initiatives: outcome measures, process measures, and balancing measures. IHI recommends a balance among the three types of measures used in QI initiative.

Measurement for improvement initiatives should not be confused with measurement for research. The comparisons in measurement for research and measurement for process improvement in QI initiatives are outlined in Table 9.8.

TABLE 9.7   QI Measures

QI Measure	Definition
Outcome measure	• Defines what the change initiative wants to achieve • The standard against which one assesses the end result of the intervention • End result of a test used to objectively determine the baseline function of a patient at the beginning of treatment and then determine treatment efficacy by using the same test at the end of treatment
Process measure	• Determines whether the parts/steps in the system are performing as the protocol planned • Process measures help to determine whether the initiative is on track with its efforts in place to improve the system
Balancing measure	• Changes made to one part of the system cause unexpected problems in other parts of the system • Help project implementers view the system from a different direction or dimension in an effort to determine whether changes made in one part of the system (through the initiation of a QI protocol) are causing problems in other parts of the system

QI, quality improvement.

Source: Adapted from Institute for Healthcare Improvement. (2015b). *Measures. Science of improvement: Establishing measures.* Author. www.ihi.org/resources/Pages/HowtoImprove/ScienceofImprovementEstablishingMeasures. aspx; Institute for Healthcare Improvement. (2020e). *Quality improvement 102: The model for improvement: Your engine for change summary sheet.* http://www.ihi.org/education/ihiopenschool/Courses/Documents/QI102 -FinalOnePager.pdf.

TABLE 9.8   Comparison of Measurement for Quality Improvement Versus Research

	Measurement for Research	Measurement for Learning and Process Improvement
Purpose	Discover and identify new knowledge	Apply new information to daily practices
Tests	One large "blind" test	Multiple sequential test cycles that are observable
Biases	Control for internal biases within the research protocol	Stabilize biases within the testing processes
Data	Gather as much data as possible during the study process	Gather just enough data that are needed to complete and start another test cycle
Duration	Study may take much needed time to complete data collection to obtain results	Short and frequent PDSA cycles accelerate improvement toward the desired outcomes
Variables	Controls as many variables as possible during study implementation	No need to control variables during the implementation process; no manipulation of the environment

PDSA, Plan–Do–Study–Act.

Source: Adapted from Institute for Healthcare Improvement. (2015b). *Measures. Science of improvement: Establishing measures.* Author. www.ihi.org/resources/Pages/HowtoImprove/ScienceofImprovementEstablishingMeasures.aspx.

Data: Change That Improves Outcomes

The third question of the Model for Improvement is "What change can we make that will result in improvement?" Data identify problems in the system and opportunities for change and guide the development of interventions needed to reach project aims (Victorian Quality Council, 2008). For example, the evaluation of a handoff process between the anesthesia providers and post-anesthesia care unit (PACU) nurses that showed an unstructured handoff process identified data to support the development of an improved handoff process that provided more structure to the communication processes between anesthesia staff and PACU nurses. Given the need for more structure in communication, project developers decided to implement a handoff checklist used in other types of handoff situations as one step to improve handoffs between anesthesia providers and PACU nurses.

Data and data analysis are the bases for identifying problems, determining change strategies, and measuring the impact of the change strategies (Langley et al., 2009). Qualitative and quantitative assessments of the implementation strategies and the resultant outcomes demonstrate how well the change initiative aim has been met. Collecting the appropriate data throughout the implementation process is essential to determining the impact and success of the interventions. The analysis of appropriate data shows the project's success and impacts on the system and ensures that the right conclusions are drawn from the interventions (2009).

SUSTAINABILITY OF IMPROVEMENT INITIATIVES

Sustainability is the extent to which a newly implemented improvement process is maintained or institutionalized within the ongoing, stable operations of an organization and integrated into the culture of the organization's ongoing clinical practice and policies (Proctor et al., 2011). Another way to describe sustainability is when the improved outcomes and new ways of working become the organizational norm (Maher et al., 2010). While a quality initiative may achieve change and improve outcomes in a given time frame, it is important to sustain or continue to achieve the desired outcomes.

In any improvement initiative, the organization needs to focus on both achieving the aims of the change initiative and sustaining the changes and desired outcomes of the improvement efforts (Mortimer et al., 2018). In many change initiatives, sustaining the change does not occur because change methods can be complex to maintain, oversight of the new processes can waiver or stop, and the human and economic resources needed to sustain the initiative may not be sufficient to maintain the project (Beer & Nohria, 2000; Silver et al., 2016a). The United Kingdom's National Health Service (NHS) found that 33% of QI projects are not sustained following evaluation 1 year after the initiative is completed (Maher et al., 2010; Silver et al., 2016a). There are a number of factors that lead to either sustainability or deterioration of organizational change that starts and can be identified at the development phase of change initiative. Factors that affect a project's sustainability can be financial, political, contextual, and leadership in nature (Buchanan & Fitzgerald, 2007).

The Institute for Innovation and Improvement developed a sustainability model that is used from the start of a QI initiative to address factors within a change initiative that affect its sustainability (Maher et al., 2010). Factors that support a project's sustainability should be in place from the beginning of the QI initiative. The NHS Sustainability Model describes three areas of focus, process, staff, and organization, along with 10 associated factors that should be identified and addressed prior to the start of a change initiative. The presence of the project factors will increase the chance of sustaining the change initiative (Maher et al., 2010) (see Table 9.9).

TABLE 9.9　NHS Sustainability Model: QI Project Factors that Maximize Sustainability

Area of Focus	Project Factors That Support Sustainability
Process	Benefits beyond helping patients
	Credibility of the evidence
	Adaptability of improved process
	Effectiveness of the system to monitor progress
Staff	Staff involvement and training to sustain the process
	Staff behaviors toward sustaining the change
	Senior leadership engagement
	Clinical leadership engagement
Organization	Fit with organizational strategic aims and culture
	Infrastructure present for sustainability
	Cost–benefit analysis to consider ongoing resource needs for staff and equipment

NHS, National Health Service; QI, quality improvement.

Source: From Maher, L., Gustafson, D., & Evans, A. (2010). *Sustainability model and guide.* https://www.england .nhs.uk/improvement-hub/wp-content/uploads/sites/44/2017/11/NHS-Sustainability-Model-2010.pdf

There is a strategic imperative to sustain the implementation processes or working methods that achieved performance improvement (Buchanan & Fitzgerald, 2007) because it shows that the change steps to achieve the desired outcomes have become part of the fabric of the system. When a QI initiative is sustained, the implementation strategies are maintained and become routinized within the system as the process used to achieve the improved outcomes aims of the change initiative.

KNOWLEDGE GENERATED FROM QUALITY IMPROVEMENT PROJECTS

In order to describe the knowledge generated from QI initiatives, it is helpful to first understand the types of knowledge that encompass scholarly activities. Boyer developed a model of scholarship that broadened the focus of scholarly activity to include activities that expand beyond traditional research projects (Boyer, 1990). Boyer's four areas of scholarship are the scholarships of discovery, integration, application, and teaching and learning. QI initiatives often apply the knowledge and findings gained from research to develop processes or protocols that are then put in place to improve health care outcomes. Therefore, the knowledge that QI generates is in the realms of application and integration of knowledge (1990). See Table 9.10.

The DNP nurse advances the scholarship of practice through the development, implementation, and evaluation of QI initiatives at the local, regional, national, or international levels (AACN, 2018; Boyer, 1990).

Dissemination of Findings of Quality Improvement Initiatives

Throughout a quality initiative, the results of the change process should be communicated to the stakeholders and organizations. There are a number of ways to disseminate findings including presentations to stakeholders, detailed reports, news releases, meetings with key people in the organization, and press conferences, to name a few. It is imperative that the findings are shared with those who are then in charge of continuing the process within the institution (Unite for Sight, 2015).

TABLE 9.10 Categories and Focus of Scholarship

Type of Scholarship	Focus of Scholarly Activity
Scholarship of discovery	Original research to advance knowledge
Scholarship of integration	Synthesizes information between disciplines, across topics within a discipline, or across time
Scholarship of application/scholarship of engagement	Involves rigor and application of discipline-specific expertise with results shared with and/or evaluated by peers
Scholarship of teaching	Systematic study of teaching and learning processes. Teaching transmits, transforms, and extends knowledge.

Source: Adapted from Boyer, E. L. (1990). *Scholarship reconsidered: Priorities of the professoriate.* The Carnegie Foundation for the Advancement of Teaching.

On a broader scale, the details of a quality initiative can be written in a scholarly paper to describe the goals, change methods, and outcomes for other organizations to review.

Models in Quality Improvement Initiatives

A model serves as a blueprint to guide the QI processes of problem identification, solution determination, evaluation of the implementation processes, and system evaluation while providing a standard format of how work flows that everyone can understand (Scoville & Little, 2014). Models guide people and systems to ensure that people get the right care, at the right time, by the right team, and in the right place and to outline best practice care and services for a person (Agency for Clinical Innovation, 2013).

In QI, the improvement team uses a model to guide the approach and steps to change within the organization and guide a rigorous evaluation process for a QI/patient safety project. A model describes the process to follow as the steps of the project unfold from identification of the problem, initiation of changes, and timing of evaluation processes to the determination of how effective the change plan has been. Finally, models provide a pathway to take ongoing findings and use them to improve the system during the implementation process and to then make further changes that lead to the goal of improved outcomes

This section describes specific models that health care organizations can use to guide QI activities and shape quality program infrastructures to improve care and outcomes for patients and organizational systems (HRSA, 2011b).

The Model for Improvement

The Model for Improvement is a change framework created by Associates for Process Improvement (API) and based on the QI work of W. Edwards Deming (1900–1993). It is an effective and a simplistic process to guide purposeful change actions through a systematic approach to improve patient care and process-based outcomes (IHI, 2015a). The Model for Improvement defines a nonlinear change process that adapts to modifications throughout the initiative and supports small tests of change to determine what improvement processes are optimal to achieve project aims (Langley, 2009).

There are five central principles that guide QI initiatives in the Model for Improvement (Langley, 2009):

1. Knowing why you need to improve something;
2. Having a feedback mechanism to identify that improvement is occurring;
3. Developing a change process that results in improvement;
4. Testing a change process (small-scale) before implementing the change (full-scale); and
5. Knowing when to implement the change process.

The first section of the Model for Improvement asks three questions that define the endpoint of a change initiative and guide the improvement initiative from the start to the end (IHI, 2015a; Langley et al., 2009). The three questions that can be answered in any order are as follows:

1. What are we trying to accomplish? (defines what does the system want to achieve)
2. How will we know that the change is an improvement? (determines the evidence needed to show that an improvement has occurred)
3. What change can we make that will result in improvement? (describes changes necessary that will cause improvement and positive change in the system)

These questions guide the improvement team to identify and describe the problems in a system and articulate outcomes that need to be improved, indicators that show whether an improvement is achieved, and the implementation plan needed to improve the desired outcomes. It is necessary to address the details of each question prior to the start of a QI initiative in order to drive change and improvements (Langley et al., 2009). The question *What are we trying to accomplish?* makes the program developers identify the problem within the system and describe the goal or the aims of the change initiative. Questions 2 and 3 of the model address the implementation plan and the data and the data analysis needed to achieve the change and show to what extent the change is accomplishing the desired goals.

The second part of the Model for Improvement employs the PDSA cycle that is the basis for small, rapid-cycle tests of change (IHI, 2020b). The PDSA cycle is a formula for change that helps project managers determine whether modifications to implementation steps are needed to project aims and outcomes (Scoville & Little, 2014). PDSA cycles are the framework for the trial and learning methodology that implements small tests of change and repeated again and again for continuous improvement as an ongoing process to test the change (ASQ, 2020). (See section The Plan–Do–Study–Act Cycle: Evaluation and Change for discussion and description of PDSA cycles.)

The Triple Aim

The IHI Triple Aim framework is an approach to optimizing health system performance. It is a framework that provides a basis for organizations and communities to transition from a health care focus to optimizing health for populations and individuals (IHI, 2015c). The Triple Aim framework is a statement of purpose to transform health care systems to better meet the needs of people and patients. The successful implementation of the Triple Aim will result in new systems that contribute to the health of populations while reducing the costs to society (Lewis, 2014).

The Triple Aim describes three dimensions that should be pursued simultaneously to ultimately improve the quality of health care, outcome measures, and cost of care: improving the patient experience of care (including quality and satisfaction); improving the health of populations; and reducing the per capita cost of health care (Berwick et al., 2008; IHI, 2015c).

The Triple Aim addresses IHI's recognition that successful health and health care systems of the future will be able to deliver excellent quality of care, at optimized costs, while improving the health of their population. The IHI believes that achieving the Triple Aim is the ultimate goal for the high-performing hospitals and health systems (IHI, 2015c; Lewis, 2014; Stiefel & Nolan, 2012). The IHI Triple Aim framework advocates a focused approach to change based on the identification of target populations: defining what a system wants to accomplish and measure; development of a project that will affect change in the system; and the implementation of a change approach that is able to adapt to local needs and conditions (IHI, 2015c).

The Lean Model

The "Lean" approach to QI and optimization of performance and management of value-producing system is a set of tools, methods, and integrated principles developed from the Toyota Production System. The motivation underlying the Lean method is to demystify the quality process so that problem-solving becomes a part of the mindset of all of the staff, not just of quality experts in the organization (Scoville & Little, 2014). The strength of Lean is fast implementation, immediate benefits regarding error reduction, and improved productivity and customer lead times, while long-term benefits include improvements in customer satisfaction, staff morale, and financial performance.

The Lean model defines value by what a patient or customer wants and maps how the value flows to the patient. The Lean approach to QI started in the manufacturing industry to streamline processes while right sizing an organization to produce a quality product in a safe, efficient, and outcomes-oriented manner (Dahlgaard-Park & Dahlgaard, 2006; Lean Enterprise Institute, 2015). While the Lean approach guarantees the proficiency of a process through making the process time efficient and cost-effective (HRSA, 2011b), its focus is on eliminating waste, avoiding superfluous processes, and reducing production time and costs while preserving value with less work. Operations that fail to create value for the end customer are deemed wasteful. The Japanese founders of Toyota listed the seven wastes as (a) transport, (b) inventory, (c) motion, (d) waiting, (e) overproduction, (f) overprocessing, and (g) defects (HRSA, 2011b).

The Lean approach to QI is a five-step process to guide the implementation of the model (Lean Enterprise Institute, 2015):

1. Identify value: Specify value from the standpoint of the end customer by product family.
2. Map the value stream: Identify all steps in the value stream for each product family, eliminating whenever possible those steps that do not create value.
3. Create flow: Make the value-creating steps occur in tight sequence so the product will flow smoothly toward the customer.
4. Establish pull: As flow is introduced, let customers pull value from the next upstream activity.
5. Seek perfection: Value is specified, value streams are identified, wasted steps are removed, and flow and pull are introduced. The process goes on indefinitely and continues until the ideal process is achieved in which perfect value is created with no waste.

Leaders in health care have adapted Lean tools and principles to obtain higher quality outcomes at a lower cost to meet the needs of the organization (Lean Enterprise Institute, 2015). The Lean approach to QI works best in process-oriented industries that have clearly defined manufacturing or supply-chain elements such as the automotive, pharmaceutical, and industrial engineering industries.

Six Sigma Model

The Six Sigma approach to quality is a performance improvement method used when there is a need for drastic changes and improvements in an organization. An organization that initiates the Six Sigma approach to QI understands that the process will be timely and expensive due to the need for radical changes within the organizational structure (Benedetto, 2002). Due to the large-scale organizational changes necessary when Six Sigma is used as the change model, small QI initiatives do not warrant the use of the Six Sigma approach. The term "Sigma" is the number of standard deviations a given process is from perfection. At the Six Sigma level, a manufacturing process is virtually error-free with approximately 3.4 defects per million opportunities (99.9996%; HRSA, 2011b; Villanova, 2020).

The Six Sigma approach to improvement is a strategy focused on changing the culture of an organization that is in need of improving its processes that fall below desired outcomes (Benedetto, 2002). The Motorola Corporation designed the Six Sigma to decrease process variations, reduce cost, and eliminate defects in the manufacturing of their products. It uses strategies and tools to limit variability and defects in business processes, with the ultimate goal of process and performance improvement.

The Six Sigma uses two models to frame improvement called DMAIC, designed to examine existing processes, and DMADV, used to develop new processes. The DMAIC process steps are similar to the IHI Model for Improvement in that both identify the problem and follow through to improving the problem. The five steps of the DMAIC model are the following:

Step 1: Define the problem. Identify the problem that affects customer or company processes.
Step 2: Measure the problem
Step 3: Analyze the problem
Step 4: Improve (solve the problem)
Step 5: Control (sustain the improvements)

The DMADV approach to change is appropriate to use when a client or customer requires an improved product or a completely new service or product. The DMADV approach is focused on creating a product that addresses the customer's requirements. The DMADV model steps are the following (Villanova, 2020):

Step 1: Define: Identify what the customer wants.
Step 2: Measure: Define metrics to collect data and record specifications.
Step 3: Analyze: Test results of the manufacturing process.
Step 4: Design: Compare the test results with customer wants and needs.
Step 5: Verify: Adjust product or service processes.

The Six Sigma methodologies are implemented over many months or years with an end result of a service or product that is aligned with what a customer wants, needs, and expects.

Lean Six Sigma Model

The Six Sigma and Lean are often used in conjunction with one another in health care initiatives. While both of them address profit maximization, the Six Sigma focuses on the customer and end product, while the Lean focuses on waste and production methods. In health care, the Lean and Six Sigma approaches to QI can reduce variability and waste and improve errors, processes, patient care, and patient satisfaction rates, which, in turn, improve outcomes (Mozammel et al., 2011).

SUMMARY

This chapter described the intersection of the DNP nurse with QI and change initiatives and the role the DNP nurse has in improving health care outcomes within a health care system. The DNP educational process equips its graduates with the background and experience to lead quality and change initiatives at the local and national levels. The DNP nurse has a transformative role in health care delivery by evaluating systems of care and leading teams that develop and implement quality initiatives that improve care delivery and improve patient outcomes. Understanding the many facets of QI and its essential role in achieving the safe and effective delivery of health care is an essential aspect of the role of the DNP nurse in the 21st century.

REFERENCES

Agency for Clinical Innovation. (2013). *Understanding the process to develop a model of Care: An ACI framework*. Author [On-line]. http://www.aci.health.nsw.gov.au/__data/assets/pdf_file/0009/181935/HS13-034_Framework-DevelopMoC_D7.pdf

Agency for Healthcare Research and Quality. (2018). *Education & training for health professionals-flowchart*. https://www.ahrq.gov/patient-safety/education/index.html

Agency for Healthcare Research and Quality. (2019). *The EvidenceNOW key driver diagram*. Author. https://www.ahrq.gov/evidencenow/tools/keydrivers/index.htm

American Association of Colleges of Nursing. (2006). *The essentials of doctoral education for advanced nursing practice*. https://www.aacnnursing.org/Portals/42/Publications/DNPEssentials.pdf

American Association of Colleges of Nursing. (2018). *Defining scholarship for academic nursing*. www.aacnnursing.org/Portals/42/News/Position-Statements/Defining-Scholarship.pdf.

American Association of Colleges of Nursing. (2021). *The essentials: Core competencies for professional nursing education*. Author. https://www.aacnnursing.org/Portals/42/AcademicNursing/pdf/Essentials-2021.pdf

American Psychological Association. (2015). *Frequently asked questions about institutional review boards*. Author [On-line]. http://www.apa.org/about/gr/science/advocacy/2007/irbs.aspx

American Society for Quality. (2020). *Project planning and implementing tools: Plan-Do-Check-Act cycle*. https://asq.org/quality-resources/pdca-cycle

Andel, C., Davidow, S. L., Hollander, M., & Moreno, D. A. (2012). The economics of health care quality and medical errors. *Journal of Health Care Finance, 39*(1), 39. PMID: 23155743.

Baily, M. A., Bottrell, M. M., Lynn, J., & Jennings, B. (2006). Special report: The ethics of using QI methods to improve health care quality and safety. *Hastings Center Report, 36*(4), S1–S40. https://doi.org/10.1353/hcr.2006.0054

Beer, M., & Nohria, N. (2000). Cracking the code of change. *Harvard Business Review, 78*(3), 133–141. PMID: 11183975.

Benedetto, A. R. (2002). Six Sigma: Not for the faint of heart. *Radiology Management, 25*, 40–53. PMID: 12800564.

Berwick, D., Nolan, T., & Whittington, J. (2008). The Triple Aim: Care, health, and cost. *Health Affairs, 27*, 759–769. https://doi.org/10.1377/hlthaff.27.3.759

Black, H. G., Goad, E. A., & Attaway, J. S. (2018). Medical errors: Extreme service failures and recoveries. *International Journal of Pharmaceutical and Healthcare Marketing, 12*(1), 15–24. https://doi .org/10.1108/ijphm-11-2016-0063

Blayney, D. W. (2008). Strengths, weaknesses, opportunities, and threats. *Journal of Oncology Practice, 4*(2), 53. https://doi.org/10.1200/JOP.0820501

Botwinick, L., Bisognano, M., & Haraden, C. (2006). *Leadership guide to patient safety.* IHI Innovation Series white paper. Institute for Healthcare Improvement. www.IHI.org

Boyer, E. L. (1990). *Scholarship reconsidered: Priorities of the professoriate.* The Carnegie Foundation for the Advancement of Teaching.

Brennan, T. A., Hebert, L. E., Laird, N. M., Lawthers, A., Thorpe, K. E., Leape, L. L., & Hiatt, H. H. (1991). Hospital characteristics associated with adverse events and substandard care. *Journal of the American Medical Association, 265,* 3265–3269. https://doi.org/10.1001/jama.1991.03460240061028

Brown, M. A., & Crabtree, K. (2013). The development of practice scholarship in DNP programs: A paradigm shift. *Journal of Professional Nursing, 29*(6), 330–337. https://doi.org/10.1016/j .profnurs.2013.08.003

Buchanan, D. A., & Fitzgerald, L. (2007). Improvement evaporation: Why do successful changes decay? In D. A. Buchanan, L. Fitzgerald, & D. Ketley (Eds.), *The sustainability and spread of organizational change* (pp. 22–40). Routledge.

Carter, M. W., Zhu, M., Xiang, J., & Porell, F. W. (2014). Investigating the long-term consequences of adverse medical events among older adults. *Injury Prevention, 20,* 408–415. https://doi.org/10.1136/ injuryprev-2013-041043

Children's Hospital of Philadelphia. (2020). *Quality improvement vs research.* https://irb.research.chop .edu/quality-improvement-vs-research

Dahlgaard-Park, S.M., & Dahlgaard, J. J. (2006). Lean production, Six Sigma quality, TQM and company culture. *The TQM Magazine, 18,* 263–281. https://doi.org/10.1108/09544780610659998

DeGirolamo, K., D'souza, K., Hall, W., Joos, E., Garraway, N., Sing, C. K., McLaughlin, P., & Hameed, M. (2018). Process mapping as a framework for performance improvement in emergency general surgery. *Canadian Journal of Surgery, 61*(1), 13–18. https://doi.org/10.1503/cjs.004417

Edgman-Levitan, S., Shaller, D., Campione, J., Zema, C., Abraham, J. R., & Yount, N. (2020, February). *The CAHPS ambulatory care improvement guide: Practical strategies for improving patient experience.* Agency for Healthcare Research and Quality. https://www.ahrq.gov/cahps/quality-improvement/ improvement-guide/improvement-guide.html

Federal Drug Administration. (2014). Institutional review boards frequently asked questions—Information sheet. U.S. Food and Drug Administration. http://www.fda.gov/RegulatoryInformation/ Guidances/ucm126420.htm

Grady, C. (2007). Quality improvement and ethical oversight. *Annals of Internal Medicine, 146*(9), 680–681. https://doi.org/10.7326/0003-4819-146-9-200705010-00156

Grady, C. (2015). Institutional review boards: Purpose and challenges. *Chest, 148*(5), 1148–1155. https://doi.org/10.1378/chest.15-0706

Grol, R., & Grimshaw, J. (1999). Evidence-based implementation of evidence-based medicine. *The Joint Commission Journal on Quality Improvement, 25*(10), 503–513. https://doi.org/10.1016/ s1070-3241(16)30464-3

Health Resources and Services Administration. (2011a). *Managing data for performance improvement.* https://www.hrsa.gov/sites/default/files/quality/toolbox/508pdfs/managingdataperformanceim provement.pdf

Health Resources and Services Administration. (2011b). *Quality improvement.* U.S. Department of Health and Human Services. https://www.hrsa.gov/sites/default/files/quality/toolbox/508pdfs/quali tyimprovement.pdf

Holm, M., Selvan, M., Smith, M., Markman, M., Theriault, R., Rodriguez, M., & Martin, S. (2007). Quality improvement or research: Defining and supervising QI at the University of Texas M. D. Anderson Cancer Center. In B. Jennings, M. Baily, M. Bottrell, & J. Lynn (Eds.), *Health care quality improvement: Ethical and regulatory issues* (pp. 144–168). Hastings Center.

Hopkins Medicine. (2015). *Evaluating quality improvement and patient safety projects.* Armstrong Institute for Patient Safety and Quality. http://www.hopkinsmedicine.org/armstrong_institute/training _services/workshops/evaluating.html

Institute for Healthcare Improvement. (2015a). *How to improve: Improvement methods.* Author. https:// www.ihi.org/IHI/Topics/Improvement/ImprovementMethods/HowToImprove/

Institute for Healthcare Improvement. (2015b). *Measures. Science of improvement: Establishing measures.* Author. www.ihi.org/resources/Pages/HowtoImprove/ScienceofImprovementEstablishingMeasures .aspx

Institute for Healthcare Improvement. (2015c). *The IHI triple aim.* Author. https://www.ihi.org/engage/ initiatives/tripleaim/pages/default.aspx

Institute for Healthcare Improvement. (2020a). *Quality improvement essentials toolkit.* http://www.ihi .org/resources/Pages/Tools/Quality-Improvement-Essentials-Toolkit.aspx

Institute for Healthcare Improvement. (2020b). *Science of improvement.* www.ihi.org/about/Pages/Sci enceofImprovement.aspx

Institute for Healthcare Improvement. (2020c). *Process mapping.* https://www.med.unc.edu/ihqi/ resources/process-mapping/

Institute for Healthcare Improvement. (2020d). *Science of improvement: Testing changes.* http://www.ihi .org/resources/Pages/HowtoImprove/ScienceofImprovementTestingChanges.aspx

Institute for Healthcare Improvement. (2020e). *Quality improvement 102: The model for improvement: Your engine for change summary sheet.* http://www.ihi.org/education/ihiopenschool/Courses/Docu ments/QI102-FinalOnePager.pdf

Institute for Healthcare Improvement. (2020f). *Science of improvement: Forming the team* http://www .ihi.org/resources/Pages/HowtoImprove/ScienceofImprovementFormingtheTeam.aspx

Institute for Healthcare Improvement. (2020g). *Science of improvement: Setting aims.* http://www.ihi.org/ resources/Pages/HowtoImprove/ScienceofImprovementSettingAims.aspx

Institute of Medicine. (1990). Medicare: A strategy for quality assurance (Vol. 1). National Academies Press.

Institute of Medicine. (2000). *To err is human: Building a safer health system.* The National Academies Press. https://doi.org/10.17226/9728.

Institute of Medicine. (2001). *Crossing the quality chasm: A new health system for the 21st century.* National Academies Press. https://doi.org/10.17226/10027

Institute of Medicine. (2003). *Health professions education: A bridge to quality.* National Academies Press.

James, B. C. (2007). Quality-improvement policy at Intermountain Healthcare. In B. Jennings, M. A. Baily, M. Bottrell, & J. Lynn (Eds.), *Health care quality improvement: Ethical and regulatory issues* (pp. 169–176). The Hastings Center.

James, J. T. (2013). A new, evidence-based estimate of patient harms associated with hospital care. *Journal of Patient Safety, 9*(3), 122–128. https://doi.org/10.1097/pts.0b013e3182948a69

Knox, L., & Brach, C. (2013). *The practice facilitation handbook: Training modules for new facilitators and their trainers.* Agency for Healthcare Research and Policy. https://www.ahrq.gov/ncepcr/tools/ pf-handbook/mod13-trainers.html

Langley, G. J., Moen, R., Nolan, K. M., Nolan, T. W., Norman, C. L., & Provost, L. P. (2009). *The improvement guide: A practical approach to enhancing organizational performance.* Jossey-Bass.

Lean Enterprise Institute. (2015). *Principles of lean.* Author. http://www.lean.org/WhatsLean/Principles. cfm

Leape, L., Berwick, D., Clancy, C., Conway, J., Gluck, P., Guest, J., Lawrence, D., Morath, J., O'Leary, D., O'Neill, P., & Pinakiewicz, D. (2009). Transforming healthcare: A safety imperative. *Quality and Safety in Health Care, 18*(6) 424–428. https://doi.org/10.1136/qshc.2009.036954

Lewis, N. (2014). *A primer on defining the triple aim.* Institute for Healthcare Improvement. http://www .ihi.org/communities/blogs/Documents/rsomgtae.4lc.1e880535-d855-4727-a8c1-27ee672f115d.33. pdf

Maher, L., Gustafson, D., & Evans, A. (2010). Sustainability model and guide. https://www.england. nhs.uk/improvement-hub/wp-content/uploads/sites/44/2017/11/NHS-Sustainability-Model-2010. pdf

Marshall, M., & Mountford, J. (2013). Developing a science of improvement. *Journal of the Royal Society of Medicine, 106*(2), 45–50. https://doi.org/10.1177/0141076812472622

Massoud, M. R. (2001). Advances in quality improvement: Principles and framework. *QA Brief, 9,* 13–17.

Marshfield Clinic. (2016). Program evaluation, including quality assurance and quality improvement: Determining the need for IRB review. https://www.marshfieldresearch.org/Media/Default/ORIP/Doc uments/Program%20Evaluation.pdf

McCarthy, D. (2008). *Case study: Is it quality improvement or research? The experiences of Intermountain Healthcare and Children's Hospital Boston.* The Commonwealth Fund [On-line]. http://

www.commonwealthfund.org/publications/newsletters/quality-matters/2008/july-august/case-study-is-it-quality-improvement-or-research-the-experiences-of-intermountain-healthcare

McDonald, K. M. (2013). Considering context in quality improvement interventions and implementation: Concepts, frameworks, and application. *Academic Pediatrics, 13*(6), S45–S53. https://doi.org/10.1016/j.acap.2013.04.013.

Melynk, B. (2013). Distinguishing the preparation and roles of doctor of philosophy and doctor of nursing practice graduates: National implications for academic curricula and health care systems. *Journal of Nursing Education, 52*(8), 442–448. https://doi.org/10.3928/01484834-20130719-01

Mittman, B., & Salen-Schatz, S. (2012). *Improving research and evaluation around continuous quality improvement in health care*. Robert Wood Johnson Foundation.

Mortimer, F., Isherwood, J., Wilkinson, A., & Vaux, E. (2018). Sustainability in quality improvement: Redefining value. *Future Healthcare Journal, 5*(2), 88–93. https://doi.org/10.7861/futurehosp.5-2-88

Mozammel, A., Mapa, L. B., & Scachitti, S. (2011). Application of Lean Six Sigma in healthcare—A graduate level directed project experience. Calumet American Society for Engineering Education.

National Ethics Committee of the Veterans Health Administration. (2002). *Recommendations for the ethical conduct of quality improvement*. National Center for Ethics in Health Care, Veterans Health Administration, Department of Veterans Affairs.

National Research Council of the National Academies (National Research Council) (2005). *Advancing the nation's health needs: NIH research training programs.*: National Academies Press.

Office for Human Research Protections. (2005). *45 CFR 46 – Protection of human subjects. Title 45 Part 46*. Department of Health and Human Services. https://www.govinfo.gov/app/details/CFR-2005-title45-vol1/CFR-2005-title45-vol1-part46/summary

O'Kane, M. (2009). Do patients need to be protected from quality improvement? In B. Jennings, M. A. Baily, M. Bottrell, & J. Lynn (Eds.), *Health care quality improvement: Ethical and regulatory issues* (pp. 89–100). The Hastings Center.

Paplham, P., & Austin-Ketch, T. (2015). Doctor of nursing practice education: Impact on advanced nursing practice. *Seminars in Oncology Nursing, 31*(4), 273–281. https://doi.org/10.1016/j.soncn.2015.08.003

Plsek, P. (1999). Innovative thinking for the improvement of medical systems. *Annals of Internal Medicine, 131*(6), 438–444. https://doi.org/10.7326/0003-4819-131-6-199909210-00009

Proctor, E., Silmere, H., Raghavan, R., Hovmand, P., Aarons, G., Bunger, A., Griffey, R., & Hensley, M. (2011). Outcomes for implementation research: Conceptual distinctions, measurement challenges, and research agenda. *Administration and Policy in Mental Health and Mental Health Services Research, 38*(2), 65–76. https://doi.org/10.1007/s10488-010-0319-7

Reid, P. P., Compton, W., Grossman, J. H., & Fanjiang, G. (2005). *Building a better delivery system: A new engineering/health care partnership*. National Academies Press.

Robert Wood Johnson Foundation. (2012). *Identifying contextual factors that impact quality improvement projects and their likelihood of success*. Author. https://www.rwjf.org/en/library/articles-and-news/2012/06/identifying-contextual-factors-that-impact-quality-improvement-p.html

Rodziewicz, T. L., & Hipskind, J. E. (2020). *Medical error prevention*. StatPearls. https://www.ncbi.nlm.nih.gov/books/NBK499956/

Rush University. (2020). *Rush university medical center non-human subject research request form*. https://redcap.rush.edu/redcap/surveys/?s=LWREMPAE4X%20

Schimpff, S. C. (2012). *The future of health-care delivery: Why it must change and how it will affect you*. Potomac Books.

Scoville, R., & Little, K. C. (2014). *Comparing lean and quality improvement. IHI white paper IHI white paper*. Institute for Healthcare Improvement. http://www.ihi.org/resources/Pages/IHIWhitePapers/ComparingLeanandQualityImprovement.aspx.

Shea, C. M., Turner, K., Albritton, J., & Reiter, K. L. (2018). Contextual factors that influence quality improvement implementation in primary care: The role of organizations, teams, and individuals. *Health Care Management Review, 43*(3), 261. https://www.ncbi.nlm.nih.gov/pmc/articles/PMC5976517/

Shojania, K. G., Duncan, B. W., McDonald, K. M., Wachter, R. M., & Markowitz, A. J. (2001). *Making health care safer: A critical analysis of patient safety practices* (Rep. No. 43). Agency for Healthcare Research and Quality.

Silver, S. A., Harel, Z., McQuillan, R., Weizman, A. V., Thomas, A., Chertow, G. M., Nesrallah, G., Bell, C.M., & Chan, C. T. (2016b). How to begin a quality improvement project. *Clinical Journal of the American Society of Nephrology, 11*(5), 893–900. https://doi.org/10.2215/CJN.11491015

Silver, S. A., McQuillan, R., Harel, Z., Weizman, A. V., Thomas, A., Nesrallah, G., Bell, C. M., & Chertow, G. M. (2016a). How to sustain change and support continuous quality improvement. *Clinical Journal of the American Society of Nephrology: CJASN, 11*(5), 916–924. https://doi.org/ 10.2215/ CJN.11501015

Slonim, A. D., & Pollack, M. M. (2005). Integrating the institute of medicine's six quality aims into pediatric critical care: Relevance and applications. *Pediatric Critical Care Medicine, 6*(3), 264–269. https://doi.org/10.1097/01.pcc.0000160592.87113.c6

Stiefel, M., & Nolan, K. (2012). *A guide to measuring the triple aim: Population health, experience of care, and per capita cost.* Institute for Healthcare Improvement White Paper. www.IHI.org

Trautman, D. E., Idzik, S., Hammersla, M., & Rosseter, R. (2018). Advancing scholarship through translational research: The role of PhD and DNP prepared nurses. *Online Journal of Issues in Nursing, 23*(2). Manuscript 2. https://doi.org/10.3912/OJIN.

Unite for Sight. (2015). *Dissemination and utility of evaluation findings.* Author [On-line]. http://www .uniteforsight.org/evaluation-course/module7

U.S. Department of Health & Human Services. (2000). *The challenge and potential for assuring quality health care for the 21st century.* Author.

U.S. Department of Health & Human Services. (2020). *Quality improvement activities FAQs, Office for human research protections.* https://www.hhs.gov/ohrp/regulations-and-policy/guidance/faq/quality -improvement-activities/index.html

Van Den Bos, J., Rustagi, K., Gray, T., Halford, M., Ziemkiewicz, E., & Shreve, J. (2011). The $17.1 billion problem: The annual cost of measurable medical errors. *Health Affairs, 30,* 596–603. https:// doi.org/10.1377/hlthaff.2011.0084

Victorian Quality Council. (2008). *A guide to using data for health care quality improvement.* Victorian Government Department of Human Services. https://aci.health.nsw.gov.au/__data/assets/pdf _file/0006/273336/vqc-guide-to-using-data.pdf

Villanova. (2020). *Six Sigma: DMADV methodology.* https://www.villanovau.com/resources/six-sigma/ six-sigma-methodology-dmadv/

Vincent, D., Johnson, C., Velasquez, D., & Rigney, T. (2010). DNP-prepared nurses as practitioner-researchers: Closing the gap between research and practice. *The American Journal for Nurse Practitioners, 14*(11/14), 28–34. Corpus ID: 29249935.

Weiserbs, K. F., Lyutic, L., & Weinberg, J. (2009). Should quality improvement projects require IRB approval? *Academic Medicine, 84*(2), 153. https://doi.org/10.1097/acm.0b013e3181939881

TEN

EVALUATION OF PATIENT CARE BASED ON STANDARDS, GUIDELINES, AND PROTOCOLS

Ronda G. Hughes

Evaluating is itself the most valuable treasure of all that we value.
It is only through evaluation that value exists: and without
evaluation the nut of existence would be hollow.
—*Friedrich Nietzsche*

INTRODUCTION

Doctor of nursing practice (DNP) nurses are often called upon to evaluate the achievement of individual, family, and population health outcomes using quality indicators of health and care. This chapter examines strategies for the evaluation of patient care based on accepted standards and guidelines. The Institute of Medicine (IOM) Roundtable on Evidence-Based Medicine (IOM, 2009b) set a goal that "by 2020, ninety percent of clinical decisions should be supported by accurate, timely, and up-to-date clinical information that reflects the best available evidence." That was a lofty goal when it has been estimated that about 20% of clinical decisions are evidence based (McGlynn et al., 2003). Of the more than $3.6 trillion annually invested in health care nationally ($11,172 per person), less than 0.1% is devoted to evaluating the relative effectiveness of the various diagnostics, procedures, devices, pharmaceuticals, and other interventions in clinical practice. In order to appreciate what standards, guidelines, and protocols represent, a review of the background and development of each will be explored so that the advanced practice nurses (APNs) can critically review these entities before adoption or translation into practice (Centers for Medicare & Medicaid Services [CMS], 2019).

The delivery and quality of health care services vary by setting, health care team, organization, and geographic location. Researchers continue to find variation associated with practice patterns, understanding of evidence, and sociodemographics of populations. Health care leaders, managers, policy makers, and practitioners have been concerned about this variation and have been actively involved in various strategies to bring and drive health care toward high-quality consistency. Many of these efforts have involved developing, implementing, and enforcing standards, guidelines, and protocols as part of evidence-based practices (EBP).

ORGANIZATIONAL FACTORS INFLUENCING PATIENT CARE

Knowing that the delivery of health care services is not perfect, and that variation is prevalent, there are numerous opportunities to improve patient care across care settings. Health care delivery is influenced by experience, patient preferences and overall health, external organizations, system features, and research evidence. Because these different influences can be considered a type of evidence and can conflict with each other, it is important to understand how they differ from one another, what is behind decisions to use one type of evidence over another, and how the difference may drive certain care delivery decisions and outcomes such as variation in patient-specific outcomes compared with population-based outcomes. It is assumed that purposeful efforts to integrate high-quality research-based evidence into clinical practice to standardize practice should obviate the need to first start with clinical experience in decision-making and the tendency to aggregate all sources of influence for decision-making into one homogeneous category (Richardson, 2015).

TYPES OF RESEARCH INFLUENCING PATIENT CARE

Research is evaluated through various mechanisms and can support or refute current or proposed standards, guidelines, and protocols. There are several major types of research that are used to influence patient care decisions. Randomized controlled trials (RCTs), a form of clinical trial or experiment type of research commonly used to test the safety and efficacy or effectiveness of health care services (e.g., a type of surgical procedure), are held by many to be the gold standard. Considering the scope of depth of clinical and health care research and the cost of conducting an RCT, other forms of research can also be successfully used to inform practice. For example, descriptive research provides data and characteristics about a population or phenomenon but does not describe what factors may have caused a situation. One example would be determining how many people within a specific population have been diagnosed and are being managed for diabetes.

There is also research that statistically assesses the relationship (or correlation) between two or more random variables. Determining a predictive relationship between the flu season and demand for visits or emergency department utilization serves to illustrate one example. Another type of research draws a sample from a larger population and makes a distinction between those with the risk factors and those without them. These two cohorts are followed over a period of time to determine the frequency and timing that the outcomes of interest occur. Additionally, qualitative research provides insight into the social processes, subcultures, experiences, and perceptions of individuals and populations that are generally not detectable through databases or other sources of information. Together, the different types of research can be used to inform the development, testing, and implementation of standards, guidelines, and protocols.

The information or research supporting practice and changes in how care is delivered varies. This information can range from a recommendation, a suggestion for practice that is not necessarily approved by expert groups, to a guideline that was the product of intensive research evidence and consensus among experts. The following section provides a brief discussion and definitions of a number of terms as a basis for discussion. These terms include standards, standard of care, guidelines, protocols, recommendations, indicators, EBP, and best practices.

Indicators

Indicators are visible signs of whether or not an intervention or program is achieving the expected outcomes or progressing in the intended direction. An indicator is a measurable surrogate (e.g., a number or percentage) that is considered representative of an outcome and can be tracked to determine whether there is an increase or decrease or an improvement or deterioration in the outcome. Quality indicators are measures of health care quality that make use of readily available hospital administrative data.

Standards

Standards are considered to be the expected level and type of care. They reflect a desired and achievable level of performance against which actual performance can be compared. Their main purpose is to promote, guide, and direct practice. According to the Healthcare Information and Management Systems Society (HIMSS), a standard is "established by consensus and approved by a recognized body, or is accepted as a de facto standard by the industry" (HIMSS, 2010, p. 113). Standards of care are developed over time or are the result of findings from clinical and health care research and can vary by state or community (Moffett & Moore, 2011).

In legal terms, a standard of care is used as the benchmark against what a clinician does in practice. If, for example, the U.S. Department of Health and Human Services (DHHS) declares a treatment procedure as not safe and effective, then the practitioners who employ such a treatment procedure can be deemed as not meeting the professionally recognized standards of health care. Professionally recognized standards are applicable to practitioners providing care and are recognized by the professional peers of a clinician/clinical group. However, this does not mean that all other treatments meet the professionally recognized standards of care. In a malpractice lawsuit, the clinician's lawyers would want to prove that the clinician's actions were aligned with the standard of care. The plaintiff's lawyers would want to show how the clinician violated the accepted standard of care and was therefore negligent (Moffett & Moore, 2011).

All industries have some form of standards by which the quality of their services or products can be judged. The American Nurses Association (ANA) states that a standard is a statement set forth by the profession and by which others can judge the profession by its service, education, and quality of practice (ANA, 2010). In another publication, the ANA says standards are authoritative statements by which the nursing profession describes the responsibilities for which its practitioners are accountable. Standards reflect the values and priorities of the profession and provide direction for professional nursing practice and a framework for the evaluation of this practice. Standards also define the nursing profession's accountability to the public and the outcomes for which registered nurses are responsible (2010).

For nurses, there are nursing standards of care, promulgated by professional organizations. For example, the ANA promotes nursing excellence through standards, a code of ethics, and credentialing. The ANA standards describe the responsibilities for which its practitioners are accountable, reflect the values and priorities of the profession, and provide direction for professional nursing practice and a framework for the evaluation of this practice. These standards also define the nursing profession's accountability to the public and the outcomes for which registered nurses are responsible.

The ANA Standards of Professional Performance describe a competent level of behavior for professional nurses, including activities related to quality of care, performance appraisal, education, collegiality, ethics, collaboration, research, and resource utilization. These standards serve as guidelines for accountability; a method to ensure patients receive high-quality care; specificity, so that the nurses know exactly what is necessary to provide nursing care; and measures that can be used to determine whether the care meets the standards. Of these standards, two in particular will be discussed for illustrative purposes (Maloney, 2016).

First, the quality of practice is defined as the registered nurse systematically enhances the quality and effectiveness of nursing practice. The measurement criteria are as follows (ANA, 2004):

1. Demonstrates quality by documenting the application of the nursing process in a responsible, accountable, and ethical manner
2. Uses quality improvement activities to initiate changes in nursing practice and the health care delivery system
3. Uses creativity and innovation to improve nursing care delivery
4. Incorporates new knowledge to initiate changes in nursing practice if desired outcomes are not achieved
5. Participates in quality improvement activities

Second, the research standard is defined as the nurse integrates research findings in practice. This is measured using the following criteria (ANA, 2004):

1. Utilizes best available evidence, including research findings, to guide practice decisions
2. Participates in research activities as appropriate to the nurse's education and position such as the following:
   A. Identifying clinical problems suitable for nursing research
   B. Participating in data collection
   C. Participating in a unit, organization, or community research committee
   D. Sharing research activities with others conducting research
   E. Critiquing research for application to practice
   F. Using research findings in the development of policies, procedures, and practice guidelines for patient care
   G. Incorporating research as a basis for learning

Nurses demonstrate the standards of care for professional nursing through the nursing process. This involves assessment, diagnosis, outcome identification, planning implementation, and evaluation. The nursing process is the foundation of clinical decision-making and encompasses all significant action taken by nurses in providing care to all patients. Accountability for one's practice as a professional rests with the individual nurse. The ANA standards of care describe a competent level of nursing care (ANA, 2004). The levels of care are demonstrated through the nursing process. Standards of care are also important if a legal dispute arises over whether a nurse practiced appropriately in a particular case.

Guidelines

Guidelines can be defined generically or specifically to clinical practice. A guideline is a description that clarifies what should be done, and how, to achieve given objectives (HIMSS, 2010, p. 55). Guidelines are developed to standardize care based on what should be considered the best available evidence and information. Most guidelines are based on research when possible. Clinical practice guidelines are a set of systematically developed statements, usually based on scientific evidence, to assist practitioners and patient decision-making about appropriate health care for specific clinical circumstances (2010, p. 21). Clinical practice guidelines are produced by government agencies, health care systems, professional organizations, and specialty centers.

Each of the many steps needed to develop guidelines can be vulnerable to bias or error; as a result, a practitioner may misinterpret the research evidence and its translation while developing a clinical practice guideline. There are various strategies to developing guidelines but no universal standard mechanism to ensure that each published guideline was developed in the best way possible (World Health Organization [WHO], 2010). Generally, the process begins with identifying and refining the subject area of a possible guideline. Next, a group (optimally versus an individual) is created to engage stakeholders and identify and assess the evidence. Again, optimally, this group summarizes, categorizes, and critically evaluates available evidence. This evaluation of the evidence is then translated into a clinical practice guideline. The guideline should then be reviewed by experts in the field and key stakeholders. After a guideline is published, it should be updated frequently to reflect new research knowledge when available.

Acknowledging that clinical guidelines were becoming more a part of clinical practice, concerns were raised with guidelines in terms of the benefits of encouraging the use of interventions proven to be successful and informing decision-making, as well as the harms of misleading decision makers because the evidence informing the guideline was thin or misinterpreted or biases may have incorrectly influenced the recommendation(s) (Woolf et al., 1999). These and many other concerns have been raised about guidelines. In a recent report, the IOM (2011a) set forth eight standards for clinical practice guidelines:

1. Establishing transparency
2. Managing conflict of interest
3. Overseeing guideline development group composition
4. Examining clinical practice guideline systematic review intersection
5. Establishing evidence foundations for and rating strength
6. Addressing articulation or recommendations
7. Providing for external review
8. Updating

As such, APNs must be careful in implementing or adapting clinical guidelines in that for many topics or situations, there are a multitude of guidelines. These guidelines may not concur with each other and most likely were developed using different processes and different sources of evidence. To address these concerns, APNs must carefully consider each guideline and evaluate the best match to their practice and patient population.

Protocols

A clinical protocol is a set of rules defining a standardized treatment program or behavior in specific circumstances (HIMSS, 2010, p. 21). A protocol is a detailed guide for approaching a clinical problem and is designed to address a specific practice situation. It is often agency specific; for example, a checklist for pressure ulcer prevention, including assessment steps and timeline for turning and repositioning patients.

Protocols exist to reduce variation in care for a specific patient population. They are generally to be adhered to in practice, particularly when the recommended actions have been scientifically studied and experts in the field have considered and advised on their application. Clinical protocols are defined as standards of care that define specific care actions that should be given to a defined patient population. Many specify how, when, and by whom a specific action should be performed. Some clinical protocols present a comprehensive plan of care, such as perioperative and postoperative care for elderly patients receiving joint replacement surgery, whereas other protocols address just one aspect of care, such as prophylactic antibiotics before joint replacement surgery.

Best Practices

A best practice describes a process or technique whose application results in improved patient and/or organizational outcomes. A best practice is something that an individual, group, or organization can apply to an action to perform significantly better than other individuals, groups, or organizations. From a nonscientific perspective, best practices can also be defined as the most efficient (least amount of effort) and effective (best results) way of accomplishing a task, based on repeatable procedures that have proven themselves over time for large numbers of people. A best practice is applicable to a particular condition or circumstance and may have to be modified or adapted for similar circumstances.

Various organizations, professional associations, and many others publish "best practices" to inform clinical decision-making. Generally, best practices are accepted, informally standardized techniques, methods, or processes that have proven themselves over time to accomplish given tasks. These practices are commonly used but are generally based on no specific formal methodology. It is assumed that if done right, using best practices will achieve a desired outcome across organizations that can be delivered more effectively and consistently.

A DNP nurse searching for best practices for any given question will usually begin with a review of the literature so that research and other sources of evidence inform best practices. It rests on the DNP nurse to evaluate the literature to determine the basis and strength of a possible intervention based on the source, reliability, and quality of the information and the methods used to define the "best practice." Although meta-analysis is considered the highest level of research evidence, clinical questions in practice do not always have research of quantity and quality to provide this level of evidence. Therefore, the DNP nurse must review what literature is available to make a judgment about what might potentially be a better or best practice in a given situation.

Evidence-Based Practice

EBP is a problem-solving approach to clinical decision-making within a health care organization that integrates the best available research evidence with the best available experiential (patient and practitioner) evidence. Both internal and external influences on practice, as well as critical thinking in the judicious application of evidence, are considered (Newhouse et al., 2007). EBP is based on research evidence about the effectiveness of interventions that are used to guide decision-making about patient care. It relies on a ranking of the multiple research studies that critically differentiate the most to the least reliable research findings. This is important because individual research findings can be misleading for a variety of reasons, ranging from poor study design to small sample size that is not generalizable (Flyvbjerg, 2006).

Even when evidence is available, many research studies have identified significant gaps between actual practice and the best possible practice. Part of this gap has been because of the lack of research evidence to inform and standardize practice to achieve predictable outcomes. Another part of this gap reflects the view that EBP discounts individual clinical skills and patient preferences (Hajjaj et al., 2010). Although in many instances there is no research evidence, the aim of EBP is to integrate current best evidence from research (when it is available) with clinical policy and practice. In doing so, clinical decision-making can be based on evidence-informed tools of what works to improve performance, narrow the gap between practice and research, and improve patient outcomes (Bates et al., 2003).

To apply EBPs, APNs need to implement the best interventions and practices that are informed by the best evidence. From the perspective of quality and safety, EBP is considered the gold standard of care. EBP can raise the bar within a clinical practice and achieve more predictable patient outcomes.

MAJOR INFLUENCES ON SHAPING AND EVALUATING HEALTH CARE

Health and Medicine Division of the National Academies of Sciences, Engineering, and Medicine

Formerly referred to as the IOM, the Health and Medicine Division (HMD) is a non-profit, private organization whose purpose is to provide national advice on issues relating to biomedical science, medicine, and health to improve health care. It relies on a volunteer workforce of scientists and other experts, operating under a rigorous, formal peer-review system. The IOM strives to provide unbiased, evidence-based, and authoritative information and advice concerning health and science policy issues. With the release of *To Err Is Human* (Kohn et al., 1999), the IOM began a series of reports on improving quality and safety of health care as well as implications for evaluating the health care and influencing national policy reimbursement policies.

In *Crossing the Quality Chasm: A New Health System for the 21st Century* (IOM, 2001), the IOM set forth six aims for health care improvement. These aims—safe, effective, timely, patient centered, efficient, and equitable—have become a standard throughout health care. In terms of other standards, the IOM also asserted that chronic diseases were best managed when using a "protocol or plan that provides an explicit statement of what needs to be done for patients, at what intervals, and by whom, and that considers the needs of all patients with specific clinical features and how their needs can be met" (IOM, 2001, p. 94).

The report, *Keeping Patients Safe: Transforming the Work Environment of Nurses* (IOM, 2004a), emphasized the evidence for nursing and set forth policy recommendations primarily regarding nurse staffing. The IOM focused their recommendations on improving patient safety through strategies that would improve the work environment for nurses. Among the many recommendations were adequate staffing, organizational support for ongoing learning and decision support, using mechanisms that promote interdisciplinary collaboration, and implementing a work design that promotes safety. Although important for patients, practitioners, and organizations, the challenge is to act upon these recommendations in lieu of sufficient evidence for specific interventions that can optimize outcomes across organizations. The IOM also recommended changes in the minimum standards for registered and licensed nurse staffing in nursing homes but only recommended them because of the lack of evidence for minimum standards in hospitals (IOM, 2004a).

In *Patient Safety: Achieving a New Standard for Care* (2004b), the IOM set forth recommendations to improve patient safety. One of the major recommendations was to better manage health information technology and data systems to enable patient safety as a standard across care delivery sites. The health information technology and data systems are needed to inform care decisions and support patient safety. To operationalize these recommendations, the IOM specified the need for common data standards for effective information sharing and utilization (IOM, 2004b).

The IOM has also addressed issues relating to evidence and how it should be used. In *Knowing What Works in Health Care: A Roadmap for the Nation* (IOM, 2008), the IOM recommended government oversight of the production of information for comparative effectiveness and to set forth high-priority topics for systematic reviews of clinical effectiveness. The IOM also recommended that methodological standards and a common language for characterizing the strength of the evidence be developed for systematic reviews (2008). Consequently, an oversight committee was developed, and millions of dollars were allocated by the federal government for comparative effectiveness research (CER) under the health care reform law passed in March 2010. The CER defined methods that compare existing health care interventions to determine what treatment works best for specific patients and what poses the greatest benefits and harms (Greenfield & Rich, 2012).

In *Finding What Works in Health Care: Standards for Systematic Reviews*, the IOM (2011b) responded to a directive from Congress to develop standards for conducting systematic reviews of the comparative effectiveness of medical and surgical interventions. These standards are intended to ensure that systematic reviews will be objective, transparent, and scientifically valid. In this report, the IOM recommended standards for the entire systematic review process, making specific recommendations on finding and assessing individual studies, synthesizing the body of evidence, and reporting systematic reviews.

The Joint Commission

Formerly called The Joint Commission on Accreditation of Healthcare Organizations (JCAHO), The Joint Commission (TJC) is a private nonprofit organization that provides elective accreditation of over 19,000 health care organizations and programs in the United States. TJC seeks to improve health care by encouraging and evaluating health care organizations. Organizations can receive accreditation only when they demonstrate the achievement of specific performance standards. Government recognizes TJC accreditation as a condition for Medicare and Medicaid reimbursement and licensure (TJC, 2020a).

TJC's standards for acute care hospitals set the precedent for standards in other settings and are quoted in the judgments of some civil malpractice cases. When there are changes in TJC's standards, they are generally consistent with changes in federal policy and precedent-setting court cases as well as changes in national concerns (e.g., sentinel events) or major reports (e.g., the IOM report, *To Err Is Human*).

Consistent with its stated mission of "improving health care for the public," TJC has set forth standards, goals, and measures to promote improvements in patient safety. To receive accreditation, health care organizations need to achieve a series of standards that represent high-quality care. TJC's National Patient Safety Goal (NPSG) highlights problematic areas in health care and describes available evidence and expert-based solutions to these problems (TJC, 2020b), if they exist. The NPSGs have become a critical method by which TJC promotes and enforces major changes in patient safety. TJC also sets forth quality improvement measures and works with the Centers for Medicare & Medicaid Services (CMS) to set forth common national hospital performance measures (CMS, 2019; TJC, 2020c).

In 1990, the JCAHO dropped its Managed Care Accreditation Program and turned its accredited managed care organizations over to the National Committee for Quality Assurance (NCQA). NCQA's first standards for managed care were published in 1991 and have been revised about every 2 years since then. The NCQA works with managed care organizations, health care purchasers, state regulators, and consumers to develop standards and performance measures that are intended to evaluate the structure and functions of medical and quality management systems in managed care organizations (see http://www.ncqa.org/tabid/59/default.aspx for information on the Health Plan Employer Data Information Set).

Centers for Medicare & Medicaid Services

As part of the DHHS, the CMS, previously known as the Health Care Financing Administration, administers the Medicare program and works in partnership with state governments to administer Medicaid, the State Children's Health Insurance Program (SCHIP), and health insurance portability standards. The CMS is also responsible for the administrative simplification standards from the Health Insurance Portability and Accountability Act of 1996 (HIPAA), quality standards in long-term care facilities, and clinical laboratory quality standards under the Clinical Laboratory Improvement Amendments (see www.cms.gov). Throughout its programs and responsibilities, the CMS exerts tremendous influence on practice standards by setting forth reimbursement policies for covered services and by developing, interpreting, implementing, and evaluating policies for professional standards review, related peer review, utilization review, and utilization control programs under Medicare and Medicaid. Hospitals must meet specific requirements and conditions established by the CMS to receive reimbursement for providing services to Medicare and Medicaid beneficiaries. These conditions include patients' rights, quality assessment and performance improvement, and utilization review.

Agency for Healthcare Research and Quality

Formerly known as the Agency for Health Care Policy and Research, the Agency for Healthcare Research and Quality (AHRQ) is also part of the HHS. The mission of the AHRQ is to improve the quality, safety, efficiency, and effectiveness of health care for all Americans. AHRQ's mission helps the DHHS achieve its strategic goals to improve the safety, quality, affordability, and accessibility of health care; ensure public health promotion and protection, disease prevention, and emergency preparedness; promote the economic and social well-being of individuals, families, and communities; and advance scientific and biomedical research and development related to health and human services. AHRQ facilitates the development of evidence through research grants and evidence-based research syntheses through its EBP centers (www. ahrq.gov/clinic/epc). Research funded by AHRQ helps people make more informed decisions and improve the quality of health care services. Quality and patient safety indicators are found on the AHRQ website (www.-qualityindicators.ahrq.gov). AHRQ works with organizations, such as the National Quality Forum, to set forth evidence-based indicators of quality (AHRQ, 2020).

After AHRQ's "near death experience" from Congress in 1995 over its release of guidelines for back surgery and patrician politics, it turned the business of developing guidelines over to nongovernmental organizations, including professional organizations. Although not directly involved in guideline development, an important repository of guidelines is maintained by AHRQ, covering a variety of topics (www.guidelines.gov).

HOW STANDARDS, GUIDELINES, AND PROTOCOLS ARE DEVELOPED

There are significant variations and several major forces in defining practice guidelines and protocols. Researchers apply various science-based methodologies to develop the research that can serve as the evidence. Experts and practitioners weigh in with their opinions based on personal experience and continue the tradition through education and reinforcement in practice settings. National health policy leaders and insurers influence minimal standards of care and what services will be reimbursed and where. The public influences what type of care is expected through public opinion, the new media, and publications. Patients and their families influence what care is provided through preferences and interactions with practitioners. When standards, guidelines, and protocols are developed, many forces come together. For example, clinical, administrative, and academic experts developed the standards of nursing practice (ANA, 2014).

Process of Developing Standards, Guidelines, and Protocols

In many instances, practice guidelines are used to convey a synthesis of the strengths and weaknesses of the research and its practice implications as well as provide a basis for improving care quality by reducing practice variations (Baker, 2001). It can take 5 years for published guidelines to be adopted into routine practice (Lomas et al., 1993). Even when guidelines exist and are broadly accepted, they are often not used in practice.

The IOM asserted that clinical guidelines should be used to guide health care decisions by practitioners and patients (Field & Lohr, 1990). Yet the strength of the guideline and its applicability to practice is dependent on appropriate interpretation of the research evidence that is developed using formal methods. These methods should include identification of the area or areas of practice where a guideline could be helpful, a synthesis of relevant research evidence, a review by a guideline development group, and an external review of the recommendations for the guidelines (Eccles & Grimshaw, 2004; Shekelle et al., 2012).

Research Evidence

Research tests innovations in laboratories and in practice. The millions of dollars that many public and private organizations invest in research provide hope that health care services can be improved. The challenge is that evidence developed through research has a tendency to "sit" in research journals and not be used in practice.

Unfortunately, there is often a disconnect between research efforts and clinical practice. To improve research being used in practice, the research evidence needs to be synthesized because only rarely should findings from one research project be integrated into practice. Conclusions from synthesized research can then be used to develop clinical practice recommendations and policy. It is then up to organizational leaders and practitioners to apply the recommendations and policy in the right setting, at the right time, and in the right manner. These steps help to form a link between research and practice.

Synthesizing and Grading the Evidence

Findings from research are published primarily in peer-reviewed research journals. Various strategies have been developed to assess the quality of the research evidence. Practitioners can find research syntheses from groups, such as EBP centers (see www.ahrq.gov/clinic/epc) and the Cochrane Collaborative (see www.cochrane.org), the peer-reviewed literature, and from information services that systematically review and evaluate the literature for specified topics and questions (AHRQ, 2020).

There are several challenges for both those doing the reviews and those reading the findings. First, these reviews and critical evaluations of research findings are dependent on the research that has been completed, which may have only some bearing on the questions at hand. Second, many of the systematic reviews and efforts to inform guidelines hold RCTs as the gold standard, where the majority of the knowledge gaps in clinical practice cannot be adequately addressed by RCTs. And third, how the research is synthesized and evaluated is dependent on the reviewers, the inclusion and exclusion criteria, and the criteria they use to evaluate the research (Timmermans & Berg, 2003).

Another mechanism to locate and utilize synthesized research findings by integrating them into practice is through health information technology, such as clinical decision support systems that are sometimes integrated into electronic medical records. Optimally, electronic decision support systems enhance clinical practice and decision-making with real-time information, but they must keep current with changes in evidence and clinical practice (Bates et al., 2003).

In practice, with particular patients, practitioners can search various sources of evidence. To effectively search EBP resources, it is helpful to decide what details are important to the clinical question at hand so that the right questions can be asked. According to Richardson (2000), a well-built clinical question includes the following components:

- The patient's disorder or disease
- The intervention or finding under review
- A comparison intervention (if applicable—not always present)
- The outcome

The acronym PICOT, from these four components, has been used to assist in remembering the steps: **P**, patient/population or problem; **I**, intervention or issue of interest; **C**, comparison intervention or issue of interest; **O**, outcome(s) of interest; and **T**, time it takes for the intervention to achieve the outcome(s) (Stillwell et al., 2010).

Several strategies have been developed to evaluate the quality of evidence and the strength of practice recommendations. The strategies have different approaches to evaluating the evidence and have strengths and limitations (Atkins et al., 2004), according to the criteria used to evaluate the evidence and the subjectivity of the reviewers using a specific strategy. The U.S. Preventive Services Task Force (USP-STF) developed a system (see Table 10.1) to stratify evidence by USPSTF (2018).

In evaluating the research evidence, the USPSTF makes recommendations for a clinical service based on a balance of risk versus benefit and the level of evidence on which the recommendation can be based. The USPSTF used the following levels to reflect the strength of the recommendation for clinical practice (USPSTF, 2018):

Grade and definition:

TABLE 10.1   U.S. Preventive Services Task Force Evidence Grading System

High	The available evidence usually includes consistent results from well-designed, well-conducted studies in representative primary care populations. These studies assess the effects of the preventive service on health outcomes. This conclusion is therefore unlikely to be strongly affected by the results of future studies.
Moderate	The available evidence is sufficient to determine the effects of the preventive service on health outcomes, but confidence in the estimate is constrained by such factors as: ■ The number, size, or quality of individual studies. ■ Inconsistency of findings across individual studies. ■ Limited generalizability of findings to routine primary care practice. ■ Lack of coherence in the chain of evidence. As more information becomes available, the magnitude or direction of the observed effect could change, and this change may be large enough to alter the conclusion.
Low	The available evidence is insufficient to assess effects on health outcomes. Evidence is insufficient because of: ■ The limited number or size of studies. ■ Important flaws in study design or methods. ■ Inconsistency of findings across individual studies. ■ Gaps in the chain of evidence. ■ Findings not generalizable to routine primary care practice. ■ Lack of information on important health outcomes. More information may allow estimation of effects on health outcomes.

Source: U.S. Preventive Services Task Force. (2018). *Grade definitions.* https://www.uspreventiveservicestaskforce.org/uspstf/grade-definitions

- Grade A: The USPSTF recommends the service. There is high certainty that the net benefit is substantial. Offer or provide this service.
- Grade B: The USPSTF recommends the service. There is high certainty that the net benefit is moderate, or there is moderate certainty that the net benefit is moderate to substantial.
- Grade C: The USPSTF recommends selectively offering or providing this service to individual patients based on professional judgment and patient preferences. There is at least moderate certainty that the net benefit is small.
- Grade D: The USPSTF recommends against the service. There is moderate or high certainty that the service has no net benefit or that the harms outweigh the benefits.
- Grade I: The USPSTF concludes that the current evidence is insufficient to assess the balance of benefits and harms of the service. Evidence is lacking, of poor quality, or conflicting, and the balance of benefits and harms cannot be determined.

Another system for rating the hierarchy of evidence is as follows (Melnyk & Fineout-Overholt, 2019):

- Level I: Evidence from a systematic review or meta-analysis of all relevant RCTs, or evidence-based clinical practice guidelines based on systematic reviews of RCTs
- Level II: Evidence obtained from at least one well-designed RCT
- Level III: Evidence obtained from well-designed controlled trials without randomization
- Level IV: Evidence from well-designed case-control and cohort studies
- Level V: Evidence from systematic reviews of descriptive and qualitative studies
- Level VI: Evidence from a single descriptive or qualitative study
- Level VII: Evidence from the opinion of authorities and/or reports of expert committees

These and many other tools can be used to evaluate the quality of a guideline and the evidence that informed the guideline. APNs evaluating guidelines and the evidence will need to select which tool to use. However, it is important to appreciate the differences in the evaluation tools for guidelines and evidence as well as the significance of a guideline in altering clinical practice and the possibility of not achieving the preferred outcome because of the challenges involved in changing clinical practice.

Comparative Effectiveness

Innovations in pharmaceuticals and therapeutic interventions have resulted in a tremendous range of treatment options for clinicians, patients, and insurers. As the state of the evidence evolves, little is known or widely understood about the relative effectiveness of these various options. Efforts to compare the effectiveness among these options for a specific condition can focus on the benefits and risks of each option or the costs and the benefits of those options. In some instances, one of the options may prove to be more effective clinically or more cost-effective for a broad range of patients. However, a key issue is determining which specific type(s) of patient(s) would benefit most from a specific option.

CER was defined by the IOM as "the generation and synthesis of evidence that compares the benefits and harms of alternative methods to prevent, diagnose, treat, and monitor a clinical condition or to improve the delivery of care. The purpose of CER is to assist consumers, practitioners, purchasers, and policymakers to make informed decisions that will improve health care at both the individual and population levels" (IOM, 2009, p. 29). The core question of CER is which treatment works best, for whom, and under what circumstances. Findings from CER can provide invaluable information for clinical and coverage-related decision-making. Although the importance of CER increases, there continue to be both technical and policy-related questions about how CER is conducted, disseminated, and utilized.

Over the past few years, the federal government has made a substantial investment in CER. The American Recovery and Reinvestment Act of 2009 provided $1.1 billion for CER, dividing that money between the Office of the Secretary in the DHHS, the National Institutes of Health, and the AHRQ. Then in March 2010, Congress passed the Affordable Care Act, which created the Patient-Centered Outcomes Research Institute, a nongovernmental body that will establish a nationwide agenda for the research, much of which will be funded by a tax imposed on health insurers. The purpose of this institute is to review evidence and produce new information on how diseases, disorders, and other health conditions can be treated to achieve the best clinical outcome for patients. One of the organizations providing leadership in the area of CER is the AHRQ.

Revising Existing Standards, Guidelines, and Protocols

Standards, guidelines, and protocols developed more than 5 years ago, and in some instances less than 5 years ago, may be out-of-date given more recent research evidence published. As research evolves with new information, guidelines need to be updated; some may need to be updated as often as every 3 years to reflect changes in empirical knowledge (Garcia et al., 2014).

Changing Practice

To implement EBPs in many organizations, decision makers need to balance the strengths and limitations of all relevant research evidence with the practical realities of the practice environment and patient population. This includes consideration of the clinical usefulness, the limitations of the available evidence, and understanding of the differentiation that exists among the multiple EBPs for the same issue. From a practical standpoint, evidence-based guidelines have to be tailored to the organization and the unique subculture(s) within.

Practitioners who want to improve the quality, safety, effectiveness, and efficiency of health care services can apply research evidence and best practices. However, practitioners are challenged to find, assess, interpret, and apply the current best evidence. Evidence is increasingly accessible through publications and information services such as electronic databases, systematic reviews, and health care journals. However, there are challenges to the successful application of the best information to changing practice.

To provide guidance on which factors practitioners should consider when determining whether research findings from a study should inform practice changes, the following have been proposed (Cone & Lewis, 2003, p. 418):

Factors related to the study in question:

1. The study should be of the highest possible quality (e.g., important and testable clinical question, prospective, large enough, randomized, blinded, controlled, minimal sources of bias).
2. The study results should be the best information available.
3. The study results should be valid and plausible.
4. The benefits of the change should outweigh the risks of implementing the change.

Factors not related to the study in question:

1. The costs of changing (or not changing) practice must be assessed.
2. The similarity of your clinical setting to that of the study.
3. The similarity of your health care system to that of the study.
4. Expert opinion regulation.

Guidelines have consistently been found to have minimal impact on changing physician behavior owing to "lack of awareness, familiarity, lack of agreement, lack of self-efficacy, lack of outcome expectancy, the inertia of previous practice, and external barriers" (Sbarbaro, 2001). There may be similar issues for nurses (Creedon, 2005; Lyerla, 2008), yet several studies have indicated that nurses are more compliant with guidelines than physicians (Erasmus et al., 2010). However, one of the most significant challenges for nurses using guidelines is that much of the nursing knowledge has not been translated into evidence-based guidelines. Also, research is needed to understand advanced practice nurses' challenges and compliance with guidelines to determine opportunities for improvement.

Determining Which Guidelines to Use in Practice

Before a guideline is adopted or translated into practice, clinicians and organizations should critically review the guideline. There are two approaches to evaluating guidelines for potential use in clinical practice. The Appraisal of Guidelines for Research and Evaluation II (AGREE) collaboration developed an evaluation instrument with 23 criteria for appraising the process used to produce clinical practice guidelines. The AGREE II Instrument addresses variability in guideline quality and assesses guidelines from the perspective of transparency and methodological rigor. The instrument is organized using six domains and 23 questions (Brouwers et al., 2010). The six domains are:

1. Scope and purpose
2. Stakeholder involvement
3. Rigor of development
4. Clarity
5. Applicability
6. Editorial independence

The other approach uses the Grading of Recommendations Assessment, Development and Evaluation (GRADE) system, which provides a framework for developing and presenting summaries of evidence and a systematic approach for making clinical practice recommendations. When using GRADE, participants decide what the clinical question is, including the population that the question applies to, the two or more alternatives, and the outcomes that matter most to those faced with the decision. A study—ideally, a systematic review—provides the best estimate of the effect size for each outcome, in absolute terms (e.g., a risk difference). Participants then rate the quality of evidence, which is best applied to each outcome, because the quality of evidence often varies between outcomes. An overall GRADE quality rating can be applied to a body of evidence across outcomes, usually by taking the lowest quality of evidence from all of the outcomes that are critical to decision-making.

GRADE has four levels of evidence—also known as certainty in evidence or quality of evidence: very low, low, moderate, and high. Evidence from RCTs starts at high quality, whereas evidence that includes observational data starts at low quality. Using GRADE, strong recommendations suggest that all or almost all persons would choose that intervention suggesting that it is not usually necessary to present both options. Weak recommendations reflect low certainty in the evidence, a close balance between desirable and undesirable consequences, substantial variation or uncertainty in patient values and preferences, and interventions require considerable resources (Alonso-Coello et al., 2016a, 2016b).

Getting Research into Practice

After the research and evidence and/or guidelines have been identified and evaluated for application to practice, getting research-based evidence into practice requires applying evidence-based recommendations at the right time, in the right place, and in the right way. Yet there are most likely several barriers to implementation, from the organizational level to the actual process of care. First, senior staff and management within the organization must be committed to change and enable that change through resource allocation and policies. Second, leaders and clinicians must be invested in making the necessary changes to implement evidence into practice. Third, it is often necessary to make changes in how care is organized and how it is delivered, which is often initially resisted. Fourth, clinicians will need skill development and training to successfully utilize the evidence in practice. Fifth, it is important to ensure clinicians have the tools they need to successfully use the evidence in practice, such as computerized decision support tools. Finally, it is important to build alliances with key partners and share ownership at the beginning of the process in ensuring the success of implementation and continued utilization of the evidence in practice. If any of these organizational-level factors are not in place and functioning, efforts to implement the evidence/guideline into practice may be thwarted or may initially be successful but fail over time.

Although evidence/guidelines standardize care across settings and practitioners, there are aspects that need to be tailored to the patient and their circumstances. Because the delivery of health care involves complex decisions, implementing evidence/guidelines will not necessarily meet individual patient needs (Titler, 2008). In practice, practitioners need to integrate the best evidence, clinical expertise, and patient preferences and values in making decisions (Richardson, 2000).

Given the importance of patient- and family-centered care, practitioners need to consider involving patients in the decision-making process. Practitioners need to be able to define each patient's unique circumstances, determine what is wrong with the patient, and assess how it is affecting the patient. Once the possible interventions and treatments are discussed with the patient, it may be adverse to recommend interventions and care management. Using a patient-centered care approach infuses the patient's preferences, values, and rights into the process of deciding which interventions to use and the appropriate management. Although this is appropriate and encouraged by policy makers and decision makers, guidelines, standards, and protocols are generally written in a way that assumes patient consent to the evidence. As such, it is important to integrate research evidence into clinical decision-making and customize it to the patient's clinical circumstances and wishes to derive a meaningful decision about interventions and care management.

Evaluating Your Practice Outcomes

As important as using evidence in practice is, it is also important to understand the impact of both non–evidence-based and EBP on care processes and outcomes. Many organizations and practitioners continue to make the mistake of implementing evidence-based or evidence-informed changes in care processes but fail to measure the impact on care process as well as patient and organizational outcomes. This is a significant failure because there is always a cost associated with changes in care processes and decision-making and thinking that implementing evidence/guidelines will result in better outcomes cannot be proven unless appropriately measured and assessed. At a basic level, outcomes should be assessed before and after a change is made.

SUMMARY

Patient and organizational outcomes can be improved and consistency in care across settings and practitioners achieved by applying evidence and clinical standards, guidelines, and protocols to practice. There are many influences on what evidence is available and how it may be used in practice. Practitioners and patients need to be actively involved in using the best evidence to inform decision-making and improve outcomes.

REFERENCES

Agency for Healthcare Research and Quality. (2020, October). *Evidence-based practice center (EPC) program overview*. https://www.ahrq.gov/research/findings/evidence-based-reports/overview/index.html

Alonso-Coello, P., Schunemann, H. J., Moberg, J., Brignardello-Petersen, R., Akl, E. A., Davoli, M., Treweek, S., Mustafa, R. A., Rada, G., Rosenbaum, S., Morelli, A., Guyatt, G. H., & Oxman, A. D. (2016a). GRADE Evidence to Decision (EtD) frameworks: A systematic and transparent approach to making well informed healthcare choices. 1: Introduction. *BMJ, 353*, i2016. https://doi.org/10.1136/bmj.i2016

Alonso-Coello, P., Oxman, A. D., Moberg, J., Brignardello-Petersen, R., Akl, E. A., Davoli, M., Treweek, S., Mustafa, R. A., Vandvik, P. O., Meerpohl, J., Guyatt, G. H., Schünemann, H. J., & GRADE

Working Group. (2016b). GRADE Evidence to Decision (EtD) frameworks: A systematic and transparent approach to making well informed healthcare choices. 2: Clinical practice guidelines. *BMJ, 353*, i2089. https://doi.org/10.1136/bmj.i2089

American Nurses Association. (2010). *Credentialing definitions.* https://www.nursingworld.org/education-events/faculty-resources/research-grants/styles-credentialing-research-grants/credentialing-definitions/#:~:text=Standard%20%E2%80%94%20Authoritative%20statement%20enunciated%20and,or%20education%20can%20be%20judged.&text=Standards%20are%20authoritative%20statements%20by,which%20its%20practitioners%20are%20accountable.

American Nurses Association. (2014). *ANA standards for excellence.* https://www.nursingworld.org/~4af2ee/globalassets/docs/ana/ethics/full-code.pdf

Atkins, D., Eccles, M., Flottorp, S., Guyatt, G. H., Henry, D., Hill, S., Liberati, A., O'Connell, D., Oxman, A. D., Phillips, B., Schünemann, H., Edejer, T., Vist, G. E., Williams, J. W., & GRADE Working Group. (2004). Systems for grading the quality of evidence and the strength of recommendations I: Critical appraisal of existing approaches. The GRADE Working Group. *BMC Health Services Research, 4*, 38. https://doi.org/10.1186/1472-6963-4-38

Baker, R. (2001). Is it time to review the idea of compliance with guidelines? *The British Journal of General Practice, 51*(462), 7. PMID: 11271891.

Bates, D. W., Kuperman, G. J., Wang, S., Gandhi, T., Kittler, A., Volk, L., Spurr, C., Khorasani, R., Tanasijevic, M., & Middleton, B. (2003). Ten commandments for effective clinical decision support: Making the practice of evidence-based medicine a reality. *Journal of the American Medical Informatics Association, 10*(6), 523–530. https://doi.org/10.1197/jamia.M1370

Brouwers, M., Kho, M. E., Browman, G. P., Cluzeau, F., Feder, G., Fervers, B., Graham, I. D., Grimshaw, J., Hanna, S. E., Littlejohns, P., Makarski, J., & Zitelsberger, L. (2010). AGREE II: Advancing guideline development, reporting and evaluation in healthcare. *CMAJ, 182*(18), E839–E842. https://doi.org/10.1503/cmaj.090449

Centers for Medicare & Medicaid Services. (2019). *National health expenditures 2018 highlights.* https://www.cms.gov/files/document/highlights.pdf

Cone, D. C., & Lewis, R. J. (2003). Should this study change my practice? *Academic Emergency Medicine, 10*(5), 417–422. http://citeseerx.ist.psu.edu/viewdoc/download?doi=10.1.1.941.7318&rep=rep1&type=pdf

Creedon, S. A. (2005). Healthcare workers' hand decontamination practices: Compliance with recommended guidelines. *Journal of Advanced Nursing, 51*(3), 208–216. https://doi.org/10.1111/j.1365-2648.2005.03490.x

Eccles, M. P., & Grimshaw, J. M. (2004). Selecting, presenting and delivering clinical guidelines: Are there any "magic bullets"? *Medical Journal of Australia, 180*(Suppl. 6), S52–S54. https://doi.org/10.5694/j.1326-5377.2004.tb05946.x

Erasmus, V., Daha, T. J., & Brug H. (2010). Systematic review of studies on compliance with hand hygiene guidelines in hospital care. *Infection Control and Hospital Epidemiology, 31*(3), 283–294. https://doi.org/10.1086/650451

Field, M. J., & Lohr, K. N. (Eds). (1990). *Clinical practice guidelines: Directions for a new program.* National Academy Press.

Flyvbjerg, B. (2006). Five misunderstandings about case-study research. *Qualitative Inquiry, 12*(2), 219–245. https://doi.org/10.1177/1077800405284363

Garcia, L. M., Sanabria, A. J., Alvarez, E. G., Trujillo-Martin, M. M., Etxeandia-Ikobaltzeta, I., Kotzeva, A., Rigau, D., Louro-González, A., Barajas-Nava, L., Díaz del Campo, P., Estrada, M., Solà, I., Gracia, J., Salcedo-Fernandez, F., Lawson, J. R., Brian Haynes, R. B., & Alonso-Coello, P. (2014). The validity of recommendations from clinical guidelines: A survival analysis. *CMAJ, 186*(16), 1211–1219. https://doi.org/10.1503/cmaj.140547

Greenfield, S., & Rich, E. (2012). Welcome to the journal of comparative effectiveness research. *Journal of Comparative Effectiveness Research, 1*(1), 1–3. https://doi.org/10.2217/cer.11.13

Hajjaj, F. M., Salek, M. S., Basra, M. K. A., & Finlay, A. Y. (2010). Non-clinical influences on clinical decision-making: A major challenge to evidence-based practice. *Journal of the Royal Society of Medicine, 103*(5), 178–187. https://doi.org/10.1258/jrsm.2010.100104

Healthcare Information and Management Systems Society. (2010). *HIMSS dictionary of healthcare information technology terms, acronyms and organizations.* Author.

Institute of Medicine. (2001). *Crossing the quality chasm: A new health system for the 21st century.* National Academies Press.

Institute of Medicine. (2004a). *Keeping patients safe: Transforming the work environment of nurses.* National Academies Press.

Institute of Medicine. (2004b). *Patient safety: Achieving a new standard for care.* National Academies Press.

Institute of Medicine. (2008). *Knowing what works in health care: A roadmap for the nation.* National Academies Press.

Institute of Medicine. (2009a). *Initial national priorities for comparative effectiveness research.* National Academies Press.

Institute of Medicine. (2009b). (US) *roundtable on evidence-based medicine.* Leadership Commitments to Improve Value in Healthcare: Finding Common Ground: Workshop Summary. National Academies Press (US). Institute of Medicine: Roundtable on Evidence-Based Medicine. https://www.ncbi.nlm.nih.gov/books/NBK52847

Institute of Medicine. (2011a). *Clinical practice guidelines we can trust.* National Academies Press. https://www.nap.edu/resource/13058/Clinical-Practice-Guidelines-2011-Report-Brief.pdf

Institute of Medicine. (2011b). *Finding what works in health care: Standards for systematic reviews.* National Academies Press.

The Joint Commission. (2020a). *About The Joint Commission.* https://www.jointcommission.org/about-us/facts-about-the-joint-commission/

The Joint Commission. (2020b). *National patient safety goals.* https://www.jointcommission.org/standards/national-patient-safety-goals/

The Joint Commission. (2020c). *Specifications manual for national hospital inpatient quality measures.* https://www.jointcommission.org/measurement/specification-manuals/electronic-clinical-quality-measures/

Kohn, L. T., Corrigan, J. M., & Donaldson, M. S. (Eds.). (1999). *To err is human: Building a safer health system.* National Academic Press.

Lomas, J., Sisk, J. E., & Stocking, B. (1993). From evidence to practice in the United States, the United Kingdom, and Canada. *Milbank Q, 71*(3), 405–410. https://doi.org/10.2307/3350408

Lyerla, F. (2008). Design and implementation of a nursing clinical decision support system to promote guideline adherence. *Computers Informatics Nursing, 26*(4), 227–233. https://doi.org/10.1097/01.ncn.0000304800.93003.b4

Maloney, P. (2016). Nursing professional development: Standards of professional practice. *Journal for Nurses in Professional Development, 32*(6), 327–330. https://doi.org/10.1097/nnd.0000000000000300

McGlynn, E. A., Asch, S., Adams, J., Keesey, J., Hicks, J., Decristofaro, A., & Kerr, E. (2003). The quality of health care delivered to adults in the United States. *New England Journal of Medicine, 348*(26), 2635–2645. https://doi.org/10.1056/NEJMsa022615

Melnyk, B. M., & Fineout-Overholt, E. (2019). *Evidence-based practice in nursing & healthcare. A guide to best practice* (4th ed.). Lippincott Williams & Wilkins.

Moffett, P., & Moore, G. (2011). The standard of care: Legal history and definitions. *Western Journal of Emergency Medicine, 12*(1), 109–112. PMID: 21691483.

Newhouse, R. P., Dearholt, S., Poe, S., Pugh, L. C., & White, K. M. (2007). Organizational change strategies for evidence-based practice. *Journal of Nursing Administration, 37*(12), 552–557. https://doi.org/10.1097/01.nna.0000302384.91366.8f

Richardson, P. E. H. (2015). David Sackett and the birth of evidence based medicine: How to practice and teach EBM. *BMJ, 8*(350), h3089. https://doi.org/10.1136/bmj.h3089

Sbarbaro, J. A. (2001). Can we influence prescribing patterns? *Clinical Infectious Diseases, 33*(Suppl. 3), S240–S244. https://doi.org/10.1086/321856

Shekelle, P., Woolf, S., Grimshaw, J. M., Schünemann, H. J., & Eccles, M. P. (2012). Developing clinical practice guidelines: Reviewing, reporting, and publishing guidelines; updating guidelines; and the emerging issues of enhancing guideline implementability and accounting for comorbid conditions in guideline development. *Implementation Science, 7*(1), 62. https://doi.org/10.1186/1748-5908-7-62

Stillwell, S. B., Fineout-Overhold, E., Melynk, B. M., & Williamson, K. M. (2010). Evidence-based practice, step by step: Asking the clinical question: A key step in evidence-based practice. *American Journal of Nursing, 110*(3), 58–61. https://doi.org/10.1097/01.naj.0000368959.11129.79

Timmermans, S., & Berg, M. (2003). *The gold standard: The challenge of evidence-based medicine and standardization in health care.* Temple University Press.

Titler, M. G. (2008). The evidence for evidence-based practice implementation. In R. G. Hughes (Ed.). *Patient safety and quality: An evidence-based handbook for nurses.* Agency for Healthcare Research and Quality (US). https://www.ncbi.nlm.nih.gov/books/NBK2659/

U.S. Preventive Services Task Force. (2018). *Grade definitions.* https://www.uspreventiveservicestask-force.org/uspstf/grade-definitions

Woolf, S. H., Grol, R., Hutchinson, A., Eccles, M., & Grimshaw, J. (1999). Potential benefits, limitations, and harms of clinical guidelines. *BMJ, 318*(7182), 527–530. https://doi.org/10.1136/bmj.318.7182.527

World Health Organization. (2010). *WHO handbook for guideline development.* https://www.who.int/hiv/topics/mtct/grc_handbook_mar2010_1.pdf

ELEVEN

EVALUATION OF INTERPROFESSIONAL HEALTH CARE TEAMS

Joanne V. Hickey

None of us is as smart as all of us. . . . We all know that cooperation and collaboration grow more important every day. A shrinking world in which technological and political complexity increase at an accelerated rate offers fewer and fewer arenas in which individual action suffices.
—*Warren Bennis*

INTRODUCTION

The historical background of team science developed from the 1950s to the 1980s when group functioning became a source of interest and was investigated by social psychologists. From the 1980s to the present, a focus of study on teams has evolved with investigations primarily conducted by industrial/organizational and human factors psychologists (Mathieu et al., 2018). Perhaps the most influential industries that have promoted team science development are aviation, military, nuclear, and space. The underlying theme of these industries has been working together effectively to promote safety and outcomes. The 1977 Tenerife air disaster, in which two Boeing 747 passenger jets (KLM and Pan Am) collided on a foggy runway resulting in 583 fatalities, was the worst air disaster in aviation history. The aviation disaster was a wake-up call for the industry to address safety issues, and now, the same industry is considered one of the safest. The U.S. military has long been a leader in developing high-caliber teams for national defense. The National Aeronautical Space Agency (NASA) has expanded team science by putting man into space for extended periods of time and planning for travel to Mars and beyond. NASA's success is due to meticulous attention to safety and team training.

The application of team science and safety came to the health care industry in the early 2000s fueled by the landmark Institute of Medicine (IOM) report (Kohn et al., 1999) entitled *To Err Is Human: Building a Safer Health System*. The nation was shocked to learn that between 44,000 and 98,000 people die each year from medical error. Since the publication of that report and subsequent IOM reports in which the importance of teams was noted, there is a national initiative that focuses on patient safety and the achievement of optimal patient/population outcomes. The focus on teams has been central to this work because most work in health care organization is conducted by teams both in the clinical and organizational/leadership areas. Team research in health care has addressed patient handoffs, multi-team systems, team coordination, and team training (Rosen et al., 2018; Traylor, 2020). Rosen et al. (2018) provide an excellent synthesis of evidence that examines teams and teamwork in health care delivery to characterize the current state of the science, including gaps. Some clinical areas have been researched more than others, such as intensive care units (ICUs), obstetrics, and surgery, while other areas are ripe for investigation. The dynamic nature and complexity of health care organizations and teams are well recognized as health professionals and other stakeholders strive to redesign health care delivery. Although team science has made substantial progress, there are still opportunities and challenges for further development.

The purpose of this chapter is to provide the reader with background information about health care teams, team science, types, development, functions, and outcomes of teams as well as core competencies for interprofessional collaborative practice (IPC). This information serves as a basis for better understanding of teams, models/frameworks for evaluating teams, and foci for evaluation.

THE ESSENTIALS: CORE COMPETENCIES FOR PROFESSIONAL NURSING EDUCATION

The American Association of Colleges of Nursing (AACN) 2021 *Essentials: Core Competencies for Professional Nursing Education* continue to underscore the importance of working in teams for advanced practice nurses and DNP graduates. Domain 6: Interprofessional Partnerships addresses this domain of practice and team membership. In addition, key concepts related to interprofessional practice including communications and diversity, equity, and inclusion as well as other concepts help elucidate the clinical competencies necessary for contemporary nursing practice. The competencies for Domain 6: Interprofessional Partnerships are found on pages 43–45 of the 2021 *Essentials* at https://www.aacnnursing.org/Portals/42/AcademicNursing/pdf/Essentials-2021.pdf.

TEAM AND RELATED DEFINITION

Putting a group of people together does not constitute a team. For example, committees, councils, and task forces are not necessarily a team. A group does not become a team simply because someone calls them a team. The difference between a group and a team is their performance together and the results. A working group's performance is a function of what its members do as individuals, while a team's performance includes both individual results and *collective work products*, defined as what two or more members must work on together (Katzenbach & Smith, 1993).

Teams vary from one to another and are defined by many, but tend to have similar concepts included. A *team* is "a small number of people with complementary skills who are committed to a common purpose, set of performance goals, and an approach for which they hold themselves mutually accountable" (Katzenbach & Smith, 1993). Another useful definition of teams is "a distinguishable set of two or more people who interact, dynamically, interdependently, and adaptively toward a common and valued goal, objective, or mission" (Salas et al., 1992; Salas & Frush, 2013).

For teams to be effective, both taskwork and teamwork must be performed successfully (Burke et al., 2003). *Taskwork* involves the performance of specific tasks that team members must complete to achieve team goals (Salas et al., 2015), while "*teamwork* focuses on the shared behaviors (what team members do), attitudes (what team members feel or believe), and cognitions (what team members think or know) for teams to accomplish these tasks" (Morgan et al., 1994; Salas et al., 2015). These are the ABCs of teamwork.

Teams view themselves, and are viewed by others, as a distinct social entity working within a larger entity (Cohen & Bailey, 1997). Hackman (2002) describes well-designed teams as those with clear goals, thought-out tasks that are conducive to teamwork, and team members with the right skills, commitment, and experiences for the task. These qualities enable structure, supportive organizational context, adequate resources, and access to coaching and support.

Teams in health care have been defined as the relationship between two or more health care professionals who interdependently care for patients (Lemieux-Charles & McGuire, 2006). Salas et al. (2015) identify a set of considerations for teamwork based on the scientific team literature to provide an integrated understanding of the major components of teamwork. The framework consists of *six processes and emergent states—cooperation, conflict, coordination, communications, coaching,* and *cognition.* In addition, *three influencing conditions* that impact the six processes and emergent states are *composition* (e.g., *team members*), *culture,* and *context.* The following defines the terms:

- *Cooperation:* the motivational drivers of teamwork driven by behaviors reflective of attitudes, beliefs, and feelings.
- *Conflict:* the perceived incompatibilities in the interests, beliefs, or views held by one or more team members.
- *Coordination:* the use of behavioral and cognitive mechanisms necessary to perform a task and transform team resources into outcomes.
- *Coaching:* leadership behaviors to establish goals and set direction that leads to and encourages team members to successful accomplishment of these goals.
- *Cognition:* a shared understanding among team members, based on team member interactions, in which the knowledge of roles, responsibilities, team objectives, and norms and knowledge of teammate knowledge, skills, and attitudes (KSA) come together for a shared mental model about the team.
- *Composition:* addresses the composition of team membership based on needed KSAs and representation of diversity to address the goals of the team.
- *Context:* characteristics and circumstances of the setting that influence behavior, its perception, and how these variables interact on achieving team outcomes.
- *Culture:* the customs, beliefs, language, rules, knowledge, collective identities, and memories developed by members of social groups (i.e., team, organization, health care) that make the environment unique and meaningful.

Salas et al. (2018) identified three teamwork competencies that are transportable (i.e., can be used irrespective of the team, setting, or task), which include coordination, communications, and adaptability. The framework and identification of transportable concepts are useful for those involved in the evaluation of health care teams. Table 11.1 provides definitions of selected terms used in team science.

TABLE 11.1 Definitions of Selected Terms Used in Team Science

Term	Definition
Collaboration	An active and ongoing partnership, often involving people from diverse backgrounds who work together to solve problems or provide services (IOM, 2015, p. xi). A complex process through which relationships are developed among health care professionals so that they effectively interact and work together for the mutual goal of safe and quality patient care (Freshman et al., 2010, p. 110).
Interdisciplinary collaboration	An interpersonal process that facilitates the achievement of goals that cannot be reached when professionals act individually.
Interprofessional collaboration	A type of interprofessional work involving various health care professionals who come together regularly to solve problems or provide services (IOM, 2015, p. xi).
Interprofessional teamwork	A type of work involving different health care professionals who share a team identity and work together closely in an integrated and interdependent manner to solve problems and deliver services (IOM, 2015, p. xi).
Leadership	The ability to coordinate the activities of team members and teams by managing the resources available to team members and facilitating team performance by communicating plans, providing information about team performance through debriefs, and providing support to team members when needed (Agency for Healthcare Research and Quality [AHRQ], 2012).
Team effectiveness	The degree to which team goals and objectives are successfully met.
Team mental models	The shared and organized understanding and mental representation of knowledge or beliefs relevant to key elements of the team's task environment (Klimoski & Mohammed, 1994).
Team processes	Interdependent acts of members that convert inputs into outputs through cognitive, verbal, and behavioral activities directed toward organizing task work to achieve collective goals. Task work involves what activities the team performs and reflects skill and member competence. By contrast, teamwork describes how they do it and relies on higher level behaviors, such as the ability to direct, align, communicate, negotiate, and monitor task work (Marks et al., 2001).
Value	Value has different meanings depending on contexts. Value in health care is expressed as the physical health and sense of well-being achieved related to the cost (IOM Roundtable on Evidence-Based Medicine, 2008).

AHRQ, Agency for Healthcare Research and Quality; IOM, Institute of Medicine.

TEAM FORMATION

Groups do not become teams or well-functioning teams automatically. Once a group meets the criteria for a team, the team develops through a series of linear phases. Team development is usually regarded as an informal process by which members attempt to create effective social structures and work processes on their own (Kozlowski & Ilgen, 2006). A number of team developmental process models are available, but the most commonly cited model is that of Tuckman (1965). The model initially included the four stages of forming, storming, norming, and performing; a fifth stage, adjourning, was later added (Tuckman & Jensen, 1977). These are the stages that small groups go through as they come together and begin to function effectively (Smith, 2005).

The *forming stage* is the team creation stage described as a time of orientation through testing. The testing helps team members identify boundaries of both interpersonal and task behaviors. Interpersonal work is around the establishment of dependency relationships with leaders, other group members, or pre-existing standards. The *storming stage* is a phase of conflict and polarization around roles and interpersonal issues with concomitant emotional response of team members around tasks. While these behaviors serve as resistance to group influence and task requirements, they provide opportunities for conflict resolution.

In the *norming stage*, resistance is overcome because of the development of in-group behaviors and cohesiveness, evolution of new standards, and adoption of new roles. Personal opinions are expressed, and norms and patterns of behavior and activities are worked out. The *performing stage* is characterized by effective interpersonal structures to accomplish the work; while roles become flexible and functional, group energy is channeled into getting the work done as a common goal. At the norming state, structural issues have been resolved, and an effective structure supports group work. Finally, in the *adjourning stage*, the focus is on dissolution or termination of roles, the completion of tasks, and reduction of dependency. If unplanned, the process of adjourning can be stressful with a component of mourning related to individual losses.

While the linear Tuckman (1965) model has stood the test of time, some have challenged the linearity in favor of models that reflect the fluctuations that groups experience. There does appear to be general support that small groups tend to follow a fairly predictable developmental path (Smith, 2005). From the perspective of evaluation, the Tuckman model can provide insight into the group process and achievement of outcomes. The developmental stage of the group is one variable in understanding and evaluating groups and team performance. Although the Tuckman model may be useful in understanding the development of a traditional stable team, it is unclear how the team formation steps apply to the nontraditional teams commonly seen in current practice.

In forming teams, the composition and roles of team members are important. The responsibilities of the team leader contribute greatly to the success of a team (see Box 11.1). The responsibilities of team members are similar to those of the leader, as found in Box 11.2.

BOX 11.1   Responsibilities of Team Leaders

- Organize the team.
- Identify and articulate clear goals (i.e., the plan).
- Assign tasks and responsibilities.
- Monitor and modify the plan; communicate changes.
- Review the team's performance; provide feedback when needed.
- Manage and allocate resources.
- Facilitate information sharing.
- Encourage team members to assist one another.
- Facilitate conflict resolution in a learning environment.
- Model effective teamwork.

Source: Agency for Healthcare Research and Quality. (2013). Pocket guide TeamSTEPPS 2.0. Team strategies and tools to enhance performance and patient safety. Author. https://www.ahrq.gov/sites/default/files/wysiwyg/professionals/education/curriculum-tools/teamstepps/instructor/essentials/pocketguide.pdf

---

BOX 11.2 Responsibilities of Team Members

- Commit to be active and engage in the work of the team.
- Put team goals ahead of your own.
- Think for yourself.
- Self-management.
- Work with minimal supervision.
- Commit to the organization and goals of the team.
- Competence in your area of expertise (that you bring to the team).
- Willingness to open and respectful communications.
- Good listener.
- Critical thinker.
- Willingness to stand up for what you believe.
- Willingness to work through conflict effectively.

Source: Ulrich, B., & Crider, N. M. (2017). Using teams to improve outcomes and performance. *Nephrology Nursing Journal, 44*(2), 141–151. https://www.proquest.com/scholarly-journals/using-teams-improve-outcomes-performance/docview/1987370695/se-2?accountid=7034

CLASSIFICATION OF TEAMS

Team taxonomies are devised for a variety of purposes such as membership, purpose, goals, and function. All types of teams have both advantages and disadvantages. The following discusses common classifications of teams.

Traditional Versus Nontraditional Teams

Teams can be classified as *traditional teams*, defined as those whose members interact through traditional meetings and consultation, and *nontraditional teams*, whose structure, methods, and work are fluid and less structured. Health care organizations include both traditional and nontraditional teams. An example of a traditional team is one that includes a number of health professionals who work together on a regular basis to provide care for a group or population of patients, such as a team that rounds on a daily basis in the ICU. The team members may include physicians, nurses, respiratory therapists, clinical pharmacists, physical therapists, dietitians, social workers, discharge planners, and others. However, more and more nontraditional teams are part of health care delivery as well. A group of two or more health providers may work together periodically to achieve mutual goals for a patient and, once completed, dissolve the team until a similar need re-emerges. An example of a nontraditional team is one in which a rehabilitation nurse, occupational therapist, and physical therapist work together on a scheduled basis to provide a common goal of ambulation therapy for a spinal cord injured patient.

A *multiteam system* is another type of team that forms in response to complex goals that require the coordinated efforts of multiple specialized teams to address focused problems of a larger problem. The multisystem team is a large-scale collaboration in response to pressing challenges in areas such as disease prevention, disaster response, and health care problems (Mathieu et al., 2001). For example, teams from different clinical specialties work in collaboration to provide integrated care for a patient. A patient diagnosed with cancer may be managed by both a surgical team and an oncology team who work collaboratively on mutually set goals for the patient. A more complex team example is seen in the response to the COVID-19 pandemic that required health care organizations to work across organizational, clinical, and community settings in new and innovative ways to respond to the complex issues caused by the pandemic. Multiteam system function is an area requiring extensive study. The current research is reviewed by Shuffler and Carter (2018).

Teams may work together across settings and communicate via electronic media such as telehealth. Technology makes it possible to connect across systems as well as globally. The models for teams continue to evolve and expand.

Classification by Functionality and Membership

Teams can be classified by how they function, which includes unidisciplinary, multidisciplinary, interdisciplinary, interprofessional, and transdisciplinary teams.

Unidisciplinary Teams

Unidisciplinary teams are composed of providers all from a single discipline, such as a group of cardiovascular nurse practitioners that provide telehealth patient visits. All team members share the same professional paradigm, skills, and training; speak a common language of health care; and function in the same role within the group.

Multidisciplinary Teams

Multidisciplinary refers to a team where members of different disciplines or professions work separately, each with their own paradigm for treatment goals, with little or no awareness of the work offered by the other disciplines (Korner et al., 2015). The assessments and consultations of each discipline are conducted separately with little or no communication among members (Columbia University, n.d.). Although members within this team contribute to the care of a patient, they often do so without knowledge of the overall specific goals or what other team members are doing. Further, the multidisciplinary team provides a "silo" approach to care, with each provider "doing their own thing" and documenting the care they give. This approach often lacks coordination, continuity of care, and a comprehensive approach to the achievement of common goals.

Interdisciplinary Teams

Interdisciplinary describes a deeper level of team member collaboration in which processes such as development of a plan of care or evaluation occur jointly, with professionals of different disciplines pooling their knowledge in an independent fashion. An interdisciplinary team can be composed of a group of professionals representing several disciplines working interdependently in the same setting and interacting both formally and informally. Team members work to achieve a common team goal, although members may conduct separate assessments. Information is communicated and problems are solved in a systematic way among team members, typically during team meetings. For the interdisciplinary team model to be successful, the team must address issues of group dynamics, clarification of roles, team unity, communications, leadership, and decision-making practices (Columbia University, n.d.).

Interprofessional Teams

Interprofessional describes the interactions among individual professionals who may represent a particular discipline or branch of knowledge, but who additionally bring their unique educational background, experiences, values, roles, and identities to the process of working across health care professions to cooperate, collaborate, communicate, and integrate care in teams to ensure that care is continuous, reliable, and evidence based (IOM, 2003). The term *interprofessional* has been used with increased frequency to refer to clinical practice. *Interprofessional team-based care* is defined as "care delivered by intentionally created, usually relatively small work groups in health care who are recognized by others, as well as by themselves, as having a collective identity and shared responsibility for a patient or group of patients (e.g., rapid response team, palliative care team, primary care team, and operating room team)" (IPEC, 2016, p. 8). The World Health Organization (WHO) defines *interprofessional care* as "when multiple health workers from different professional backgrounds work together with patients, families, carers, and communities to deliver the highest quality of care" (WHO, 2010). The term *interprofessional* includes only those classified as a "professional" and thus excludes potential collaborators such as patients, family members, community health workers (CHWs), and others who might have information and knowledge of the work at hand; this limitation is counterintuitive to patient-centered care.

The Interprofessional Education Collaborative Expert Panel (IPEC) defines *interprofessional teamwork* as "the level of cooperation, coordination, and collaboration characterizing the relationships between professions in delivering patient-centered care" (IPEC, 2016, p. 8).

Transdisciplinary Teams

Transdisciplinary is a specific form of interdisciplinary work in which boundaries between and beyond disciplines are transcended and knowledge and perspectives from different scientific disciplines, as well as nonscientific sources, are integrated. Transdisciplinary is the newest term in the disciplinarity nomenclature and is undergoing the process of consensus building around a definition. The prefix "trans" means to go across something. By going across, beyond, and over disciplinary boundaries, a process emerges to assemble the disciplines in new ways and to recombine disciplinary knowledge and information for the creation of new knowledge (Choi & Pak, 2006). There is interest in transdisciplinary teams because of the complexity of current health care problems and the belief that only transdisciplinary thinking and problem-solving can adequately address these challenges. For example, transdisciplinary teams of molecular scientists, biologic engineers, geneticists, ethicists, and others are needed to solve such complex questions related to stem cell and personal health issues.

Community Health Workers and Others as Teams Members

The term *community health workers* refers to individuals anchored in the community who provide care and services that influence patient care and health care delivery. They include many different job titles and roles such as lay health worker, peer advisor, community health advocate, promotora, and others (Institute for Clinical and Economic Review, 2013). CHWs receive a minimal amount of training (e.g., 2–6 weeks), but are members of the community at large and have an appreciation and respect for the ethnic, linguistic, cultural, experiential connections and social determinants of health of the population from which they come (Brooks et al., 2014). CHWs work as members of the health care team to increase the team's cultural competence by helping team members understand the beliefs, culture, and values of the patient that influence the patient's acceptance and adherence to a health care plan. As trusted members of the same community from which the patient comes, CHWs assist the patient in achieving health care goals from preventive through treatment stages. For example, CHWs assist the patient in understanding treatment options, take the patient to appointments as needed, and run errands, such as getting a needed prescription at the local pharmacy. Their work contributes greatly to delivering patient-centered care. A growing body of evidence suggests that the implementation of a CHW program produces meaningful and measurable results (Brooks et al., 2014). With the growing number of aged persons and persons with chronic diseases in the United States, as well as the cultural and ethnic diversity, the focus on chronic disease management and home care is expected to continue to grow along with the need for CHWs to decrease readmission and emergency department visits, increase patient adherence, improve health and wellness, and reduce cost. Members of the interprofessional team must learn how to incorporate CHWs into the team and work effectively with them to achieve optimal outcomes for patients and communities.

Other occupations and disciplines that provide services in the community also impact patient and population health outcomes. Others include insurers, exercise and alternative health modality providers, local elected officials, social service agencies, schools, fire department, and police department. All of the resources from these occupations and disciplines are available to teams for collaboration to building healthy communities. In addition, advocating for inclusion of other members of the public is important because of the contemporary changes in how health care is being defined, and the opportunity to engage the public is supported and termed *participatory engagement*. (Tebes & Thai, 2018).

Value of Teams

The pursuit of multidisciplinary work and teamwork is important for several reasons, including the following (Choi & Pak, 2006):

- To resolve real-world problems
- To resolve complex problems
- To provide different perspectives about a problem
- To create a comprehensive prospective theory-based hypothesis for research
- To develop consensus around clinical definitions and guidelines for complex diseases and conditions
- To provide comprehensive services such as health care and health education

The current research and literature overwhelmingly acclaim the value of teams, in particular interdisciplinary and interprofessional health care teams, as the primary approach and best practice to improve teamwork and patient/population outcomes. Both models are used across the continuum of care including ICUs, long-term care facilities, geriatric acute and chronic care units, transitional care units, and community-based clinics and facilities. As one delves into the literature to find and examine the supporting evidence for such claims, the results are mixed. The complexity of health care teams and their relationship to improved health care outcomes is daunting to untangle, with researchers developing new models to find causality between teams and outcomes in a dynamic and ever-changing health care system.

THEORETICAL PERSPECTIVES OF HEALTH CARE TEAMS

Knowledge about team science and teamwork has developed dramatically over the years, resulting in a voluminous body of literature about teams, while the research and literature focused on health care teams has evolved since the early 2000s. Since the 1950s, the social, organizational, and business/management sciences have investigated teams from a variety of discipline-specific perspectives, resulting in a number of theoretical models to view teams such as how teams are organized, how they work, and how they achieve outcomes. One can evaluate team function based on group dynamics, effectiveness, efficiency, interpersonal communications, satisfaction, and outcomes. What has been learned about teams from other disciplines has provided a foundation upon which to build health care team science.

Sociologic Influence

Team behavior through the conceptualization of group processes was strongly influenced by sociologic studies of hierarchical differentiation (Ingersoll & Schmitt, 2004). The primary focus of research was on a group's social structure and its influence on team communications and problem-solving (Farrell et al., 1986, 1988), and proposed guidelines to counteract poor team decision-making processes with the following: (a) emphasize open, honest, and direct communications; (b) facilitate team development through orientation of new team members and team retreats; (c) focus on the team's mission statement, goals, policies, and procedures; (d) acknowledge effective individual and teamwork; and (e) identify team processes that lead to poor decision-making with a focus on finding more effective decision-making processes (Ingersoll & Schmitt, 2004).

Organizational Influence

Organizational research has focused on organizational structure, organizational culture, team performance, and learning organizations. Team structure is the fundamental characteristic of teams, and structure includes size, membership, leadership, identification, and distribution. Weick and Roberts (1993) examined high-reliability organizations (HROs) that espoused to be nearly error-free operations. They found that HROs integrate highly developed mental models and processes that all members follow, which are a reflection of overlapping knowledge and performance standards. Another example of organizational theory is that of learning organizations. Senge (1990), in addressing systems thinking, noted that team learning is vital because teams, not individuals, are the fundamental learning unit in modern organizations. Still another area of interest is organizational culture and its influence on interprofessional teamwork, team effectiveness, and patient/organizational outcomes (Korner et al., 2015).

Business/Management Influence

Micro- and macrosystem theory are other paths of organizational investigation of business and management. A *microsystem* refers to a small team of people working together as one unit to get jobs done (Ogrinc et al., 2018, p. 63). In aviation, the microsystem is the flight crew and air traffic controllers. In health care, it is the health care team. Microsystem theory focuses on the frontline component of service delivery. Ogrinc et al. (2018) investigated high-performance clinical microsystems and identified characteristics that led to excellent systemic outcomes. These characteristics include: leadership and the culture of the microsystems; macroorganizational support of the microsystem; a focus on patients and staff; interdependence of care teams; easy access to information and information technology; a focus on process improvement; and high-level performance patterns (Ogrinc et al. 2018).

A *macrosystem* refers to the overarching structure above the microsystem, such as the organization or the system. A macrosystem includes the policies, procedures, culture, and leadership that oversee the microsystems. Interactions between the microsystem and macrosystem affect performance and outcomes at both levels.

Finally, the generic logic model of input–process–output (IPO) is used as a framework to study teamwork effectiveness and outcomes. The IPO model describes the impact of input (e.g., organizational culture, team composition, communication patterns, task design) and the processes of teams (e.g., communication, coordination, collaboration, cooperation, leadership) on the team's outputs (team performance, cost-effectiveness, quality of care, treatment outcomes, and patient safety; Korner et al., 2015). The parsimony of the model allows for flexibility. Because of the inherent complexity in understanding the multiple variables that influence team outcomes and effectiveness, researchers usually select a few variables of interest in the model to study which variables do not provide the big picture of teams.

HOW TEAMS WORK

The work of teams is complex, and the magnitude of complexity increases with greater numbers and type of team members, the level of complexity of the work, and contextual–environmental factors. Teams are dynamic with complex internal and external interactions. Internal interactions occur within the team and include member-to-member and member-to-team interactions. External factors include interactions with the patient/family, other teams, and the organization; elements of the organization; oversight committees; and the overall health care delivery system.

Teams are ever changing as they undergo multiple transitions in their development, work, and goals responding to the dynamic needs of patients, organizations, and the health care system requiring adaptability. A one-time snapshot of a team does little to capture the immense complexity and dynamics of the team, which suggests the need to study teams over time, to create multiple snapshots. In addition, current research methodologies are generally ineffective at enlightening investigators about the complex interactive processes and outcomes of teams. Most studies provide insight about a few variables of interest by reporting relationships among selected variables, but do not address causality or outcomes. The state of the science on health care teams is "messy," although it provides some direction for evaluation of teams.

Teamwork

The concept of teamwork has evolved over time. *Teamwork* refers to the actual behaviors (e.g., exchange of information), cognitions (e.g., shared mental models), and attitudes (e.g., cohesion) that make interdependent performance possible (Salas et al., 2008). "*Teamwork* is an adaptive, dynamic, and episodic process that encompasses the thoughts, feelings, and behaviors among team members while they interact toward a common goal. Teamwork is necessary for effective team performance as it defines how tasks and goals are accomplished in a team context" (Salas et al., 2015, p. 600). According to Xyrichis and Ream (2008), *teamwork* in health care is "a dynamic process involving two or more health care professionals with complementary backgrounds and skills, sharing common health goals, and exercising concerted physical and mental effort in assessing, planning, or evaluating patient care" (p. 238). Teamwork occurs by using a number of strategies such as interdependent collaboration, open communications, shared decision-making, and generated value-added patient, organizational, and staff outcomes (Xyrichis & Ream, 2008). *Team-based care* is defined "as an approach to health care whereby a group of people work together to accomplish a common goal, solve a problem, or achieve a specified result" (IOM, 2015, p. xii). The principles of team-based health care include shared goals, clear roles, mutual trust, effective communications, and measurable processes and outcomes (Mitchell et al., 2012).

Teaming

Stable traditional teams are becoming less common in health care. The concept of teaming has been added to the nomenclature of teamwork in a knowledge economy. *Teaming* is defined as the activity of working together. Unlike the traditional concept of a team, teaming is an active process rather than a static entity. It is a way of collaboratively working that brings people together to generate new ideas, find answers, and solve problems. Teaming is further described as: blending ways of relating to people; listening to other points of view; coordinating action; and making shared decisions. It is a dynamic process of working that provides the necessary coordination and collaboration without the luxury (or rigidity) of stable team structure. In health care, many teams come together for a circumscribed purpose, accomplish the task, and disband until the need arises again for their special expertise. There is an ebb and flow to the teamwork. The work may take minutes or occur over a short and circumscribed time. Teaming has been described as teamwork on the fly, involving coordination and collaboration without the benefit of stable team structures. For example, many operations within hospitals and clinics require flexible staffing and make stable team composition rare (Edmondson, 2012).

Different competencies and leadership styles are required to work in these contemporary teams. Critical is the ability to act in the moment because there is no time to build a foundational relationship of familiarity with others through sharing of personal history and prior experience and experiential work. The new competencies include sharing crucial knowledge quickly and being able to quickly learn by asking pointed questions clearly and frequently. This is particularly important because teaming is the engine of organizational learning and involves bringing people together to generate new ideas and make decisions, often about complex problems. Teaming is integral to any enterprise and is critical when any of the following conditions exist: work requires people to juggle multiple objectives with minimal oversight; need to shift from one situation to another while maintaining high levels of communication and tight coordination; need to integrate perspectives from different disciplines; collaboration required across dispersed locations; preplanned coordination is impossible or unrealistic due to the rapid changing nature of the work; and complex information must be processed, synthesized, and used quickly (Edmondson, 2012).

Weinberg et al. (2011) describe *collaborative capacity* as the likelihood that providers, no matter how brief their exchange, will collaborate as if they were members of a conventional team, even in the absence of a formal team structure. They recommend a "shift in emphasis from teams with their requirements for clear group boundaries and stable membership over time to collaborative capacity, which emphasizes the ability of providers to engage in teamwork which includes sharing interdependent tasks with norms of respectful and helpful interaction and engaging in joint collaborative decision making" (Weinberg et al., 2011). For the evaluator, understanding team structure and processes is important in evaluating outcomes.

TEAM EFFECTIVENESS

Team effectiveness refers to an evaluation of the results of performance by the team (Lemieux-Charles & McGuire, 2006). A major focus in health care is outcomes and what factors contribute to achievement of superior outcomes. Collaboration is a frequently addressed concept in the literature and is identified as a key variable in teamwork that contributes to superior outcomes. Weaver et al. (2013) noted that while teamwork is not synonymous with collaboration, although these terms are often used interchangeably, it is the broader concept and includes many elements such as collaboration, common goals, and mental models.

The need for greater interprofessional collaboration has been emphasized since the 1970s (IOM, 2010). A growing body of research notes the potential for collaboration among teams composed of diverse individuals to generate successful solutions to complex, knowledge-driven problems (Singh & Fleming, 2010; Wuchty et al., 2007). Researchers have also emphasized the importance of building interprofessional teams and establishing collaborative cultures to identify and sustain continuous quality improvement of care (Kim et al., 2010; Pronovost et al., 2008). Other evidence of the benefits of teamwork and team effectiveness has emerged and includes increased learning and development of people and organizations, better utilization of resources and planning, minimization of unnecessary costs, improved job performance work quality, increased discussion among participants, networking, professional development, and positive effect on career (Choi & Pak, 2006).

Many studies have examined interdisciplinary teams and collaboration in relationship to patient outcomes in a variety of settings, such as nursing homes, long-term care facilities, acute/critical care units, rehabilitation, and primary care, as well as with specific populations, such as geriatrics, the chronically ill, and others (Boaro et al., 2010; Korner, 2010; Meier & Beresford, 2010; Neumann et al., 2010; Pezzin et al., 2011; Pyne et al., 2011). What is clear is that much still needs to be learned about team effectiveness and its impact on health care delivery, especially with nontraditional teams.

Health care teams are complex dynamic entities working in complex dynamic environments. Marks et al. (2001) noted that the framework of team processes and outcomes is multidimensional, and team behavior is constantly changing. The changing nature of a team and team member behavior is tempered by the developmental level of the team and the work of the team that transitions between existing goals and new goals, including evolving processes. A single snapshot of a team provides little information in understanding how teams work in the achievement of outcomes.

A Cochrane systematic review (Zwarenstein et al., 2009) addressed IPC and health outcomes. The review suggested that practice-based interprofessional collaboration can improve health care processes and outcomes, but because of the limitations of the literature (e.g., small number of studies, sample sizes, problems with conceptualization and measurement of collaboration, and heterogeneity of interventions and settings), it was not possible to draw generalizable conclusions about the key elements of IPC and its effectiveness (Zwarenstein et al., 2009). In a 2017 Cochrane update, nine new IPC studies were reviewed. The authors concluded that because of the low to very low level of evidence found, there is not sufficient evidence to draw clear conclusions on the effects of IPC interventions. Nevertheless, due to the difficulties health professionals encounter when collaborating in clinical practice, it is encouraging that research on the number of interventions to improve IPC has increased since this review was last updated. While the field of IPC is developing, further rigorous, mixed-method studies are required. Future studies should focus on longer acclimatization periods before evaluating newly implemented IPC interventions and use longer follow-up to generate a more informed understanding of the effects of IPC on clinical practice (Reeves et al., 2017). Box 11.3 provides a list of characteristics of high-performance teams.

Research is slowly evolving regarding teams and interdisciplinary practice teams and how they affect patient outcomes. Table 11.2 provides a list of variables related to health care teams that have been investigated. These variables have been extracted from multiple studies and have been organized into arbitrary categories. Each category is mutually exclusive from the other categories, although variables from a number of categories may be examined during a particular evaluation. From a cursory review of the list, it is clear that there are multiple perspectives that can be used to examine and evaluate teams.

Barriers to Teams

In the health care arena, there are many barriers to establishing and maintaining high-performance teams and team effectiveness. Some barriers cut across all practice areas while others are specific to particular areas of practice and environments. Barriers to interprofessional teamwork and collaboration are included in Table 11.3.

Durbin (2006) notes that local customs (e.g., culture) may be the most difficult barrier to overcome. In addition, resistance comes from many sources such as hospital administration (concern about added cost), unit administrator (change in authority and control), bedside staff (must learn new ways of interacting with a team), and private physicians (altered authority gradient for patient management and decisions). Both taskwork (e.g., technical) competency and teamwork competency are necessary to achieve high performance in interdisciplinary teams.

BOX 11.3   Characteristics of High-Performing Teams

- Members with clear roles and responsibilities
- Members with a clear, valued, and shared vision

  - A common purpose
  - An engaging purpose
  - A leader who promotes the vision with the appropriate level of detail

- Members share a mental model
- Team optimizes resources
- Strong team leadership
- Engage in a regular discipline of feedback

  - Regularly provide feedback to one another and as a team
  - Establish and revise team goals and plans
  - Differentiate between higher and lower priorities
  - Have mechanisms for anticipating and reviewing issues of team members
  - Periodically diagnose team effectiveness, including its results, processes, and vitality (including morale, energy, and retention)

- Develop a strong sense of collective trust, team identity, and confidence

  - Manage conflict by effectively confronting one another
  - Have a strong sense of team orientation
  - Trust other team members' intentions
  - Believe strongly in the team's collective ability to succeed
  - Develop collective efficacy
  - Have a high degree of psychological safety

- Create mechanisms to cooperate, coordinate, and generate ongoing collaboration

  - Identify teamwork and task requirements
  - Ensure that the team has the right mix of competencies through staffing and development
  - Distribute and assign work thoughtfully
  - Consciously integrate new team members
  - Involve the right people in decisions in a flexible manner
  - Examine and adjust the team's physical workplace to optimize communication and coordination

- Manage and optimize performance outcomes

  - Communicate often and at the right time to ensure that fellow team members have the information they need in order to contribute
  - Use closed-loop communication
  - Learn from each performance outcome
  - Continually strive to learn

Source: Agency for Healthcare Research and Quality. (2015). TeamSTEPPS 2.0. https://www.ahrq.gov/teamstepps/instructor/fundamentals/index.html

Taskwork or technical competency is based on professional training, education, and experience as well as licensure and certification. Teamwork competency is based on education and the KSA about interdisciplinary work. In addition, competency may be defined differently in each discipline.

TABLE 11.2　Perspectives for Evaluating Health Care Teams

Group Process Perspective
- Interactions of team members
- Accomplishment of tasks
- Engagement in team activities
- Engagement in team development activities
- Analytical skills
- Decision-making processes (e.g., shared, hierarchal)
- Competition between and among members
- Team norms

Communications Perspective
- Open, honest, and direct communications
- Constructive feedback
- Effective conflict resolution

Cohesiveness Perspective
- Commitment to mutual purpose
- Understanding and commitment to team mission, goals, policies, and procedures
- Orientation of new members
- Supporting of team members
- Shared team mental model

Leadership Perspective
- Hierarchal versus shared leadership
- Interchange of leadership and followership (person with the most knowledge for particular project leads)
- Leadership development opportunities available to all members
- Organizational support for team

Individual Team Member Perspective
- Values
- Attitudes
- Autonomy
- Motivation
- Personal and professional development
- Confidence building
- Self-monitoring
- Emotional intelligence

Team Development Perspective
- Crew resource management or TeamSTEPPS®
- Culture of learning
- Individual and group competency development

High-Performance Perspective
- Shared vision
- Clear roles and responsibilities
- Clear and transparent communications
- Mutual respect
- Trust
- Cohesiveness
- Collaboration
- Collaborative capacity
- Cooperation
- Expectation of accountability of all members for outcomes
- Appreciation of expertise and contribution of each discipline
- Interdisciplinary working together
- Individual and team effectiveness
- Shared decision-making
- Team members supportive of team decisions and each other
- Use of common mental models
- Coordination of care

Structural Perspective
- Vertical versus horizontal
- Shared versus hierarchal authority
- Hierarchal leadership
- Transformational leadership
- Appropriate team memberships (e.g., disciplines represented) and how this contributes to outcomes

Satisfaction Perspective
- Patient/family satisfaction with team
- Individual team members satisfied with team
- Others external to the team such as employer, administrator, or funder

Patient Outcome Perspective
- Length of stay (LOS)
- Mortality
- Morbidity/complications
- Functionality (e.g., social, intellectual, activities of daily living [ADLs], instrumental ADLs)
- Cost of care
- Service utilization

Safety and Quality Perspective
- Justculture
- Root cause analysis

TABLE 11.3 Barriers to Effective Team Performance

Inconsistency in team membership or wrong members on team	Conflict that is unresolved
Lack of time	Lack of coordination and follow-up
Lack of information sharing	Distractions
Lack of coaching	Lack of organizational support
Defensiveness	Unreasonable workload
Conventional or narrow thinking	Misinterpretation of cues
Complacency	Lack of role clarity
Varying communication styles	Turf issues
Hierarchy issues (gender, power, socialization, education, status, and cultural differences between professions and individuals)	Lack of payment system to reward interdisciplinary work

Source: Agency for Healthcare Research and Quality. (2015). TeamSTEPPS 2.0. https://www.ahrq.gov/teamstepps/instructor/fundamentals/index.html

Dysfunction and Failure of Teams

Health care teams can be dysfunctional and fail for many reasons. The list of barriers provided in Table 11.3 provides some insights. Dysfunction leads to team failure. Understanding why and how teams fail is critical to understanding corrective interventions to support high-performance teams. Dysfunctional teams can have a negative impact on work relationships, decrease productivity and effectiveness, and, if not managed, can jeopardize the organization (Lencioni, 2002). Lencioni (2002) identified five dysfunctions of a team: absence of trust, fear of conflict, lack of commitment, avoidance of accountability, and inattention to results. Functional conflict, according to Amason (1996), is a productive part of the team process when it supports the goals of the group, while dysfunctional conflict hinders team performance and requires intervention to refocus the team. The team leader must be able to distinguish between the two forms of conflict and intervene to address dysfunctional conflict.

Blackmore and Persaud (2012) identified five critical domains important to optimize team functioning: a common team goal, the ability and willingness to work together to achieve team goals, decision-making, communications, and relationships. Characteristics of behaviors for each domain are provided as well as a description of functional and dysfunctional teams and improvement strategies. The five domains are recurrent domains, as reported in the literature, related to interprofessional teams and need to be linked to patient and population outcomes through more research.

EDUCATION FOR INTERPROFESSIONAL COLLABORATIVE PRACTICE

People do not come to teams knowing how to practice in teams; effective team member functioning requires teamwork education. *Team training* is defined as "a learning strategy comprising a set of tools and methods that learners use to systematically acquire teamwork knowledge, skills, and attitudes (KSAs)" (Hughes et al., 2016; Salas et al., 2008). Educational strategies to keep teams and organizations functioning within industry-accepted safety standards include crew resource management (CRM), Team-STEPPS, and core competencies for IPC. Each strategy is discussed briefly in this section.

Interest in team-based education for U.S. health professionals is not new. At the first IOM conference entitled "Interrelationships of Educational Programs for Health Professionals," 120 leaders from allied health, dentistry, medicine, nursing, and pharmacy considered key questions about promoting interprofessional education. The conference report was entitled *Educating for the Health Team* (IOM, 1972), while another report, *Health Professions Education: A Bridge to Quality* (IOM, 2003), underscored the need for all health professionals to be competent in working in teams.

A systematic review of the literature from the past decade was conducted directed at interventions to improving team effectiveness within health care organization to identify the "evidence base" levels of research (Buljac-Samardzic et al., 2020). The review concluded that the number of studies on team interventions has increased exponentially. However, the research focused on certain interventions, settings, and/or outcomes. CRM, TeamSTEPPS®, and simulation-based training seem to provide the greatest opportunities for reaching the improvement goals in team functioning (Buljac-Samardzic et al., 2020). Table 11.4 provides the KSA characteristics of effective team training.

Crew Resource Management

Strategies to keep teams and organizations functioning within industry-accepted safety standards have been developed and include CRM, also known as team

TABLE 11.4 Team Training—Attitudes, Behaviors, and Cognitions That Influence Teamwork

	Competencies
Attitudes	● Cohesion ● Commitment to teamwork ● Trust ● Psychological safety ● Collective efficacy
Behaviors	● Communication ● Coordination ● Planning ● Performance monitoring ● Backup behaviors ● Handoffs ● Providing feedback
Cognitions	● Knowledge stock ● Knowledge of task structure ● Shared understanding of team member roles ● Situation awareness ● Implicit team coordination ● Transactive memory systems

Source: Salas, E. (2015). Team training essentials: A research-based guide. Routledge.

cooperation training. CRM was first introduced in response to safety outcomes in the aviation industry after the Tenerife disaster and has been applied to a number of industries, disciplines, and settings such as military training and operating rooms. CRM is designed to shift an individual focus toward shared responsibilities. The training encompasses a wide range of tools and techniques such as check-list, debriefings, and simulation to enhance communications, situational aware-ness, problem-solving, decision-making, teamwork, and optimal use of all available resources (e.g., equipment, procedures, people) to promote and enhance efficiency and safety (Rosenbaum, 2019).

TeamSTEPPS®

The Agency for Healthcare Research and Quality (AHRQ, 2015) in collaboration with the Department of Defense (DoD) developed a team training curriculum called TeamSTEPPS® designed to educate health professionals and others in teamwork and patient safety. It is an evidence-based system designed to improve communica-tions, team leadership, situation monitoring, and mutual support for effective team-work skills among health care professionals and others. TeamSTEPPS® provides a source of ready-to-use multimedia materials and a training curriculum to success-fully integrate teamwork principles into all areas of an organization and health care system. The curriculum includes a number of resources such as validated instru-ments, slides, and an evidence-based detailed curriculum. More information is available at their website: www.teamstepps.ahrq.gov/

Core Competencies for Interprofessional Collaborative Practice

As a response to the continued call for interprofessional education (IPEC) from the IOM and multiple other sources, the Interprofessional Education Collabora-tive was formed to set standards for interprofessional education and practice. Six national professional education associations (i.e., nursing, osteopathic medicine, pharmacy, dentistry, medicine, and public health) were represented. An additional 60 other professions have participated on Institute teams. The updated version (IPEC, 2016) builds on the IPEC (2011) report that provided key operational defi-nitions and principles that guided the identification of four core competencies and related sub-competencies. The four IPEC core competencies and sub-competencies are included in Exhibit 11.1.

In summary, team education is imperative for team members to learn how to work effectively in teams. Salas (2015) noted that attitudes, behaviors, and cog-nitions (ABCs) change within an individual or team as a result of team training. Cognitive and behavior change are the goals of team training that translates into improved outcomes.

MEASUREMENT METHODS FOR TEAMS

The choice of method to measure depends on the area of interest and the psycho-metric characteristics of the instrument. The three major methods used when con-sidering methods of measurement of team performance include surveys, direct or

---

Exhibit 11.1

**Interprofessional Collaborative Practice Core Competencies
With Related Sub-Competencies**

Core Competency 1: Work with individuals of other professions to maintain a climate of mutual respect and shared values. (values/ethics for interprofessional practice [VE])

VE Sub-competencies:

VE1. Place the interests of patients and populations at the center of interprofessional health care delivery and population health programs and policies, with the goal of promoting health and health equity across the life span.

VE2. Respect the dignity and privacy of patients while maintaining confidentiality in the delivery of team-based care.

VE3. Embrace the cultural diversity and individual differences that characterize patients, populations, and the health care team.

VE4. Respect the unique cultures, values, roles/responsibilities, and expertise of other *health professions* and the impact these factors can have on health outcomes.

VE5. Work in cooperation with those who receive care, those who provide care, and others who contribute to or support the delivery of prevention and health services and programs.

VE6. Develop a trusting relationship with patients, families, and other team members (Canadian Interprofessional Health Collaborative, 2010).

VE7. Demonstrate high standards of ethical conduct and quality of care in one's contributions to team-based care.

VE8. Manage ethical dilemmas specific to interprofessional patient-/population-centered care situations.

VE9. Act with honesty and integrity in relationship with patients, families, communities, and other team members.

VE10. Maintain competence in one's own profession appropriate to scope of practice.

Core Competency 2: Use the knowledge of one's own role and those of other professions to appropriately assess and address the health care needs of patients and to promote and advance the health of populations. (Roles/Responsibilities [RR])

RR Sub-competencies:

RR1. Communicate one's roles and responsibilities clearly to patients, families, community members, and other professionals.

RR2. Recognize one's limitations in skills, knowledge, and abilities.

RR3. Engage diverse professionals who complement one's own professional expertise, as well as associated resources, to develop strategies to meet specific health and health care needs of patients and populations.

RR4. Explain the roles and responsibilities of other care providers and how the team works together to provide care, promote health, and prevent disease.

RR5. Use the full scope of knowledge, skills, and abilities of professionals from health and other fields to provide care that is safe, timely, efficient, effective, and equitable.

RR6. Communicate with team members to clarify each member's responsibility in executing components of a treatment plan or public health intervention.

RR7. Forge interdependent relationships with other professions within and outside of the health system to improve care and advance learning.

RR8. Engage in continuous professional and interprofessional development to enhance team performance and collaboration.

RR9. Use unique and complementary abilities of all members of the team to optimize health and patient care.

(continued)

RR10. Describe how professionals in health and other fields can collaborate and integrate clinical care and public health interventions to optimize population health.

Core Competency 3: Communicate with patients, families, communities, and professionals in health and other fields in a responsive and responsible manner that supports a team approach to the promotion and maintenance of health and the prevention and treatment of disease. (Interprofessional Communication [CC])

CC Sub-competencies:

CC1. Choose effective communication tools and techniques, including information systems and communication technologies, to facilitate discussions and interactions that enhance team function.

CC2. Communicate information with patients, families, community members, and health team members in a form that is understandable, avoiding discipline-specific terminology when possible.

CC3. Express one's knowledge and opinions to team members involved in patient care and population health improvement with confidence, clarity, and respect, working to ensure common understanding of information and treatment and care decisions, and population health programs and policies.

CC4. Listen actively and encourage ideas and opinions of other team members.

CC5. Give timely, sensitive, instructive feedback to others about their performance on the team, responding respectfully as a team member to feedback from others.

CC6. Use respectful language appropriate for a given difficult situation, crucial conversation, or interprofessional conflict.

CC7. Recognize how one's own uniqueness (experience level, expertise, culture, power, and hierarchy within the health team) contributes to effective communication, conflict resolution, and positive interprofessional working relationships (University of Toronto, 2008).

CC8. Communicate consistently the importance of teamwork in patient-centered care and population health programs and policies.

Core Competency 4: Apply relationship-building values and the principles of team dynamics to perform effectively in different team roles to plan, deliver, and evaluate patient-/population-centered care and population health programs and policies that are safe, timely, efficient, effective, and equitable. (Teams and Teamwork [TT])

TT Sub-competencies:

TT1. Describe the process of team development and the roles and practices of effective teams.

TT2. Develop consensus on the ethical principles to guide all aspects of teamwork.

TT3. Engage health and other professionals in shared patient-centered and population-focused problem-solving.

TT4. Integrate the knowledge and experience of health and other profession to inform health and care decisions, while respecting patient and community values and priorities/preferences for care.

TT5. Apply leadership practices that support collaborative practice and team effectiveness.

TT6. Engage self and others to constructively manage disagreements about values, roles, goals, and actions that arise among health and other professionals and with patients, families, and community members.

TT7. Share accountability with other professions, patients, and communities for outcomes relevant to prevention and health care.

TT8. Reflect on individual and team performance for individual, as well as team, performance improvement.

TT9. Use process improvement strategies to increase the effectiveness of interprofessional teamwork and team-based services, programs, and policies.

TT10. Use available evidence to inform effective teamwork and team-based practices.

TT11. Perform effectively on teams and in different team roles in a variety of settings.

Source: Interprofessional Education Collaborative. (2016). Core competencies for interprofessional collaborative practice: 2016 update. Author.

video-recorded observations, and sociometric badges (Traylor, 2020). Each method has advantages as well as disadvantages that should be understood.

Surveys that include checklists (i.e., yes–no response), anchored questionnaires (i.e., Likert scales), and self-reports involve asking team members to rate themselves, the team, and/or their organization on various items to measure individual attitudes and opinions (Keebler et al., 2014). Surveys can measure communications, leadership, coordination, and other key team elements within and across settings. While they are inexpensive to administer, collect, and analyze, surveys provide only a snapshot of one individual's perspective of team performance.

Direct observation methods measure team performance in real time. Often external raters, who must be trained for interrater reliability, are used, which adds objectivity to the measurement (Rosen et al., 2018). Most of these observational tools are used in specific clinical settings such as surgery and focus on individual and team levels of analysis (Mishra et al., 2009). Observation methods are usually summative, completed at the end of an observation, and do not capture the moment-to-moment changes in performance. The direct observation method can also be used to rate performance on video recordings.

A *sociometric badge* (commonly known as a "sociometer") is a wearable electronic badge capable of automatically measuring the amount of face-to-face interaction, conversational time, speech rhythm and intonations, physical proximity to other people, and physical activity levels, using social signals derived from vocal features, body motion, and relative location (Olguin & Pentland, 2007). The badge enables objective and automatic measurements about spatiotemporal distributions of active face-to-face interactions consistent with reality, but does not measure. What it does not provide is active listening, body language, or brief conversation important to interprofessional collaboration (Ito-Masui et al., 2020). The use of a sociometer that requires technology support to collect and interpret data incurs a higher cost. Although not used as frequently as other measurement methods, sociometric badges show promise for future research.

Measurement Instruments

Validated instruments are one method to conduct an evaluation of selected aspects of team performance. In 2012, the National Center for Interprofessional Practice and Education assembled and launched a web-based collection of existing IPE and IPC measurement instruments (IPEC, 2016). Review of the instruments shows that some are specific to a population (pediatrics) or clinical practice (surgery), while others are more generic to interprofessional practice and assess teamwork, cooperation, coordination, communications, and other key elements related to teams. The information provided at the site includes: instrument description; instrument type and content; resource link; focus of assessment (who or what is being assessed); notes for data sources and content; instrument length; item format; scoring; language; instrument access; and psychometrics. This website is updated periodically with new instruments added based on established criteria. The website also provides a helpful primer to guide individuals in the selection of valid instruments. As of this writing, there are 23 instruments included in the website. Access to instruments may be open access (13), subscription (8) viewed in a journal article, and copyrighted (2) needing permission of the author. Table 11.5 provides

TABLE 11.5 Examples of Measurement Instruments for Interprofessional Teams Elements

Name of Instrument	Purpose
Assessment for Collaborative Environments (ACE-15)	To help faculty and administrators conduct a rapid assessment of the quality of interprofessional teamwork in clinical sites
Assessment of Interprofessional Team Collaboration Scale (AITCS)	A diagnostic instrument to evaluate the level of interprofessional collaboration among a variety of health care teams
Collaborative Practice Assessment Tool (CPAT)	Assesses collaborative practice among caregiving team members, patients, and clients
Communication and Teamwork Skills (CATS) Assessment	Measures communication and team skills of health care providers (i.e., situational awareness, coordination, communication, and cooperation)
Healthcare Team Vitality Instrument (HTVI)	Measures team "vitality" in hospital settings; measures the individual's perceptions of environmental support structures, engagement and empowerment, patient care transitions, and team communication
TeamSTEPPS Team Assessment Questionnaire and Team Performance Observation Tool (TAQ-TPOT)	Part of TeamSTEPPS curriculum to improve quality, safety, and efficiency of health care. It includes the TAQ—collects individual team members' perceptions of team foundation, functioning, performance, skills, leadership, climate/atmosphere, and identity—and the T-POT—collects objective observations of team structure, leadership, situational monitoring, mutual support, and communication

examples of selected instruments. See website at https://nexusipe.org/advancing/assessment-evaluation?f%5B0%5D=sm_field_who_assessed%3A3&sort_by=label

When there is not a validated instrument appropriate for the planned team evaluation, then it is necessary to collect the desired information through other sources such as an evaluation protocol that asks questions about the area of interest. Even when a validated instrument is used, it becomes *only one source of data* for an evaluation.

PLANNING AN EVALUATION OF A TEAM

With this background information about team science and key elements related to team effectiveness, how is a Doctor of Nursing Practice (DNP) nurse going to evaluate a team? As with the content on planning an evaluation in Chapter 8, there are options for how to proceed based on the area of interest about teams. Chapter 8 provides a basic framework for evaluation of a program or project. The steps of the evaluation include: (a) *purpose and scope*; (b) *design and methodology*; (c) *data collection, acquisition, and management*; (d) *data analysis and interpretation*; (e) *project management*; and (f) *dissemination*. Although these steps are listed as separate entities, there is a back-and-forth approach to these processes as the work progresses. One step is never considered completed because of the dynamic nature of the evaluation process. Table 11.6 provides a list of activities and questions/focus to consider in planning an evaluation.

TABLE 11.6 Activities and Questions/Focus to Consider in Evaluating Health Care Teams

Activities	Questions and Focus
1. Purpose and Scope	
• Determine the purpose(s) of the evaluation. • Determine the scope (boundaries) and focus of the evaluation. • Learn all you can about the team. • Describe the team; refine as new information becomes available. • Focus the evaluation. • Negotiate your role. • Establish timeline for the evaluation.	• What are the purposes of the evaluation? • What is the scope of the evaluation? • Who is requesting it and how will the report be used? • Investigate the historical background of the team: Why was it formed, has its purpose changed over time, where is it developmentally, what is the composition, to whom does it report, and so on? • How would you succinctly describe the team? • Based on the purpose, intended use, and characteristics of the team, how will you narrow the focus of the evaluation? • How will you participate in the evaluation? To whom are you responsible? Will you be given access to the people and information that you need to conduct the evaluation?
2. Design and Methodology	
• Determine design based on purpose (e.g., examine patient outcomes; examine team communication processes). • Determine the best methods based on purpose, available resources, culture, etc. • Design a plan for evaluating the team. • Decide what to measure and observe. • Determine how to measure areas of interest. • Determine any associated costs with the evaluation.	• Do you have an overall plan? • What will you measure and observe? • Do you have a written plan? • What will the evaluation cost? • Are you clear about your roles and responsibilities?
3. Data Collection, Acquisition, and Management	
• Construct or purchase instruments. • Set deadlines for data collection. • Make sure that your data collection plan is implemented properly (fidelity). • Determine what data to collect and where it will be found. • Plan how the data will be acquired and entered.	• How will you collect the data? • What resources are available to you for data collection (e.g., people, technology)? • Do you have a written timeline for data collection (e.g., Gantt chart)? • Address interrater reliability if others are collecting data.

(continued)

TABLE 11.6 Activities and Questions/Focus to Consider in Evaluating Health Care Teams (*continued*)

Activities	Questions and Focus
4. Data Analysis and Interpretation	
• Determine who and how data will be analyzed. • Involve the team in reviewing the data and its interpretation. • Determine recommendations based on data analysis and interpretations.	• Who is responsible for data analysis? • Is there a plan for data analysis? • Is the analysis free of bias? • Who is responsible for data interpretation?
5. Project Management	
• The evaluator responsible for the project is also responsible and accountable for all activities and leadership for implementation of the evaluation. • Determine personnel and their responsibilities. • Provide needed resources as negotiated with the person(s) requesting the evaluation. • Develop policies and procedures for evaluation implementation. • Provide a plan for data storage and security. • Manage the agreed upon timeline using a Gantt chart or other means.	• Has an overall plan of all activities and timeline for the evaluation been developed? • Has it been communicated to all involved in the evaluation? • Have team assignments been assigned and clarified with team members including responsibilities and expectations? • Have the data been collected and stored for accuracy and security? • Is the timeline being followed?
6. Dissemination	
• Determine the format for reporting your findings. • Meet with the team leader and/or staff to verify factual information. • Present the report (e.g., written and/or report) to designated audiences. • Return any documents or other resources used for the evaluation to owner. • Come to closure.	• How will you verify with the team leader or team members that your facts are correct? • How will you disseminate a report of the evaluation and your findings (informal, formal, memo, email, written, oral, etc.) and to whom? • How you will come to closure with the project?

In this section, the same six steps discussed earlier will be followed with a focus on evaluation of teams. The information provided is applicable regardless if the DNP nurse is an internal or external evaluator to the organization. The reader is referred to Chapter 8 for further discussion of planning an evaluation.

Purpose and Scope

In order to conduct a useful evaluation of team effectiveness, the DNP nurse (i.e., evaluator) must clearly understand the purpose and scope of the evaluation to be able to set the specific focus and boundaries (i.e., scope) for a doable evaluation. This information comes from the person or persons requesting the evaluation (e.g., director, chief nurse or executive officer, board, committee, or another initiator).

The purpose or purposes of the evaluation are varied and may include: the impact of the team on quality indicators or patient outcomes, or cost; examination of team processes in relation to compliance with evidence-based practice guidelines and best practices; comprehensiveness of care; team group dynamics; leadership practices; or team member(s) and patient satisfaction with care delivered. Another way to focus the evaluation is from the perspective of problems. What are the specific problems with the team that are to be addressed? The problem approach also helps to identify desired evaluation outcomes and helps to set the evaluation criteria to be used to evaluate performance. Because information from an evaluation may be used for decision-making, it is helpful to know who is going to receive the information and how the information will be used (e.g., team redesign, continued funding of the team, improvement in patient outcomes). All of this information helps to shape the evaluation process.

The DNP nurse may or may not have knowledge of the team and should take the time to conduct a comprehensive assessment of the team. Even if the evaluator thinks they know the team, take a fresh unbiased look at the team from the eyes of an evaluator. Examples of areas to consider are: historical background of the team (e.g., When was it formed? For what purpose? Who started the team?); the setting in which the team functions and how it is tied to the organizational structure; focus of the teamwork; changes in the purpose of the team over time; team membership; longevity of each member on the team; the team's organizational structure; leadership; how work gets done; and developmental stage of the team. This information can be gathered through discussions, observations, and review of written materials. When necessary information has been collected, the evaluator will be able to describe the team and categorize it according to type, developmental level, work patterns and processes, and outcomes.

Once the DNP nurse has collected the information and formulated a description of the team, the evaluator can begin to clarify the rationale and objectives for the evaluation and narrow the scope. This should lead to a brief written outline of purpose, rationale, objectives, and scope, which should be shared with the person or persons requesting the evaluation to verify and clarify a common focus of the evaluation. This is also a time to negotiate the evaluator role. Be clear about the expectations, responsibilities, deliverables, timeline, and the person to whom the evaluation is reported. Verify access to information and people for the conduct of the work and determine what the team members have been told about the evaluation and who provided that information. In addition, identify the contact person who will act as facilitator if issues occur in the conduct of the evaluation. Discuss what format the final report should take and who should receive it. Finally, the conditions under which the work will be done should be addressed. If the evaluator is an outside consultant, conditions of work and compensation are addressed through a contract. If the evaluator is internal to the organization, how will this work be calculated into their current workload? Is there anyone available to help or provide support for data gathering? These and other questions need to be addressed prospectively to avoid misunderstandings later.

Design and Methodology

In selecting an appropriate design and evaluation methods, the evaluator should further refine and double-check the description of the team, the rationale for the team, and the goals/objectives of the evaluation. This may seem redundant, but as the evaluator continues to work and plan, there may be new information and subtle changes in direction that influence the approach, including what questions and observations need to be completed in order to get to the heart of the evaluation. The evaluator should also clarify the outcomes on which to focus (e.g., processes, outcomes) and put the details in writing for clarity of communication. A clear understanding of how the resultant information will be used is important to maintain congruency between purposes and collected information.

The next step in the evaluation is to develop a detailed, step-by-step written plan of activities, data to be collected, methods of collection, timeline for collection, and sources of data. To map the evaluation process in a concise and efficient format, a written plan should be created or a logic model framework used to guide the evaluation. Knowledge of the organization/system and team will help to determine activities. The evaluator should decide what to measure and observe including contextual characteristics, team composition, team member characteristics, processes, patient outcomes, or costs. The variables selected must be operationally defined to determine how they can best be measured. For example, to investigate team communication patterns, the evaluator must first define communication patterns. The definition might include verbal interactions among team members, verbal interactions of team members with bedside staff nurses, written documentation of the plan of care, or exchange of information at team conferences. How the concept is operationalized will drive options for measurement. For example, verbal interactions among team members could be investigated by observation of team members at work, by a questionnaire, or both. The evaluator must decide what method or methods of measurement are available to measure performance and which will best meet the objectives of the evaluation. If there is cost associated with measurement, such as the purchase of instruments, these costs need to be included in a budget for approval by the sponsor of the evaluation.

The DNP nurse must be knowledgeable about the current team science of evaluation of teams. Understanding the state of the science in health team evaluation will help to maintain realistic expectations of what can be accomplished from an evaluation.

Data Collection, Acquisition, and Management

In this phase, the evaluator constructs or purchases instruments, creates an evaluation protocol to evaluate performance based on accepted standards and criteria, and sets timelines for data collection, acquisition, and management. Depending upon the evaluation's purposes and objectives, the evaluator may create an investigator-developed data collection instrument, purchase validated instruments, or use a combination of both. If any instruments are purchased, be sure that the intended purpose of the instrument and the purpose of the evaluation are congruent. For example, the TeamSTEPPS Team Assessment Questionnaire (AHRQ, 2016) provides a comprehensive view of team performance. Regardless if the instruments are evaluator created or purchased, the DNP nurse must follow a timeline for data collection. If another person is assisting with data collection, the DNP nurse will need to orient that person to the instrument and data collection process to ensure interrater reliability.

Data acquisition has to do with gaining possession of the desired data. This means that the evaluator needs to know what data are required, location/source of the data, the process for extracting the data, and appropriate storage of data. See Table 8.1 for location and sources of data. Chapter 8 also addresses data extraction, storage, and management.

Data Analysis and Interpretation

Data analysis is conducted once data are collected and organized in a usable format. Quantitative data may be entered into a spreadsheet of statistical analysis programs such as the Statistical Package for Social Sciences (SPSS) if it has not been previously entered. Qualitative data may be analyzed using content analysis or other qualitative data analysis methods. Data analyzed should be related clearly to the objectives outlined for the evaluation. As the evaluator analyzes the data, they must keep an eye on opportunities for quality improvement of team effectiveness around the areas evaluated. Are there any national standards or benchmarks that may be useful to frame the data collected? The evaluator should think about recommendations that may assist the decision-makers who will receive the report regarding the team.

Project Management

The section on project management presented in Chapter 8 is generic and applies to all evaluation. The reader is directed to the project management section in Chapter 8 for further information.

Dissemination

Once data analysis is completed and findings are formulated, the evaluator may wish to meet with the team leader and/or team members to discuss and follow up on the findings if such a meeting has been approved by the initiator of the evaluation. Meeting with team members is directed at transparency and provides the opportunity to correct any factual information that was reported as incorrect.

The final step in the evaluation process is dissemination of the findings of the evaluation in both written and oral reports. Content on dissemination of findings has been provided in Chapter 8 in the section on dissemination.

SUMMARY

This chapter was designed to assist the DNP nurse in the evaluation of teams based on a comprehensive understanding of the current state of health care team science and how the science of team evaluation has been investigated. As most of the work in health care delivery, as well as other aspects of life, is conducted in teams, it is paramount to know how effective teams work to achieve desired outcomes and what makes teamwork successful. However, evaluating teams is no easy process. Both teams and everything done in the health care arena are dynamic, complex, and ever changing on an increasingly rapid timeline. Attempting to evaluate such interrelated dynamic and complex entities within the context of setting and organizational and team culture is challenging.

Team performance includes both taskwork and teamwork at multiple levels and individuals harmonizing together to conduct the work of the organization through team efforts. In addition, because of the limited current knowledge about team functioning and facilitating structural components, it is not always clear as to identifying standards and criteria for acceptable team performance measures and how to collect, analyze, and interpret data. Also recognized is that an evaluation of a team at one time point provides only a snapshot of team effectiveness at one time point, and not a clear picture of how well the team is functioning overall.

Further development in team science and methodology will advance the science to better understand how teams contribute to team effectiveness and health care outcomes with the precision and clarity desired to appreciate the value provided by teams. The challenges to evaluate dynamic teamwork and performance in an equally dynamic and ever-changing health care systems are great. The varying nature of teams has changed from traditional models to nontraditional models of teaming across unit, organizations, and multisystems. Given the dynamic nature of teamwork and team evaluation, the DNP nurse will continue to be challenged to conduct meaningful evaluations of teams.

REFERENCES

Agency for Healthcare Research and Quality. (2012). *TeamSTEPPS instructor guide glossary.* http://www.ahrq.gov/professionals/education/curriculum-tools/teamstepps/instructor/reference/glossary.html

Agency for Healthcare Research and Quality. (2015). *TeamSTEPPS 2.0 fundamentals.* https://www.ahrq.gov/teamstepps/instructor/fundamentals/index.html

Agency for Healthcare Research and Quality. (2016). *TeamSTEPPS.* U.S. Department of Health and Human Services. http://teamstepps.ahrq.gov/

Amason, A. C. (1996). Distinguishing the effects of functional and dysfunctional conflict on strategic decision making: Resolving a paradox for top management teams. *Academy of Management Journal, 39*(1), 123–148. https://doi.org/10.2307/256633

American Association of Colleges of Nursing. (2021). *The essentials: Core competencies for professional nursing education.* Author. https://www.aacnnursing.org/Portals/42/AcademicNursing/pdf/Essentials-2021.pdf

Blackmore, G., & Persaud, D. D. (2012). Diagnosing and improving functioning in interdisciplinary health care teams. *The Health Care Manager, 18*(3), 195–207. https://doi.org/10.1097/HCM.0b013e3182619d48

Boaro, N., Fancott, C., Baker, R., Velji, K., & Andreoli, A. (2010). Using SBAR to improve communication in interprofessional rehabilitation teams. *Journal of Interprofessional Care, 24*(1), 111–114. https://doi.org/10.3109/13561820902881601

Brooks, B. A., Davis, S., Frank-Lightfoot, L., Kulbok, P. A., Poree, S., & Sgarlata, L. (2014). *Building a community health worker program: The key to better care, better outcomes, & lower costs.* CommunityHealth Works.

Buljac-Samardzic, M., Doekhie, K. D., & van Wijngaarden, J. D. H. (2020). Interventions to improve team effectiveness within health care: A systematic review of the past decade. *Human Resources for Health, 18*(2), 1–42. https://doi.org/10.1186/s12960-019-0411-3

Burke, C. S., Wilson, K. A., & Salas, S. (2003). Teamwork at 35,000 feet: Enhancing safety through team training. *Human Factors and Aerospace Safety, 3*(4), 287–312. https://doi.org/10.4324/9781315259482-17

Canadian Interprofessional Health Collaborative. (2010). *A national interprofessional competency framework.* http://ipontherun.ca/wp-content/uploads/2014/06/National-Framework.pdf

Choi, B. C. K., & Pak, A. W. P. (2006). Multidisciplinarity, interdisciplinarity, and transdisciplinarity in health research, services, education and policy: 1. Definitions, objectives, and evidence of effectiveness. *Clinical & Investigative Medicine, 29*(6), 351–364. https://www.proquest.com/scholarly-journals/multidisciplinarity-interdisciplinarity/docview/196425990/se-2?accountid=7034

Cohen, S. G., & Bailey, D. R. (1997). What makes teamwork: Group effectiveness research from the shop floor to the executive suite. *Journal of Management, 23*(4), 238–290. https://doi .org/10.1177/014920639702300303

Columbia University. (n.d.). *Types of teams.* https://ccnmtl.columbia.edu/projects/sl2/mod03_multi_1b.html

Durbin, C. G. (2006). Team model: Advocating for the optimal method of care delivery in the intensive care unit. *Critical Care Medicine, 34*(Suppl 3), S12–S17. https://doi.org/10.1097/01. CCM.0000199985.72497.D1

Edmondson, A. V. (2012). *Teaming: How organizations learn, innovate and compete in the knowledge economy.* Jossey-Bass.

Farrell, M. P., Heinemann, G. D., & Schmitt, M. H. (1986). Informed roles, rituals and humor in inter-disciplinary health teams: Their relation to stages of group development. *International Journal of Small Group Research, 2*(2), 143–162. https://doi.org/10.1080/13561820120068980

Farrell, M. P., Schmitt, M. H., & Heinemann, G. D. (1988). Organizational environments of interdis-ciplinary health care teams: Impact on team development and implications for consultation. *International Journal of Small Group Research, 4*(1), 31–54. https://doi.org/10.1080/13561820120068980

Freshman, B., Rubino, L., & Chassiakos, Y. R. (2010). *Collaboration across the disciplines in health care.* Jones and Bartlett Publishers.

Hackman, J. R. (2002). *Leading teams: Setting the stage for great performances.* Harvard Business School Press.

Hughes, A. M., Gregory, M. E., Joseph, D. L., Sonesh, S. C., Marlow, S. L., Lacerenza, C. N., & Salas, E. (2016). Saving lives: A meta-analysis of team training in healthcare. *Journal of Applied Psychology, 101*(9), 1266–1304. https://doi.org/10.1037/apl0000120

Ingersoll, G. L., & Schmitt, M. (2004). Interdisciplinary collaboration, team functioning, and patient safety. In A. Page (Ed.), *Keeping patients safe: Transforming the work environment of nurses* (pp. 341–383). National Academies Press.

Institute for Clinical and Economic Review. (2013). *An action guide on community health workers (CHWs): Guidance for organizations working with CHWs.* The New England Comparative Effective-ness Public Advisory Council.

Institute of Medicine. (1972). *Educating for the health team.* National Academy of Sciences.

Institute of Medicine. (2003). *Health professions education: A bridge to quality.* National Academies Press.

Institute of Medicine. (2010). *The future of nursing: Leading change, advancing health.* National Acad-emies Press.

Institute of Medicine. (2015). *Measuring the impact of interprofessional education on collaborative prac-tice and patient outcomes.* National Academies Press.

Institute of Medicine Roundtable on Evidence-Based Medicine. (2008). *Learning healthcare system con-cepts.* The National Academies Press.

Interprofessional Education Collaborative. (2016). *Core competencies for interprofessional collaborative practice: 2016 update.* Author.

Interprofessional Education Collaborative Expert Panel. (2011). *Core competencies for interprofessional collaborative practice: Report of an expert panel.* Author.

Ito-Masui, A., Kawamoto, E., Nagai, Y., Takagi, Y., Ito, M., Yano, K., Imai, H., & Shimaoka, M. (2020). Feasibility of measuring face-to-face interactions among ICH healthcare professional using wearable sociometric badges. *American Journal of Respiratory and Critical Care Medicine, 201*(2), 245–247. https://doi.org/10.1164/rccm.201904-0779LE

Katzenbach, J. R., & Smith, D. K. (1993, March–April). The discipline of teams. *Harvard Business Review,* 111–120. https://hbr.org/

Keebler, J. R., Dietz, A. S., Lazzara, E. H., Benishek, L. E., Almeida, S. A., Toor, P. A., King, H. B., & Salas, E. (2014). Validation of a teamwork perceptions measure to increase patient safety. *British Medical Journal Quality & Safety, 23,* 718–726. https://doi.org/10.1136/bmjqs-2013-001942

Kim, M. M., Barnato, A. E., Angus, D. C., Fleisher, L. A., & Kahn, J. M. (2010). The effect of multidis-ciplinary care teams on intensive care unit mortality. *Archives of Internal Medicine, 170*(4), 369–376. https://doi.org/10.1001/archinternmed.2009.521

Klimoski, R. J., & Mohammed, S. (1994). Team mental model: Construct or metaphor? *Journal of Man-agement, 20*(2), 403–437. https://doi.org/10.1177/014920639402000206

Kohn, L. T., Corrigan, J. M., & Donaldson, M. S. (Eds.). (1999). *To err is human: Building a safer health system.* National Academy Press.

Korner, M. (2010). Interprofessional teamwork in medical rehabilitation: A comparison of multidis-ciplinary and interdisciplinary team approach. *Clinical Rehabilitation, 24*(8), 745–755. https://doi .org/10.1177/0269215510367538

Korner, M., Wirtz, M. A., Bengel, J., & Goritz, A. S. (2015). Relationship of organizational culture, teamwork and job satisfaction in interprofessional teams. *BMC Health Services Research, 15*, 243. https://doi.org/10.1186/s12913-015-0888-y

Kozlowski, S. W. J., & Ilgen, D. R. (2006). Enhancing the effectiveness of work groups and teams. *Psychological Science in the Public Interest, 7*(3), 77–124. https://doi.org/ 10.1111/j.1529-1006.2006.00030.x

Lemieux-Charles, L., & McGuire, W. L. (2006). What do we know about health care team effectiveness? A review of the literature. *Medical Care Research and Review, 63*(3), 263–300. https://doi.org/10.1177/1077558706287003

Lencioni, P. (2002). *The five dysfunctions of a team.* Jossey-Bass.

Marks, M. A., Mathieu, J. E., & Zaccaro, S. J. (2001). A temporally based framework and taxonomy of team processes. *Academy of Management Review, 26*(3), 356–376. https://doi.org/10.5465/amr.2001.4845785

Mathieu, J. E., Marks, M. A., & Zaccaro, S. J. (2001). Multiteam systems. In N. Anderson, D. S. Ones, H. K.. Sinangil, & C. Viswesvaran (Eds.), *Handbook of industrial, work, and organizational psychology* (Vol. 2, pp. 289–313). SAGE.

Mathieu, J. E., Wolfson, M. A., & Park, S. (2018). The evolution of work team research since Hawthorne. *American Psychologist, 73*(4), 308–321. https://doi.org/10.1037/amp0000255

Meier, D. E., & Beresford, L. (2010). Palliative care in long-term care: How can hospital teams interface? *Journal of Palliative Medicine, 13*(2), 111–115. https://doi.org/ 10.1089/jpm.2009.9898

Mishra, A., Catchpole, K., & McCulloch, P. (2009). The Oxford NOTECHS System: Reliability and validity of a tool for measuring teamwork behaviour in the operating theatre. *Quality & Safety in Health Care, 18*, 104–108. https://doi.org/10.1136/qshc.2007.024760

Mitchell, P., Wynia, M., Golden, R., McNellis, B., Okun, S., Webb, C. E., Rohrbach, V., & Von Kohorm, I. (2012). *Core principles & values of effective team-based health care* (Discussion Paper). Institute of Medicine. www.iom.edu/tbe

Morgan, B. B., Salas, E., & Glickman, A. S. (1994). An analysis of team evolution and maturation. *Journal of General Psychology, 120*(3), 277–291. https://doi.org/10.1080/00221309.1993.9711148

Neumann, V., Gutenbrunner, C., Fialda-Moser, V., Christodoulou, N., Varela, E., Giustine, A., & Delarque, A. (2010). Interdisciplinary team working in physical and rehabilitation medicine. *Journal of Rehabilitation Medicine, 42*(1), 4–8. https://doi.org/10.2340/16501977-0483

Ogrinc, G. S., Headrick, L. A., Barton, A. J., Dolansky, M. A., Madigosky, W. S., & Miltner, R. S. (2018). *Fundamentals of health care improvement: A guide to improving your patients' care.* Joint Commission Resources & Institute for Healthcare Improvement.

Olguin, D. O., & Pentland, A. (2007). *Sociometric badges: State of the art and future applications.* IEEE 11th International Symposium on Wearable Computers, Boston, MA.

Pezzin, L. E., Feldman, P. H., Mongoven, J. M., McDonald, M. V., Gerber, L. M., & Peng, T. R. (2011). Improving blood pressure control: Results of home-based post-acute care interventions. *Journal of General Internal Medicine, 26*(3), 280–286. https://doi.org/10.1007/s11606-010-1525-4

Pronovost, P. J., Berenholtz, S. M., Goeschel, C., Needman, D., Hyzy, R., Welsh, R., Roth, G., Bander, J., Morlock, L., & Sexton, J. B. (2008). Improving patient safety in intensive care units in Michigan. *Journal of Critical Care, 23*(2), 207–221. https://doi.org/10.1016/j.jcrc.2007.09.002

Pyne, J. M., Fortney, J. C., Curran, G. M., Tripathi, S., Atkinson, J. H., Kilbourne, A. M., Hagedorn, H. J., Rimland, D., Rodriguez-Barradas, M. C., Monson, T., Bottonari, K. A., Asch, S. M., & Gifford, A. L. (2011). Effectiveness of collaborative care for depression in human immunodeficiency virus clinics. *Archives of Internal Medicine, 171*(1), 23–31. https://doi.org/10.1001/archinternmed.2010.395

Reeves, S., Pelone, F., Harrison, R., Goldman, J., & Zwarenstein, M. (2017). Interprofessional collaboration to improve professional practice and healthcare outcomes. *Cochrane Database of Systematic Reviews, 2017*(6), CD000072. https://doi.org/10.1002/14651858.CD000072.pub3

Rosen, M. A., Diaz Granados, D., Dietz, A. S., Benishek, L. E., Thompson, D., Pronovost, P. J., & Weaver, S. (2018). Teamwork in healthcare: Key discoveries enabling safer, high-quality care. *American Psychologist, 73*(4), 433–450. https://doi.org/10.1037/amp0000298

Rosenbaum, L. (2019, February 14). Divided we fall. *New England Journal of Medicine, 380*(7), 684–688. https://doi.org/10.1056/NEJMms1813427

Salas, E. (2015). *Team training essentials: A research-based guide.* Routledge.

Salas, E., Diaz Granados, D., Klein, C., Burke, C. S., Stagl, K. C., Goodwin, G. F., & Halpin, S. M. (2008). Does team training improve team performance? A meta-analysis. *Human Factors, 50*(6), 903–933. https://doi.org/10.1518/001872008X375009

Salas, E., Dickinson, T. L., Converse, S. A., & Tannenbaum, S. J. (1992). Toward an understanding of team performance and training. In R. W. Swezey & E. Salas (Eds.), *Teams: Their training and performance* (pp. 3–29). Ablex.

Salas, E., & Frush, K. (2013). *Improving patient safety through teamwork and team training*. Oxford University Press.

Salas, E., Reyes, D. L., & McDaniel, H. H. (2018). The science of teamwork: Progress, reflections, and the road ahead. *American Psychologist*, 73(4), 593–600. https://doi.org/10.1037/amp0000334

Salas, E., Rosen, M. A., Burke, C. S., & Goodwin, G. F. (2008). The wisdom of collectives in organizations: An update of the teamwork competencies. In E. Salas, G. F. Goodwin, & C. S. Burke (Eds.), *Team effectiveness in complex organizations: Cross-disciplinary perspectives and approaches* (pp. 39–790). Psychology Press.

Salas, E., Shuffler, M. L., Thayer, A. L., Bedwell, W. L., & Lazzara, E. H. (2015). Understanding and improving teamwork in organizations: A scientifically based practical guide. *Human Resource Management*, 54(4), 599–622. https://doi.org/10.1002/hrm.21628

Senge, P. M. (1990). *The fifth discipline*. Doubleday Currency.

Shuffler, M. L., & Carter, D. R. (2018). Teamwork situated in multiteam systems: Key lessons learned and future opportunities. *American Psychologist*, 73(4), 390–406. https://doi.org/10.1037/amp0000322

Singh, J., & Fleming, L. (2010). Lone inventors as sources of breakthroughs: Myth or reality? *Management Science*, 56(1), 41–56. https://doi.org/10.1287/mnsc.1090.1072

Smith, M. K. (2005). *Bruce W. Tuckman—Forming, storming, norming and performing in group*. The Encyclopedia of Informal Education. www.infed.org/thinkers/tuckman.htm

Tebes, J. K., & Thai, N. D. (2018). Interdisciplinary team science and the public: Steps toward a participatory team science. *American Psychologist*, 73(4), 549–562. https://doi.org/10.1037/amp0000281

Traylor, A. (2020, June 6). Studying teams in healthcare. In E. Thomas (Director), *Quality Improvement Series (Class)*. University of Texas Health Science Center at Houston.

Tuckman, B. W. (1965). Developmental sequence in small groups. *Psychological Bulletin*, 63(6), 384–399. https://doi.org/10.1037/h0022100

Tuckman, B. W., & Jensen, M. A. C. (1977). Stages of small-group development revisited. *Group and Organizational Studies*, 2(4), 419–427. https://doi.org/10.1177/105960117700200404

Ulrich, B., & Crider, N. M. (2017). Using teams to improve outcomes and performance. *Nephrology Nursing Journal*, 44(2), 141–151. https://www.proquest.com/scholarly-journals/using-teams-improve-outcomes-performance/docview/1987370695/se-2?accountid=7034

University of Toronto. (2008). *Advancing the interprofessional education curriculum 2009. Curriculum overview. Competency framework*. University of Toronto, Office of Interprofessional Education.

Weaver, S. J., Feitosa, J., Salas, E., Seddon, R., & Vozenilek, J. A. (2013). The theoretical drivers and models of team performance and effectiveness for patient safety. In E. Salas & K. Frush (Eds.), *Improving patient safety through teamwork and team training* (pp. 3–26). Oxford University Press.

Weick, K. E., & Roberts, K. H. (1993). Collective mind in organizations: Heedful interrelating on flight decks. *Administrative Science Quarterly*, 38(3), 357–381. https://doi.org/10.2307/2393372

Weinberg, D. B., Cooney-Miner, D., Perloff, J. N., Babington, L., & Avgar, A. C. (2011). Building collaborative capacity: Promoting interdisciplinary teamwork in the absence of formal teams. *Medical Care*, 49(8), 716–723. https://doi.org/10.1097/MLR.0b013e318215da3f

World Health Organization. (2010). *Framework for action on interprofessional education & collaborative practice*. Author. http://whqlibdoc.who.int/hq/2010/WHO_HRH_HPN_10.3_eng.pdf

Wuchty, S. B., Jones, F., & Uzzi, B. (2007). The increasing dominance of teams in production of knowledge. *Science*, 316(5827), 1036–1039. https://doi.org/10.1126/science.1136099

Xyrichis, A., & Ream, E. (2008). Teamwork: A concept analysis. *Journal of Advanced Nursing*, 61(2), 232–241. https://doi.org/10.1111/j.1365-2648.2007.04496.x

Zwarenstein, M. J., Goldman, M. J., & Reeves, S. (2009). Interprofessional collaboration: Effects of practice-based interventions on professional practice and healthcare outcomes. *Cochrane Database of Systematic Reviews*, 3(3), CD000072. https://doi.org/10.1002/14651858.CD000072.pub2

EVALUATION OF SIMULATION TO SUPPORT ONGOING COMPETENCY OF THE HEALTH CARE WORKFORCE

Kristen Starnes-Ott and M. Roseann Diehl

Attention comes first, learning after attention is focused. And learning is
primarily action.
—Dewey et al. (in Bricken, 1991)

INTRODUCTION

Simulation in health care education and training is widespread and has continued to grow and evolve rapidly over the past two decades. The Institute of Medicine (IOM) has recognized deficiencies in the current model of health care education and recommends the use of technology to improve performance and clinical decision-making (Henneman & Cunningham, 2005). Simulation has emerged as one means of achieving this goal, with over 40 years of research and thousands of individual reports citing simulation-based education (SBE) as a powerful educational intervention (McGaghie et al., 2012). Simulation growth has been complex, has lacked consistency, and has reported a multitude of methods to express data. Simulation has grown through both research about simulation (e.g., technology, impact, outcomes) and research that uses simulation (e.g., human factors, teamwork, clinical performance evaluation, decision-making; Gaba, 2007).

The very concept of simulation is nebulous at best and represents a spectrum of physical and computer modeling. Gaba (2007) defines *simulation* as a "technique, not a technology, to replace or amplify real experiences with guided experiences often immersive in nature, that evoke or replicate aspects of real world in a fully interactive manner." Simulation includes devices, trained individuals, lifelike virtual environments, and contrived social situations that mimic problems, events, or conditions (Gaba, 2007; Issenberg et al., 2004).

This chapter intends to inform and assist DNP students and graduates in developing and evaluating simulation-based curricula using best-practice methods. Simulation is an ever-changing, innovative domain of health care education and practice. Therefore, evaluation of simulation curricula at all levels of health care education and practice is crucial.

SIMULATION DOMAINS IN NURSING

Research has consistently demonstrated that simulation creates statistical improvements in knowledge/skill, critical thinking and/or confidence). Simulation has been endorsed by the International Nursing Association for Clinical Simulation and Learning (INACSL Standards Committee, 2016a), advanced practice nursing (Alexander et al., 2015; Parry & Fey, 2019), educators (Anderson & Leflore, 2008; McLaughlin et al., 2008), and students. Multiple studies suggest high levels of student satisfaction but with the risk of anxiety or intimidation (Ansen, 2015).

Simulation is effective and highly recognized in four domains: (a) assessment, (b) education and teaching, (c) research, and (d) systems integration (Palaganas & Rock, 2015). Simulation used in teaching should be supportive, nonjudgmental, and respectful. It does not preclude constructive feedback but does allow exploration without penalty. Learners should be reminded that participant performance during simulation does not always reflect the full capabilities of individuals during actual patient care. Simulation systems integration can have an overarching influence on organizational outcomes. Simulation is a tool that can have a powerful impact when it is used to improve the systems in which nurses work, whether it is patient flow, transfer of care, policies in an organization, or organizational culture. System-based improvements may address quality, safety, risk management, enterprise improvement, resilience, or other system-side desired attributes. The Society for Simulation in Healthcare (SSH) defines this fourth domain as a simulation program demonstrating consistent, planned, collaborative, integrated and iterative application of simulation-based teaching methodologies and assessment activities with systems engineering and risk management principles to achieve excellence in clinical care, enhanced patient safety, and improved metrics across health care (Deutsch & Palaganas, 2015).

BRIEF HISTORY OF SIMULATION

Simulation in health care had its early beginnings in aviation when flight simulation began in the early 20th century and with the emergence of Crew Resource Management (CRM) in the late 1970s. The majority of simulators that are presently available represent a history of multiple universities and corporations working independently and parallel to each other with differing motivations (Slone & Lampotang, 2015a, 2015b). The first partial-task trainer "Resusci-Anne" emerged in the 1940s, created by Laerdal for cardiopulmonary resuscitation (CPR) training. It was not until the mid-1960s when the first full-body manikin simulator was created called "Sim One" to help teach anesthesiology residents at the University of Southern California. This technology was ahead of its time as manikin-based simulators did not gain momentum until the 1990s (see Figure 12.1). The Institute of Medicine's (1999) landmark report, *To Err is Human: Building a Safer Health System,* emphasized patient safety, establishing momentum for simulation education. Simulators currently used today reflect a mix of manual input, physiological modeling, and state-of-the-art–based modeling (Slone & Lampotang, 2015a, 2015b).

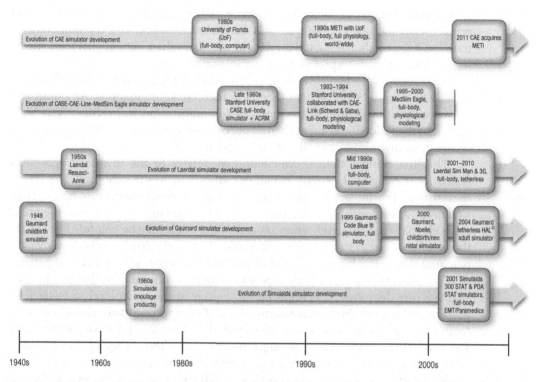

Figure 12.1 Manikin simulator development timeline.

ACRM, Anesthesia Crisis Resource Management; CAE, Canadian Aviation Electronics; CASE, Comprehensive Anesthesia Simulated Environment; METI, Medical Education Technologies Inc.; PDA, personal digital assistant.

Source: Data from Slone, F. L, & Lampotang, S. (2015a). History of modern-day mannequins. In J. C. Palaganas, J. C. Maxworthy, C. A. Epps, & M. E. Mancini (Eds.), *Defining excellence in simulation programs* (pp. 185–190). Wolters Kluwer.

OVERVIEW OF SIMULATION EDUCATION

Framing Theory That Supports Simulation Education

Linking simulation learning experiences with a theoretical foundation with intentionality helps to provide a consistent structure to base curricula. Simulation-based learning is a type of experiential education; therefore, any theory related to how humans learn and acquire expertise could be valid. An organizational model of evaluation should provide theoretical support for quality performance improvement across domains. The Shared Mental Model (Mathieu et al., 2000), also known as the team mental model, has been used as a basic framework to assess the impact on attitudes and behaviors toward communication and collaboration in complex environments. The model is underpinned by the process of *macrocognition*, which is defined as "the internalized and externalized high-level mental processes employed by teams to create new knowledge during complex, one-of-a-kind collaborative problem-solving" (Letksy, 2008).

The shared mental model inputs include information such as a description of the problem, team member expertise, organizational structure, roles and responsibilities of team members, and projected events and future information. These inputs are identified during team formation. This input leads to four distinct but nonsequential stages of collaboration: knowledge construction, collaborative team problem-solving, team consensus, and outcome evaluation and revision. When a team has a strong shared mental model, the members share similar characteristics in regard to how they interpret and process information (Gardner et al., 2017).

It is important when designing and implementing simulation experiences to directly tie a model with content themes to theoretical foundations. An example of themes surrounding health care provider communication and teamwork is highlighted in the following content themes of communication, error, information management, teamworking, and situational awareness.

The first content theme, *communication,* relates to the theory of egocentric heuristics (Chang et al., 2010), which describes how health care providers greatly overestimate the impact of their words during a patient handoff or how a crisis situation was understood or retained by other team members. Therefore, the use of methods that encourage reflection on communication may be helpful. The second theme of *error* relates to agency theory (Gordon et al., 2017). This describes the potential that exists for the shifting of professional responsibility because patients or other providers may not have access to all needed information that can be used to judge care decisions. It is important to engage at the macrolevel to foster joint professional responsibility and teamworking. This approach may also challenge a "shift work" mentality among providers and, therefore, may improve patient safety. The third theme, *information management,* relates to the theory of "coordination costs" (Arora et al., 2008), which describes how macro and meso systems are needed to manage increasingly complex health care organizations and a "bundle care" approach to maintain patient safety. The fourth theme, *teamworking,* can be related to several social science theories concerning the diffusion of responsibility and supports techniques that combat apathy and team self-monitoring (Hautz et al., 2020). The final theme, *situational awareness,* relates to Reason's three-bucket model (Reason, 2004). This model views the risk for error or human performance deficiencies (HPD) in any given situation in terms of three buckets pertaining to the professional, the task, and the environment, respectively. The three-bucket model is very similar to the process improvement approach of identifying what system level (e.g., macro, meso, micro) has been impacted or has failed. By considering the potential for error in each situation, health care providers can use this system to consider the inherent risk of a given situation (Suliburk et al., 2019).

The application of these theoretical elements supports and guides teaching in each of the five exemplar content areas, as well as deepening understanding that may lead to further theoretical developments in this area, as is depicted in Figure 12.2.

Simulation-Based Education Characteristics of Best Practice

It is well documented that SBE promotes participant/learner acquisition and maintenance of cognitive knowledge, behaviors, and skills leading to increased competence (McGaghie et al., 2011). Simulation participants enthusiastically endorse learning using simulation technology. Issenberg and McGaghie (2013) identified 12 characteristics of simulation that have become evident from research and practice (see Box 12.1). Historically, immediate feedback is the most important and frequently cited characteristic of SBE to promote effective learning. Five of these unique characteristics will be highlighted because they pertain to learning and

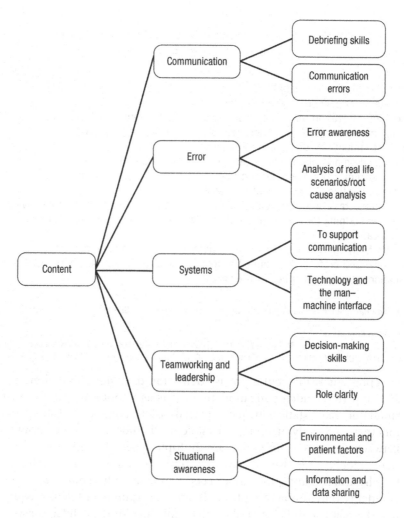

Figure 12.2 Application of theory in simulation.

Source: Gordon, M., Darbyshire, D., & Baker, P. (2012). Non-technical skills training to enhance patient safety: A systematic review. *Medical Education, 46*(11), 1042–1054. https://doi.org/10.1111/j.1365-2923.2012.04343.x. Reprinted with permission.

evaluation and include feedback, fidelity, experiential learning, deliberate practice, and reflective practice.

Immediate *feedback* in the form of debriefing post simulation is an extremely valuable tool that seeks to highlight the rationale behind participant/learner actions using a structured or semistructured discussion between participants and a facilitator (Morrison & Deckers, 2015, p. 500). Participants express their feelings about the simulated experience and their performance and receive feedback from facilitators and peers. Quality debriefing and debriefing with good judgment have been shown to promote insight, improve learner performance, and slow decay in skills over time (Issenberg & McGaghie, 2013).

Fidelity, by definition, refers to the degree to which an electronic device accurately reproduces its effect (Merriam-Webster, 2020). Simulation uses the term fidelity to describe the degree to which a simulator accurately reproduces its effect

---

BOX 12.1 Twelve Characteristics and Best Practices for Simulation-Based Education

1. Feedback (core characteristic)
2. Deliberate practice (core characteristic)
3. Curriculum integration (enhances learning and complements curricula)
4. Outcome measurement (yields more reliable data, validating actions)
5. Appropriate fidelity for curricula (core characteristic)
6. Skill acquisition and maintenance (enhances aptitude and readiness)
7. Mastery learning (core characteristic from deliberate and reflective practice)
8. Transfer to practice (T1 of translational science[a])
9. Team training (task and team-related skills practiced in a consequence-free environment)
10. High-stakes training (emerging research validates using simulation for reproducibility and standardization)
11. Instructor training (SBE is not easy, and instructors learn through real-time experience)
12. Educational and professional context (effective use of SBE requires more research and publication into best practices as it evolves)

---

[a]T1 refers to translational science applied to health care educational research. See information later in this chapter.

SBE, simulation-based education.
Source: McGaghie, W. C., Issenberg, S. B., Petrusa, E. R, & Scalese, R. J., (2010). A critical review of simulation-based medical education research: 2003–2009. *Medical Educator, 44*, 50–63. https://doi.org/10.1111/j.1365-2923.2009.03547.x

or represents reality, but a precise definition does not exist (Slone & Lampotang, 2015a, p 184). Fidelity in simulation exists as a continuum from low-fidelity–type simulators (e.g., static body parts, partial-task trainers) to high-fidelity–type simulators (e.g., full-body manikins, physiologically modeled, and computer-controlled). Between these two end points are multiple types of manikins with variable functions. Fidelity can also be viewed in three distinct dimensions that often overlap: (a) physical fidelity (physical aspects of human body replicated), (b) environmental fidelity (environment replicated), and (c) equipment fidelity (equipment works like the real thing; Paige et al., 2018). All three of these fidelity aspects can affect how deeply immersed the participant is in the simulated experience (Slone & Lampotang, 2015a, 2015b). For example, a simulated scenario using only a patient's vital signs on a monitor with only verbal interaction might be low fidelity in relation to realism or conceptual aspects, depending on how deep the participant is immersed into the simulated experience. On the other hand, a full-manikin scenario in a mock operating room might be high-fidelity in the technology aspect, but if the scenario lacks realism and is poorly designed, then it might reflect low fidelity in the conceptual aspect. All types of fidelity are important to simulation and learning (Kim et al., 2016). Fidelity (technical and conceptual) must be accurately matched to learning outcomes.

Experiential learning is another foundational characteristic of simulation. Simulation creates an immersive, engaging, active learning environment where participants can make mistakes without fear of reproach (Ackermann et al., 2009). Simulation participants/learners are able to practice various psychomotor and cognitive skills, transfer these skills into the clinical setting, and enhance patient care (Jeffries et al., 2012). Experiential learning has been reported to improve with the degree of simulated reality. The experiential nature of simulation is complex, interactive, and a true social experience (Dieckman et al., 2007). Therefore, as part of the social practice of simulation, participants/learners are asked to "suspend disbelief" as part of experiential learning in simulated curricula, creating a "fiction contract." These two phrases, coined by Dieckman et al. (2007), provide the learner with an acknowledgment that simulation is not exactly real life but an attempt to make sure the simulation setting is as true to real experience as possible. As a result of this fiction contract and experiential learning, participant stress is often reported (Ghazali et al., 2019). Stress during simulation should not inhibit the participants' ability to learn and grow from the experience (INACSL Standards Committee, 2016b). Participants should be educated and aware that this is a normal part of the simulated experience and that this is a safe learning environment.

Kolb's theory of experiential learning (2015) is often used to provide theoretical justification for the legitimacy of using simulation in educational curricula (Diehl, 2016; Kolb, 2015). Kolb's perspective combines one's experience, perception, cognition, and behavior as a continuous process (Figure 12.3). Experiential learning, as exemplified in Kolb's theory, also cites an explicit need for reflection, another inherent characteristic of simulation, which is generally accomplished through debriefing.

Deliberate practice is another foundational and powerful characteristic at the heart of simulation, where the learner, as an active participant, is engaged in repetitive performance of psychomotor or cognitive skills in a focused domain (simulated experiences) specifically designed to improve performance (Ericsson & Harwell, 2019). Informative feedback in this setting can result in increasingly better skills performance. The settings are safe and nonthreatening, allowing the anxiety of the learner to be reduced so that confidence can grow (Dieckman et al., 2007). Deliberate practice has been shown to be one of the more effective combinations of coaching and practice. See Box 12.2 for further information on features of deliberate practice (reprinted from McGaghie et al., 2010).

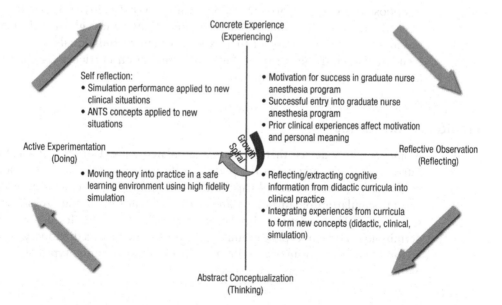

Figure 12.3 Application of Kolb's theory in simulation education.

Source: Data from Kolb, D. A. (2015). *Experiential learning experience as the source of learning and development* (2nd ed.). Pearson Education.

BOX 12.2   Nine Features of Deliberate Practice

1. Highly motivated learners/participants
2. Well-defined learning objectives/tasks
3. Appropriate level of difficulty for the learner
4. Focused, repetitive practice
5. Meaningful, reliable measurements
6. Informative feedback from facilitators, faculty, simulator
7. Feedback that promotes error correction, improved self-monitoring/
   awareness
8. Performance standard improvement reaching mastery
9. Advancement to next level/task unit

Source: McGaghie, W. C., Issenberg, S. B., Petrusa, E. R, & Scalese, R. J., (2010). A critical review of simulation-based medical education research: 2003–2009. *Medical Educator,* 44(1), 50–63. https://doi.org/10.1111/j.1365-2923.2009.03547.x

Reflective practice is an integral part of the simulation experience and has been cited as the most important part (Ruth-Sahd, 2003). Every simulated experience is a concrete experience that offers an opportunity for reflection as a means of self-examination (Morrison & Deckers, 2015, p. 500). The point is to review the simulation and possibly connect it to past practice with the intent of improving future practice and self-understanding (Ruth-Sahd, 2003). Postsimulation activities such as self-reflection and debriefing embody methods of reflective practice. Giving participants/learners time to self-reflect and/or provide debriefing techniques can improve participant/learner future performance and confidence. Several studies examining accuracy of self-reflection demonstrated that higher performing participants in simulated clinical scenarios more accurately rated their own performance as opposed to poor performers' self-evaluations (Diehl, 2016). Reflective practice research supports the concept that accurate self-awareness gleaned through practice and systematic analysis of that experience allows individuals to monitor their own progress and can easily be built into simulation curricula (Issenberg, 2006; Morrison & Deckers, 2015, p. 500).

Simulation Modalities

A *simulator* is a device that presents a simulated patient or part of a patient and interacts with the actions of the participant/learner (Gaba, 2007). Simulators currently have a wide variety of capabilities and applicable situations in health care. Several simulation organizations are working toward clarifying cross-disciplinary taxonomies. The Society of Simulation in Healthcare (2012) formed a Simulation Terminology and Concepts Committee in an effort to create a dictionary. A copy can be found on the website www.ssih.org. A list of most common types of simulation, with examples, is presented in Table 12.1.

TABLE 12.1 Most Common Types of Simulation Modalities

Simulation Modality	Description	Examples
Augmented reality	A type of virtual reality in which equipment with synthetic/virtual is superimposed/used with real-world objects (Bauman, 2010)	• Stethoscope with virtual/simulated heart sounds is used with a standardized patient
Boot camps	Intense course to expose an individual to a cadre of procedural skills, algorithms for diagnosis and management, along with integration of behavioral skills, communication, leadership (Hales & Tuttle, 2015; Kubin & Fogg, 2010)	• Anesthesia update (new equipment, scenarios, new protocols, nontechnical skills) • Pediatric critical care (airway management stations, new equipment, central lines, scenarios)
Embedded simulation persons (ESP). Also known as confederates, actors, scenario guides, simulation actors, simulated persons, standardized participants	Live individual who was coached to interact with simulation learners/participants to help improve the affective fidelity component of simulation (Dieckman et al., 2007; Sanko et al., 2015; Walker & Weidner, 2010).	• Health care team members (surgeon, circulating nurse, nurse's aide) • Family members • Difficult health care situations • Difficult people
In situ	Simulation that takes place in an actual clinical area where participants would normally function (Couto et al., 2015; Lockman et al., 2015; Owei et al., 2017)	• Cardiac arrest team training • New equipment • New clinical protocols or refreshers
Interprofessional education (IPE)	Multiprofessional exercise/often using simulated environments where various providers (two or more professions) are learning side by side to improve collaboration and quality of care (Hammick et al., 2008; INACSL Standards Committee, 2016c; Palaganas & Rock, 2015)	• Modules focused on involvement from a range of professional groups (e.g., diabetes, stroke, trauma) • Advanced cardiac life support with different provider roles and stations
Hybrid simulation	Using one type of simulation to enhance another, ultimately using more than one simulation modality, often includes a manikin and SP (Issenberg et al., 2004; Schocken & Gammon, 2015; Kneebone, 2005)	• Live preoperative SP with a mannequin for intraoperative phase of scenario
Just-in-time training	Simulation training conducted just prior to a potential intervention (Monachino & Tuttle, 2015)	• Low-volume, high-risk skills (e.g., CPR, endotracheal intubation, or central venous catheter dressing changes)

(continued)

TABLE 12.1 Most Common Types of Simulation Modalities (*continued*)

Simulation Modality	Description	Examples
Manikin-based (full-body with a variety of fidelity options). Often referred to as high-fidelity simulation (HFS; Issenberg, 2006)	Computer-controlled, programmable to create a patient case/scenario/situation with physiological modeling incorporated (e.g., heart sounds, breath sounds, pulses) (McGaghie et al., 2010; Slone & Lampotang, 2015a, 2015b).	• Patient-focused clinical scenarios (low to high fidelity) • Basic patient assessment (listening to breath and heart sounds)—low fidelity • General anesthesia induction sequence (practice before entering clinical environment) • Acute hypotension in an emergency department patient • Intraoperative airway fire with entire operative team • High-risk, low-exposure scenarios for students or experienced clinicians
Mixed-reality humans (MRH)	Combines a manikin or partial-task trainer with a virtual reality experience (Hwang et al., 2009)	• Affective skills and team training (manikin + virtual team members on screen) • Central line training (partial-task trainer + screen to show more detailed anatomy)
Objective Structured Clinical Examination (OSCE)	Simulated stations that are carefully structured to assess performance competency prior to patient care (Heine & Ferguson, 2015)	• Assessment skills • Procedural skills
Procedural simulation (often utilizes a partial-task trainer to statically reproduce anatomic regions) (Issenberg & Scalese, 2008)	Teaches technical skills and knowledge related to clinical procedures incorporating immediate feedback/debriefing (Arora et al., 2011; Hashimoto & Phitayakorn, 2015)	• Peripheral nerve block practice • Intubation • Neuraxial block practice • Central line insertion
Standardized patients (SPs)	Live individuals coached to portray a patient with a specific condition or act a certain way. (Bokken, 2009; Ericsson et al., 1993; Lowens & Gliva-McConvey, 2015). SPs can also be used with other simulation modalities such as partial-task trainers and manikins (Kneebone, 2005)	• Physical interview/assessments • Preoperative assessment
Team-based	Simulated teaching approach using small groups often multi-disciplinary (Michaelson & Manning, 2008)	• Cardiac arrest • ACLS • Acute complex situations

(continued)

TABLE 12.1 Most Common Types of Simulation Modalities (*continued*)

Simulation Modality	Description	Examples
Virtual reality	Computer-based simulation applications conducted in a virtual reality environment (Bauman & Ralston-Berg, 2015)	• Virtual anatomy programs where a cadaver is not available • Situations that would allow only a few students to experience

SIMULATION AND EVALUATION

Evaluation using simulation can take many shapes depending on the purpose of simulation education, intended learning outcomes, and simulation modality used. It is important to remember that *evaluation* is a "systematic process, purposeful, and planned" (Palaganas & Rock, 2015). Evaluation seeks to expand the evaluator's knowledge so that informed decisions can be made and can open the door to a greater understanding of what is already known and the impact of simulation on a larger community.

Creating an Evaluation Plan: Considerations

The process of curriculum development leading to evaluation begins with an idea, rationale, or curricular need. Often a formal needs assessment is structured and sent out to stakeholders and can be helpful to allow buy-in for the planned simulation curriculum. Learning objectives and outcomes need to be constructed as well as an implementation timeline. Specific simulation curricular development and design (e.g., scenarios, skill planning) is performed at this point and often takes the most time to stage the details depending on the fidelity of the simulation event. Once completed, a pilot or test run of the planned simulated curriculum is performed. This approach is akin to the Plan–Do–Study–Act (PDSA) cycle. Any glitches should be corrected and tweaked prior to going "live" with the simulated curriculum (Palaganas & Rock, 2015).

Evaluation and feedback close the loop in the curriculum development cycle, helping developers to identify whether the goals and objectives were met (Kolb, 2015). This evaluation process must be built from the beginning of the curricular development timeline. Ideally, the individual who will design the evaluation, collect the data, perform the analysis, and generate the report will be on the development team. Evaluation data can be collected from various sources, including the participants/learners, faculty, and other facilitators. This information can be used to report back to educational stakeholders. A written report can be helpful and presented to the administration and other parties that have remote involvement/interest in the simulation curriculum.

Educational Evaluation and Policy Implications

As with organizational models, educational evaluation models should guide the quality improvement process. Examples of educational program evaluation models include Kirkpatrick's approach, the Logic Model, and the Context/Input/Process/

Product (CIPP; Frye & Hemmer, 2012). (A more detailed Kirkpatrick discussion can be found under Program Evaluation.) The effectiveness of a simulation program, as with all educational modalities, depends greatly on how well it is planned and executed. Any simulation program must have a policy for quality improvement and a plan for a systematic quality/performance improvement process that is not limited to assessment of learner outcomes and achievement and course evaluation by course participants (Johnson & Auguston, 2015). It is helpful to have a written plan that explains the evaluation process and strategy (Jeffries & Battin, 2012). The first step is to create a statement of purpose and evaluation philosophy. Think about why you are gathering information, what the objectives are, and whom the data will be gathered for. Who will be responsible for writing, updating, and approving the evaluation plan? Is it one individual or a small group that can be held accountable for planning, implementing, and evaluating? This individual or group should have buy-in and be able to obtain support from leaders at every level of the organization. It is helpful to examine the relationship between those accountable and the larger organizational structure. How will the relationship between the simulation team and the larger organization develop, and who will be responsible for team building and meeting program benchmarks?

What time frame will this written evaluation plan span, decisions to utilize formative and/or summative evaluation, and how frequently will data be evaluated? A typical time frame is 1 to 2 years for a comprehensive cycle to evaluate all aspects of a simulation program. What categories or dimensions will be measured (Person 2013)? Like an evaluation plan, any systematic evaluation plan should be linked to organizational/departmental mission and vision. The organizational mission and vision should be integrated into the simulation program's evaluation plan so that simulation evaluation priorities are considered to be as important as other organizational priorities.

If just starting an evaluation plan, start small. A balanced scorecard is a simplistic method to identify categories when an evaluator is overwhelmed or unsure about where to begin an evaluation plan. A balanced scorecard examines four perspectives in an organization: (a) customer, (b) learning and growth, (c) financial, and (d) internal business process perspective. This is an excellent strategy because of its simplicity (Kaplan & Norton, 1996).

Once evaluation categories have been identified, specific measures need to be examined. One to three measures should be chosen for each category. There may be many items/processes a program wants to evaluate, monitor, or understand for purposes for improvement. Therefore, prioritization is important. Definitions of what is measured or performance indicators provide clarity and consistency (Lloyd, 2008, p. 92). It may be helpful to create a flowchart or overview with a timeline and frequency of evaluation at all levels.

Once simulated curricula have been designed, a pilot study or a "dry run" with all parties involved is recommended to see if it works as intended. If the simulated events are summative in nature, then focusing on consistency and internal validity is extremely important (Palaganas & Rock, 2015).

Collected data need to be analyzed in order to be meaningful. Data analysis can be divided into two categories: tools that analyze measurement and tools that identify root causes and design improvements; see Table 12.2 (Jordan et al., 2001). Finally, the analyzed data need to be interpreted, communicated, and disseminated. This can be done verbally in a narrative format with tables and graphs or in some combination (Russ-Eft & Preskill, 2001).

TABLE 12.2 Data Analysis Tools	
Measurement Data Analysis	**Root Causes and Design Improvements**
• Run chart • Statistical analysis • Control chart/statistical process control • Matrices, contingency tables • Flowcharts • Decision trees, historical timelines • Scatter plots of relationships between variables	• Affinity diagram • Brainstorming • Cause and effect/fishbone diagram • Failure mode and effect analysis • Histogram • Pareto analysis • Storyboarding • Gap analysis

Source: Jordan, G., Prevette, S., & Woodward, S. (2001). Analyzing, reviewing, and reporting performance data. In Training Resources & Data Exchange Performance-Based Management Special Interest Group (Eds.), *The performance-based management handbook* (Vol. 5, pp. 1–76). Oak Ridge Institute for Science and Education.

Implementing a Simulation Program Evaluation

Evaluating a simulation program allows leadership, staff, and other stakeholders to examine the success, worth, and potential areas for improvement. All simulation programs should be continuously evolving and incorporating evaluation information to justify actions. For example, properly executed program evaluations can gain support for program enhancements, updating curricular content, improving technical assistance, and simulation accreditation (Ball, 2017; Johnson & Auguston, 2015). Evaluations should be solicited not only from learners, but also from faculty, staff, and other stakeholders, as deemed necessary. Specific types of information evaluated may vary, but some common characteristics of simulation program evaluation exist (see Exhibit 12.1).

Kirkpatrick's four-level evaluation model is commonly used as an evaluation framework in SBE and can be applied to both participants and programs. Level 1 examines "reaction" to the learning activity. For example, how well did the participants like the simulation, room, food, facilitators, and so forth? Level 1 data are easy to obtain by simply employing a postsimulation evaluation. Level 2 examines "learning" by asking information about how knowledge/skill improved as a result of the simulation activity. Examples include using a pretest/posttest design or direct observation, self-assessment. However, just because a participant perceives that their knowledge has increased does not necessarily yield application of what they have learned. Level 3 examines "behavior" by addressing transfer of knowledge/skills/behaviors into their practice; for example, the observation of nursing students applying simulation lab content into their clinical rotations. The clinical educators completed a brief survey related to student observations. Other performance measures can be assessed, as well as utilizing self-assessment surveys. Level 4 "results" examine the impact of the educational experience on the organization (e.g., significant clinical outcomes, improved exam scores). Often, these types of data are more difficult and complex to obtain and are not available for 6 or more months after completion of the educational program (Johnson & Auguston, 2015). See also Chapter 3.

The most important step in planning an evaluation is to identify for whom the information is intended. For example, an evaluation intended for the dean will look very different than one intended for program faculty or designers. Once

---

Exhibit 12.1

How to Evaluate a Simulation-Based Educational Program

Getting started

- Find out who will be reading the evaluation. Know your audience.
- What information would be meaningful?
- Talk to other stakeholders.
- What is the overall evaluation approach (e.g., objectives, processes, participants, or combination)?

General evaluation content

- Nature of simulation topic/content. (Did it evolve from a needs assessment? Delphi process? Faculty request? Student request?)
- What was the intended purpose of the simulated activity: (a) education, (b) training, (c) performance assessment, (d) clinical rehearsal, and (e) research?
- Did the program meet the learning outcomes designed? Were there measurable objectives?
- Did the type of simulation equipment meet the needs of the program? Technical difficulties?
- Was there a prebrief for participants/learners, faculty, staff?
- Was there a debrief or feedback session for participants/learners, faculty, staff?
- Simulation space/environment?
- What simulation pilot testing was performed before going live?
- Did the assessment tools used meet the needs of the program? Validity testing?
- Did the students receive appropriate standardized experience? Reliability testing?
- How did the simulation program run live? Smoothly? Any glitches?
- Were there enough support staff/faculty to meet the needs of the program?
- What was the perceived learners'/participants' experience? (observational) from faculty/administrators? What were the results of participant program evaluations?
- What aspects were positive and also in need of improvement?

Future needs directions

- What areas of improvement would enhance the program? Resource optimization?
- Areas of potential research or academic scholarship that could be disseminated

Source: Cook, D. A. (2010). Twelve tips for evaluating educational programs. *Medical Teacher, 32*(4), 296–301. https://doi: .org/10.3109/01421590903480121; Gaba, D. M. (2007). The future vision of simulation in healthcare. *Simulation in Healthcare, 2*, 126–135. https://doi:.org/10.1097/01.SIH.0000258411.38212.32; Kardong-Edgren, S. E., Boese, T., & Howard, V. M. (2015). The INACSL standards of best practice. *Defining Excellence in Simulation Programs*, 17–24.

---

the intended audience has been established, the next step is to ask what would be meaningful evaluation information to the audience. The answers to these first two questions influence everything that follows (Cook, 2010). Different program data collected will be more or less valuable in different situations. Seek out how the evaluation information will be used (e.g., program effectiveness, areas for improvement, optimizing resource allocation). Also, is this a formative or summative evaluation? Summative evaluations typically come at the end or near the end of a program or course (a single time point), whereas formative feedback tends to be ongoing (at intervals; Cook, 2010).

It is important, at this point, to distinguish between program evaluation and assessment. A *program evaluation* focuses on programs as opposed to an *assessment*, which focuses on learners. Learners are assessed to determine how well the learner is doing, and programs are evaluated to determine merit or worth (Wilkes & Bligh,

1999). Next, it is important to obtain input from stakeholders who will be using the data (e.g., faculty, administration) and those who are providing the data (e.g., participants, students). Consider one of three approaches or combine them, depending on the focus of the program evaluation: (a) objectives oriented, (b) process oriented, and (c) participant oriented. The *objectives-oriented* approach is probably the best known. Examine defined goals/objectives of the simulation program and determine whether they have been met. Using only this approach can promote tunnel vision and may miss capturing developments that arose unexpectedly and many other important issues.

In the *process-oriented approach,* a variety of data is collected at the very inception of the idea for the simulation educational program and tends to be comprehensive in nature. A limitation is that data may be missing or not collected, and data collection can become resource intensive. This approach also requires foresight. Once a program is underway, it is often too late to go back and collect or examine data.

A *participant-oriented approach* seeks to determine how the people involved perceived the program and typically employs their written or verbal evaluations at the time of the program or shortly thereafter. Triangulation or the inclusion of multiple perspectives is key, especially when trying to capture data from a large program. The evaluator should examine input from not only learners/participants but also faculty and staff.

The final area to include in an evaluation is recommendations for improvement or programmatic needs that would facilitate improvement. Information can originate from those directly involved in the simulation program (e.g., participants, learners, faculty, staff) or other stakeholders as well as from the evaluation itself. These areas for improvements should be written and tracked so that simulation-based educational programs can grow and evolve using meaningful data and organized methodology. Areas of potential research or other academic scholarship should also be identified related to any simulation-based program. Finally, the evaluator should plan a written evaluation that is shared with all stakeholders, whether it includes a formal or informal verbal presentation or not (Palaganas & Rock, 2015).

Evaluation of Simulation Facilitators and Educators

Regular and timely evaluations of educators will help a program maintain and improve quality. Qualified faculty/facilitators should undergo systematic training (Feldman et al., 2012). How this training should occur is beyond the scope of this chapter; however, evaluation from program staff can gain information about operational and logistical support and is foundational for successful simulation programming. Feedback from staff (if applicable) should be conducted at regular intervals (e.g., written, verbal, group meeting). Feedback should address program support, technical challenges, and needs for future programming. The act of soliciting and potentially implementing staff suggestions also contributes significantly to morale (Palaganas & Rock, 2015).

Evaluations from faculty/facilitators help determine whether necessary support to facilitate curriculum delivery is not only being received but also perceived. Faculty evaluations collect information pertaining to simulation hardware, simulation staff support, challenges, content of simulation curricula, and needs for future simulation curricula. Faculty evaluations can be collected informally at the end of a simulation course by way of a huddle/postbrief. In addition, a formal written evaluation is also circulated quarterly for more concrete evaluation data (Johnson & Auguston, 2015).

Evaluation of Simulation Curricula

Simulation provides extra rigor when evaluating psychomotor, cognitive, and affective domains, essential to nursing practice (Kardong-Edgren et al., 2010). Participant evaluations of any simulation curricula or event should be conducted; however, there is often a lack of validity and reliability in currently available instruments to assess participant perception of SBE effectiveness. One nursing-related participant evaluation of SBE effectiveness has emerged as evidence of an example that has demonstrated validity and reliability and has been reevaluated and updated (Leighton et al., 2015). See Exhibit 12.2 for a summary of prebriefing and debriefing constructs to evaluate nursing simulations.

Exhibit 12.2

Participant Evaluation Items for Simulation-Based Education

Nursing-related participant evaluation items for simulation-based education (use with rating scale: "Do Not Agree, Somewhat Agree, Strongly Agree")

Prebriefing focused

- Prebriefing increased my confidence
- Prebriefing was beneficial to my learning

Learning focused

- I am better prepared to respond to changes in my patient's condition
- I developed a better understanding of the pathophysiology
- I am more confident of my nursing assessment skills
- I felt empowered to make clinical decisions
- I developed a better understanding of medications (leave blank if no medications in scenario)
- I had the opportunity to practice my clinical decision-making skills

Confidence focused

- I am more confident in my ability to prioritize care and interventions
- I am more confident in communicating with my patient
- I am more confident in my ability to teach patients about their illness and interventions
- I am more confident in my ability to report information to the health care team
- I am more confident in providing interventions that foster patient safety
- I am more confident in using evidence-based practice to provide nursing care

Debriefing focused

- Debriefing contributed to my learning
- Debriefing allowed me to verbalize my feelings before focusing on the scenario
- Debriefing was valuable in helping me improve my clinical judgment
- Debriefing provided opportunities to self-reflect on my performance during simulation
- Debriefing was a constructive evaluation of the simulation

Source: Leighton, K., Ravert, P., Mudra, V., & Macintosh, C. (2015). Updating the simulation effectiveness tool: Item modifications and reevaluation of psychometric properties. *Nursing Education Perspectives, 36*(5), 317–323. https://doi.org/10.5480/15-1671

TYPES OF OUTCOME EVALUATION IN SIMULATION

Outcomes-based education has become a focus in health care education with an increasing need to provide evidence that learning has occurred. However, simulation does not always reflect how one will perform in a real clinical situation, even though research does reflect correlation of simulation scores and clinical evaluation of performance (McGaghie et al., 2009; Mudumbai et al., 2012). Participant evaluation can be divided into two different categories: formative and summative. Formative evaluation assesses learning during the teaching process and supports personal and professional growth toward an outcome (e.g., quizzes, question and answer, discussions, debriefing, immediate feedback). *Summative evaluation* assesses learning at the conclusion of specified curriculum and focuses on the outcome or achievement of a specific objective (e.g., final exam, high-stakes testing, pass–fail grading; Palaganas & Rock, 2015; INACSL Standards Committee, 2016c). Rudolph et al. (2008) published the following four-step model of formative assessment: (a) identify performance gaps linked to predetermined objectives, (b) share feedback with the learner describing the gap, (c) explore why the gap exists relative to learner frames and emotions that might contribute to performance level, and (d) assist in closing performance gaps using discussion or targeted instruction about principles and skills relevant to performance (Rudolph et al., 2008).

Summative assessments collect, analyze, and provide feedback data about learners to the organization/decision makers so that a decision can be made on the competence of the learner (Smith & Ragan, 1999). Simulation, as an evaluation methodology, can provide reliable, reproducible data through a consistent testing environment, skill selection, and expected level of expertise (Boulet et al., 2011; Willhaus et al., 2014). Summative assessments should follow predetermined criteria that, if met, demonstrate a level of competence (Palaganas & Rock, 2015). The type of summative assessment must be identified at the start of planning curricula. During the development of summative activities, bias must be addressed. Review the assessment tool development section later in this chapter.

Evidence-Based Assessment Tools in Simulation

Assessment tool development is time-consuming and difficult and should follow a clearly defined scientific process for validity and reliability testing. A plethora of assessment tools already exist. It may therefore be more efficient and evidence-based to use currently available assessment tools with acceptable psychometrics rather than to try to create your own (Kardong-Edgren et al., 2010).

Simulation assessment standards have been elevated far above simply examining participant self-efficacy, self-confidence, or whether simulation provides meaningful learning outcomes. Self-assessment data to assess competency offer little or no reliable indicators and should not be used. No correlation exists between participant/learner self-evaluation and external reviewer evaluation (Diehl, 2016). The value of learning to use simulation with control groups is also not advised as SBE has been well established (Kardong-Edgren et al., 2010).

Assessment Tool Validity and Reliability Testing

Simulation used for assessment must be rigorously structured and evaluated at all levels. Individuals who are developing an assessment tool should match and select the most appropriate and realistic simulation modality with the aim of making an accurate assessment.

Any assessment activity should have validity and reliability testing plans built into tool usage and evolution (Todd et al., 2008). Data generated by assessment activities must be analyzed and appropriately managed confidentially. Review Box 12.3 for a step-by-step simulation assessment tool development guide. The heart of assessment tool development and testing is validity and reliability, discussed in previous chapters. These are also characteristics to keep in mind when choosing assessment tools.

Types of Simulation Assessment Tools

Overall, two types of assessment tools are used in simulation designed to observe learners/participants and rate performance: (a) checklists and (b) global-rating scales. These two types of assessment tools are most often used to assess procedural skills, critical decision-making, team skills, and communication. Assessment tools are typically scored using checklists (e.g., done or not done), weighted checklists, where some items are more critical than others, and rating scales, with each item

---

BOX 12.3   Simulation Development and Assessment Guide: Step by Step

Simulation-Based Education Assessment Tool

Step-by-Step Development Guide
1. What is the topic/skill to be assessed?
2. What are the learning objectives/outcomes of the simulation curriculum?
3. Who are the learners? (professions)
4. What level of learning/specialties are the learners? (i.e., preclinical, pregraduation)
5. Does this type of learning require simulation? Or would it be enhanced using simulation?
6. What are ideal behaviors/performances/expectations? Be specific.
7. What measures would be identified as passing or appropriate for level of education and training?
8. What type of simulation modality best fits to help meet learning objectives/needs of the learners to the potential ideal performance goal? Is facilitator adhering to Standards of Best Practice in Simulation? (https://www.inacsl.org/inacsl-standards-of-best-practice-simulation/)
9. Perform a structured literature search using large databases to locate an assessment tool that may have already been developed for the specific curricular need.
10. If an existing tool is located, what aspects of this assessment need to be revised? Does this change validity/reliability of tool? If so, then ongoing reevaluation of this revised tool will need to be performed to ensure progress toward validity/reliability.
11. Invite stakeholders to review adjusted assessment tool prior to going live with the tool.
12. Assessors should be adequately trained on using any chosen assessment tool to establish a level of interrater reliability.
13. Conduct postusage assessment tool evaluation from faculty or raters.
14. Finalize tool revision and reutilize repeating these steps to enhance validity/reliability.

Source: INACSL Standards Committee. (2016, December). INACSL standards of best practice: SimulationSM debriefing. *Clinical Simulation in Nursing, 12*(S), S21–S25. https://doi.org/10.1016/j.ecns.2016.09.008; McGaghie, W. C., Issenberg, S. B., Petrusa, E. R, & Scalese, R. J., (2010). A critical review of simulation-based medical education research: 2003–2009. *Medical Educator, 44,* 50–63. https://doi.org/10.1111/j.1365-2923.2009.03547.x; Todd, M., Manz, J., Hawkins, K., Parsons, M., & Hercinger, M. (2008). The development of a quantitative evaluation tool for simulation in nursing education. *International Journal of Nursing Education Scholarship, 5*(1), Article 41.1–17. https://doi.org/10.2202/1548-923x.1705.

assigned points on a scale (Palaganas & Rock 2015). *Checklist items* are statements or questions that reflect observable behaviors structured into a list that could be identified as done or not done. (See example of a checklist in Table 12.3.)

There is another version of a checklist in which the behaviors/skills are weighted as more important for success than others. This often requires input from stakeholders in deciding what items are of key importance. A Delphi process, where several rounds of expert input are conducted, can help distill these items to an optimal set of 20 or fewer (Leighton et al., 2015; Todd et al., 2008). Weighted checklists have also been found to discriminate between low- and high-ability performance (Murray et al., 2002). Another type of checklist can have "yes," "no," and a column for possible "partial accomplishment"; for example, if a student is prompted or asked a question or given a hint (Kim et al., 2016).

Global-rating scales are used to rate how well performance was during a static procedure or actions in a static/simulated setting (e.g., how well the learner assessed the patient for hypotension). These types of scales can be useful for standardized patients, hybrid simulations, and manikin-based simulation. There is a spectrum of response options or numerical points (e.g., a Likert scale). Some global-rating scales have an end point of a certain total score or certain critical behaviors that need to be observed in order to meet criteria/learning outcomes (Iramaneerat et al., 2009). A global-rating scale can have an overall pass/fail as an evaluation measure at the conclusion of the evaluation. Another option is to have a certain level on the Likert scale serve as the passing threshold. For example, if a 5-point scale is

TABLE 12.3   Example of a Checklist Assessment Tool

Intravenous Catheter (IV) Insertion in Awake Patient

Checklist Item	Performed Correctly	Not Performed/Performed Incorrectly
Explains procedure to patient and allows for questions	1	0
Selects appropriate equipment	1	0
Primes appropriate IV fluid	1	0
Inspects patient for potential placement sites	1	0
Prepares skin with alcohol	1	0
Verbally prepares patient for skin penetration	1	0
Inserts IV catheter successfully into intended vein	1	0
Applies dressing appropriately	1	0
Minimal passing score is 6/8. Total score:		
Comments		

Source: Palaganaos, J. C., & Rock, L. K. (2015). Simulation-enhanced interprofessional education: A framework for development. In J. C. Palaganas, J. C. Maxworthy, C. A. Epps, & M. E. Mancini (Eds.), *Defining excellence in simulation programs.* Wolters Kluwer.

used, then passing (meeting expectations) would occur at a score of 3 or 4. It truly depends on the learning outcomes and level of learner as to what performance is expected (Kneebone, 2005).

When choosing a rating scale, decide what type of behaviors or skills are being evaluated. Most global-rating scales use a Likert-type scale with 5 rating levels. These levels can be behaviorally descriptive or use the spectrum of agree to disagreement with the observed behavior or skill (Kneebone, 2005; Palaganas & Rock, 2015). One of the most difficult situations to evaluate are emergencies, crisis-simulated scenarios, and nontechnical skills, including crisis resource management skills and behaviors. These are dynamic, rapidly changing, and time-dependent manikin-based, team-oriented interactions. It is difficult to have a single best action, so a globalrating scale is useful (see example in Exhibit 12.3).

ALIGNING SIMULATION RESOURCES WITH LEADERSHIP GOALS

Historically, the roles of nurse leaders have been focused primarily on initiatives to improve quality and patient safety, reduce costs, and develop a strong clinical leadership team. In our ever-changing health care environment, nursing leaders are now considered operational and strategic thought leaders. This renewed focus aligns with the Institute for Healthcare Improvement's quadruple aim, which focuses on improving patient care and population health, reducing cost, and developing a more resilient workforce (Bowles et al., 2019). Nurse leaders today bring these aims forward with the implementation of various professional development opportunities

Exhibit 12.3

Example of Global Rating Scale

Anesthesia Crisis Resource Management (ACRM) Behaviors Global Rating Scale					
	1	2	3	4	5
Acquisition of available information					
Calls for help appropriately					
Reevaluates situation					
Utilizes resources effectively					
Communicates problem clearly					
Manages conflict (if required)					
Overall performance	1	2	3	4	5

Source: Murray, D., Boulet, J., Ziv, A., Woodhouse, J., Kras, J., & McAllister, J. (2002). An acute care skills evaluation for graduating medical students: A pilot study using clinical simulation. *Medical Education, 36*(9), 833–841. https://doi.org/10.1046/j.1365-2923.2002.01290.x

for the nursing workforce, which include investing in simulation education to improve productivity and increase teamwork standardization.

Historically, it has been a challenge to measure the impact of simulation from an institutional leadership viewpoint. The nurse leader must appreciate the importance of simulation education and team training to continue to meet the needs of a dynamic health care setting and a changing nursing workforce. A group of nationally known simulation leaders convened a summit in 2018 and 2019 to discuss current and future trends in simulation (Bryant et al., 2020). The outcomes of the summit suggested that it was time to move beyond knowledge acquisition to long-term retention of knowledge and transfer of learning in a clinical setting while linking to patient safety outcomes.

Nursing leaders will need to work closely with simulation experts to gain a shared mental model and vision of what outcomes are to be achieved and how they will align with the organization's strategic mission and vision. Additionally, nursing leaders will need to continue to invoke the following leadership principles in establishing a simulation program: (a) realize the risk and the reward, (b) remain relevant, (c) trust the team, (d) have grit, and (e) start somewhere. Although these "leadership pearls" are demonstrated in many aspects of health care leadership, they are especially important when direct patient outcomes that are difficult to measure are the focus as they relate to simulation. It is imperative that nursing leadership understand simulation pedagogy, underpinning theory, and be able to articulate the value to others on the leadership team.

TRANSLATIONAL SCIENCE APPLIED TO SIMULATION EDUCATION

Translational research, as it applies to simulation education, has traditionally not been applicable because it is not defined as a biomedical or basic science. Dougherty and Conway (2008) identified three phases in which translational science progressed from bench to bedside. McGaghie et al. (2010) applied these phases to medical education research and then to simulation-based medical education research (McGaghie et al., 2011; see Table 12.4).

The first translational step in this process (T1) moves basic laboratory discoveries to clinical research and knowledge. The second step (T2) translates clinical knowledge obtained from research into more effectiveness at the patient-care level. The third step (T3) focuses on health care delivery benefits at the patient-care level and translates this into public and policy makers improving societal health (Dougherty & Conway, 2008; McGaghie et al., 2010). Simulation education research has reached the T1 translational research level when results demonstrate learner skill and knowledge improvement in simulation laboratory settings. The T2 level has been reached when measurable improvements in clinical knowledge, skill, and behaviors are used in patient-care settings (e.g., basic life support [BLS], advanced cardiac life support [ACLS]). The T3 level has been reached when measured improvement in the population health from simulation education and training is noted (McGaghie et al., 2010, 2011). For example, enhanced recovery after surgery (ERAS) protocols are in place. Currently simulated nursing education and continuing education utilize this translational science framework at the T1 level (Adamson et al., 2013).

TABLE 12.4 Translational Science Application in Simulation Education Research

	T1	T2	T3
Translational Science Phase Related to Simulation	Use the simulation laboratory to study cognitive, psychomotor, and affective behavior and skills in individuals and teams applicable to clinical environment. Monitor educational progress before application to clinical setting. (Example: Practice of cardiopulmonary resuscitation using simulated scenarios in the laboratory and then applying them in a real code situation.)	Transfer cognitive, psychomotor, affective skills in individual and teams into the clinical environment as potential patient-care practices. (Example: Effective CPR practices and improved patient outcomes prompt national organizations to standardize practice nationwide.)	Transfer patient practice outcomes learned to public as protocols and established practices. (Example: A local hospital requires all nurses employed to comply with American Heart Association standards during resuscitation.)

Source: McGaghie, W. C., Issenberg, S. B., Petrusa, E. R், & Scalese, R. J., (2010). A critical review of simulation-based medical education research: 2003–2009. Medical Educator, 44, 50–63. https://doi.org/10.1111/j.1365-2923.2009.03547.x; McGaghie, W. C., Issenberg, S. B., Cohen, E. R., Barsuk, J. H., & Wayne, D. B. (2011). Does simulation-based medical education with deliberate practice yield better results than traditional clinical education? A meta-analytic comparative review of the evidence. *Academic Medicine, 86*, 706–711. https://doi.org/10.1097/acm.0b013e318217e119

McGaghie et al. (2011) identified five translational science challenges and gaps in simulation that may fuel future research: (a) identifying clinical problems where simulation and deliberate practice could be effective, (b) measuring clinical data that would set a benchmark for T3 outcomes in simulation-based research, (c) acknowledging which clinical problems can and cannot be studied beyond the T2 level (e.g., end-of-life care), (d) educating public leaders and society about simulation education and its impact on patient outcomes, and (e) establishing and exercising leadership related to clinical performance competency and the value of simulation in this process to reach T3 goals (McGaghie et al., 2011).

Other areas where simulation has changed and impacted nursing care include applications in telemedicine and telehealth that have merged in their common use of technology and theory application. Locsin (2001) built on Watson's Human Caring Theory to add that technology and caring are harmoniously aligned. The Locsin Theory proposes that technological competency is caring in nursing rather than a modality through which nurses provide care. Although telehealth has been in place for many rural areas of the nation, it is now one of the predominant methods for primary care. Totten et al. (2020) demonstrate the value of the use of telehealth and telepresence technology over the continuum of care in various health care settings.

Although the focus of telemedicine is disease diagnosis and disease curative, telehealth incorporates a holistic approach to health care delivery from a distance for health promotion, prevention, and cure. For example, providers should learn telehealth processes and practices to conduct virtual group education opportunities and use of smartphone applications to deliver community/public health nursing.

SUMMARY

Simulation-based health care education has demonstrated that results achieved through a simulated approach can transfer to improved downstream patient-care practices and improved patient outcomes and address the rising public health needs (McGaghie et al., 2010, 2011). Simulation can transfer not only knowledge, but also behaviors into the clinical setting, decreasing errors and complications leading to improved patient outcomes (Motola et al., 2013). Simulation technologies and telehealth resources will become even more important, as was learned during the 2020–2021 COVID-19 pandemic. Simulation education and practice applications and resources will be critical to educate, train, and provide needed patient care for many years to come.

REFERENCES

Ackermann, A. D., Kenny, G., & Walker, D. (2009). Simulator programs for new nurses' orientation. *Journal for Nurses in Staff Development, 23*(3), 136–139. https://doi.org/10.1097/01 .nnd.0000277183.32582.43

Adamson, K. A., Kardong-Edgren, S., & Willhaus, J. (2013). An updated review of published simulation evaluation instruments. *Clinical Simulation in Nursing, 9*(9), e393–e400. https://doi.org/10.1016/j. ecns.2012.09.004

Alexander, M., Durham, C. F., Hooper, J. I., Jeffries, P., Goldman, N., & Kardong-Edgren, S. (2015). NCSBN simulation guidelines for prelicensure nursing programs. *Journal of Nursing Regulation, 6*, 39–42. https://doi.org/10.1016/S2155-8256(15)30783-3

Anderson, M., & Leflore, J. (2008). Playing it safe: Simulated team training in the OR. *AORN Journal, 87*(4), 772–779. https://doi.org/10.1016/j.aorn.2007.12.027

Ansen, W. (2015). Assessment in healthcare simulation. In J. C. Palaganas, J.C. Maxworthy, C. A. Epps, & M. E. Mancini (Eds.), *Defining excellence in simulation programs* (pp. 509–532). Wolters Kluwer.

Arora, S., Aggarwal, R., Sirimanna, P., Moran, A., Grantcharov, T., Kneebone, R., & Darzi, A. (2011). Mental practice enhances surgical technical skills. *Annals of Surgery, 253*(2), 265–270. https://doi .org/10.1097/sla.0b013e318207a789

Arora, V. M., Johnson, J. K., Meltzer, D. O., & Humphrey, H. J. (2008). A theoretical framework and competency-based approach to improving handoffs. *Quality and Safe in Health Care, 17*(1), 11–14. https://doi.org/10.1136/qshc.2006.018952

Ball, S. (2017) Evaluating educational programs. In R. Bennett, & M. von Davier (Eds.), *Advancing human assessment. Methodology of educational measurement and assessment.* Springer. https://doi. org/10.1007/978-3-319-58689-2_11

Bauman, E. (2010). Virtual reality and game-based clinical education. In K. B. Gaberson & M. H. Oermann (Eds.), *Clinical teaching strategies in nursing education* (3rd ed., pp. 183–212). Springer Publishing Company.

Bauman, E., & Ralson-Berg, P. (2015). Virtual simulation. In J. C. Palaganas, J. C. Maxworthy, C. A. Epps, & M. E. Mancini (Eds.), *Defining excellence in simulation programs* (pp. 241–251). Wolters Kluwer.

Bokken, L. (2009). *Innovated use of simulated patient for educational purposes* (Doctoral dissertation). Datawyse, Maastricht University, Maastricht, Netherlands.

Boulet, J. R., Jeffries, P. R., Hatala, R. A., Korndorffer, J. R., Jr., Feinstein, D. M., & Roche, J. P. (2011). Research regarding methods of assessing learning outcomes. *Simulation in Healthcare, 6*(Suppl.), S48–S51. https://doi.org/10.1097/SIH.0b013e31822237d0

Bowles, J. R., Batcheller, J., Adams, J. M., Zimmermann, D., & Pappas, S. (2019). Nursing's leadership role in advancing professional practice/work environments as part of the quadruple aim. *Nursing Administration Quarterly, 43*(2), 157–163. https://doi.org/10.1097/NAQ.0000000000000342

Bricken, W. (1991). Training in VR. In T. Feldman (Ed.), *Virtual Reality '91: Impacts and applications.* Proceedings of the First Annual Conference on Virtual Reality. London, UK.

Bryant, K., Aebersold, M. L., Jeffries, P. R., & Kardong-Edgren, S. (2020). Innovations in simulation: Nursing leaders' exchange of best practices. *Clinical Simulation in Nursing, 41*, 33–40. https://doi.org/10.1016/j.ecns.2019.09.002

Chang, V. Y., Arora, V. M., Lev-Ari, S., D'Arcy, M., & Keysar, B. (2010). Interns overestimate the effectiveness of their hand-off communication. *Pediatrics, 125*(3), 491–496. https://doi.org/10.1542/peds.2009-0351

Cook, D. A. (2010). Twelve tips for evaluating educational programs, *Medical Teacher, 32*(4), 296–301. https://doi.org/10.3109/01421590903480121

Couto, T. B., Kerrey, B. T., Taylor, R. G., FitzGerald, M., & Geis, G. L. (2015). Teamwork skills in actual, in situ, and incenter pediatric emergencies: performance levels across settings and perceptions of comparative educational impact. *Simulation in Healthcare, 10*, 76–84. https://doi.org/10.1097/sih.0000000000000081

Deutsch, E. S., & Palaganas, J. C. (2015). SSH accreditation standards. In J. C. Palaganas, J. C. Maxworthy, C. A. Epps, & M. E. Mancini (Eds.), *Defining excellence in simulation programs* (pp. 2–7). Wolters Kluwer.

Dieckman, P., Gaba, D., & Rall, M. (2007). Deepening the theoretical foundations of patient simulation as social practice. *Simulation in Healthcare, 2*(3), 183–193. https://doi.org/10.1097/sih.0b013e3180f637f5

Diehl, M. R. (2016). *A novel use of the anesthetists' non-technical skills (ANTS) instrument to measure congruence of graduate nurse anesthesia student self-evaluation and faculty evaluation.* https://twu-ir.tdl.org/handle/11274/8751

Dougherty, D., & Conway, P. H. (2008). The 3Ts road map to transform US health care. *JAMA, 299*(19), 2319–2321. https://doi.org/10.1001/jama.299.19.2319

Ericsson, K. A., & Harwell, K. W. (2019). Deliberate practice and proposed limits on effects of practice on acquisition of expert performance: Why the original definition matters and recommendations for future research. *Frontiers in Psychology, 10*, 2396. https://doi.org/10.3389/fpsyg.2019.02396

Ericsson, K. A., Krampe, R., T., & Tesch-Romer, C. (1993). The role of deliberate practice in the acquisition of expert performance. *Psychological Review, 100*(3), 363–406. https://doi.org/10.1037//0033-295X.100.3.363

Feldman, M., Lazzara, E. H., Vanderbilt, A. A., & DiazGranados, D. (2012). Rater training to support high-stakes simulation-based assessments. *Journal of Continuing Education in the Health Professions, 32*(4), 279–286. https://doi.org/10.1002/chp.21156

Frye, A. W., & Hemmer, P. A. (2012). Program evaluation models and related theories: AMEE guide no. 67. *Medical Teacher, 34*(5), e288–299. https://doi.org/10.3109/0142159X.2012.668637

Gaba, D. M. (2007). The Future vision of simulation in healthcare. The Journal of the Society for Simulation in Healthcare, 2*(2), 126–135. https://doi.org/ 10.1097/01.SIH.0000258411.38212.32

Gardner, A. K., Scott, D. J., & AbdelFattah, K. R. (2017). Do great teams think alike? An examination of team mental models and their impact on team performance. *Surgery, 161*(5), 1203–1208. https://doi.org/10.1016/j.surg.2016.11.010

Ghazali, D. A., Breque, C., Sosner, P., Lesbordes, M., Chavagnat, J. J., Ragot, S., & Oriot, D. (2019). Stress response in the daily lives of simulation repeaters. A randomized controlled trial assessing stress evolution over one year of repetitive immersive simulations. *PLoS One, 14*(7), e0220111. https://doi.org/10.1371/journal.pone.0220111

Gordon, M., Darbyshire, D., & Baker, P. (2012). Non-technical skills training to enhance patient safety: A systematic review. *Medical Education, 46*(11), 1042–1054. https://doi.org/10.1111/j.1365-2923.2012.04343.x

Gordon, M., Fell, C. W., Box, H., Farrell, M., & Stewart, A. (2017). Learning health 'safety' within non-technical skills interprofessional simulation education: a qualitative study. *Medical Education Online, 22*(1), 1272838. https://doi.org/10.1080/10872981.2017.1272838

Hales, R. L., & Tuttle, S. A. (2015) Boot camps. In J. C. Palaganas, J. C. Maxworthy, C. A. Epps, & M. E. Mancini (Eds.), *Defining excellence in simulation programs*. Wolters Kluwer.

Hammick, M., Freeth, D., Koppel, I., Reebes, S., & Barr, H. (2008). A best evidence systemic review of interprofessional education. *Medical Teacher, 29*, 735–751. https://doi.org/10.1080/0142159 0701682576

Hashimoto, D. A, & Phitayakorn, R. (2015). Procedural training. In J. C. Palaganas, J. C. Maxworthy, C. A. Epps, & M. E. Mancini (Eds.), *Defining excellence in simulation programs* (pp. 227–234). Wolters Kluwer.

Hautz, S. C., Oberholzer, D. L., Freytag, J., Exadaktylos, A., Kammer, J. E., Sauter, T. C., & Hautz, W. E. (2020). An observational study of self-monitoring in ad hoc health care teams. *BMC Medical Educator, 20*(1), 201. https://doi.org/10.1186/s12909-020-02115-3

Heine, N., & Ferguson, D. (2015). Management of standardized patient programs. In J. C. Palaganas, J. C. Maxworthy, C. A. Epps, & M. E. Mancini (Eds.), *Defining excellence in simulation programs*. (pp. 391–422) Wolters Kluwer.

Henneman, E. A., & Cunningham, H. (2005). Using clinical simulation to teach patient safety in an acute/critical care nursing course. *Nurse Educator, 30*, 172–177. https://doi .org/10.1097/00006223-200507000-00010

Hwang, Y., Lampotang, S., Gravenstein, N., Luria, I., & Lok, B. (2009). Integrating conversational virtual humans and mannequin patient simulators to present mixed reality clinical training experiences. Proceedings of the 8th IEEE International Symposium in Mixed and Augmented Reality (pp. 197–198). http://ieeexplore.ieee.org/xpls/abs_all.jsp?arnumber=5336466&tag=1

INACSL Standards Committee. (2016a, December). INACSL standards of best practice: SimulationSM simulation design. *Clinical Simulation in Nursing, 12*(S), S26–S29. https://doi.org/10.1016/ j.ecns.2016.09.005

INACSL Standards Committee. (2016b, December). INACSL standards of best practice: SimulationSM participant evaluation. *Clinical Simulation in Nursing, 12*(S), S26–S29. https://doi.org/10.1016/ j.ecns.2016.09.009.

INACSL Standards Committee. (2016c, December). INACSL standards of best practice: SimulationSM simulation-enhanced interprofessional education (sim-IPE). *Clinical Simulation in Nursing, 12*(S), S34–S38. https://doi.org/10.1016/j.ecns.2016.09.011.

Institute of Medicine. (1999). The err is humans: Building a safer health system. National Academy Press.

Iramaneerat, C., Myford, C. M., Yudkowsky, R, & Lowenstein, T. (2009). Evaluating the effectiveness of rating instruments for a communication skills assessment of medical residents. *Advances in Health Sciences Education, 14*, 575–594. https://doi.org/10.1007/s10459-008-9142-2

Issenberg, S. B. (2006). The scope of simulation-based healthcare education. *Simulation in Healthcare, 1*(4), 203–208. https://doi.org/10.1097/01.sih.0000246607.36504.5a

Issenberg, S. B., & McGaghie, W. C. (2013). Looking to the future. In W. C. McGaghie (Ed.), *International best practices for evaluation in the health professions*. Radcliffe Publishing Ltd. National League for Nursing

Issenberg, S. B., McGaghie, W. C., Petrusa, E. R., Gordon, D. L., & Scalese, R. J. (2004). *Features and uses of high-fidelity medical simulations that lead to effective learning: A BEME systematic review (BEME Guide No. 4)*. Association for Medical Education in Europe.

Issenberg, S. B., & Scalese, R. J. (2008). Simulation in health care education. *Perspectives in Biology & Medicine, 51*(1), 31-46. https://doi.org/10.1353/pbm.2008.0004

Jeffries, P. R., & Battin, J. (2012). Developing successful health care education simulation centers: The consortium model. Springer.

Jeffries, P. R., Rodgers, B., & Adamson, K. (2012). NLN Jeffries simulation theory: Brief narrative description. *Nursing Education Perspectives, 36*(5), 292–293. https://doi.org/10.1097/ 00024776-201509000-00004

Johnson, G., & Auguston, J. L. (2015). Writing and implementing a strategic plan. In J. C. Palaganas, J. C. Maxworthy, C. A. Epps, & M. E. Mancini. (Eds.), *Defining excellence in simulation programs* (pp. 364–375). Wolters Kluwer.

Jordan, G., Prevette, S., & Woodward, S. (2001). Analyzing, reviewing, and reporting performance data. In Training Resources & Data Exchange performance-based Management Special Interest Group (Eds.), *The performance-based management handbook* (*Vol. 5*, pp. 1–76). Oak Ridge Institute for Science and Education.

Kaplan, R., & Norton, D. (1996). *The balanced scorecard*. Amazon.com.

Kardong-Edgren, S., Adamson, K., & Fitzgerald, C. (2010). A review of currently published evaluation instruments for human patient simulation. *Clinical Simulation in Nursing, 6*(1), 25–35. https://doi.org/10.1016/j.ecns.2009.08.004

Kim, J., Park, J., & Shin, S. (2016). Effectiveness of simulation-based nursing education depending on fidelity: A meta-analysis. *BMC Medical Education, 16,* 152. https://doi.org/10.1186/s12909-016-0672-7

Kneebone, R. (2005). Evaluating clinical simulations for learning procedural skills: A theory-based approach. *AAMC Academic Medicine Journal of the Association of American Medical Colleges, 80*(6), 549–553. https://doi.org/10.1097/00001888-200506000-00006

Kolb, D. A. (2015). *Experiential learning experience as the source of learning and development* (2nd ed.). Pearson Education.

Kubin, L., & Fogg, N. (2010). Back-to-basics camp: An innovative approach to competency assessment. *Journal of Pediatric Nursing, 25,* 28–32. https://doi.org/10.1016/j.pedn.2008.07.004

Leighton, K., Ravert, P., Mudra, V., & Macintosh, C. (2015). Updating the simulation effectiveness tool: Item modifications and reevaluation of psychometric properties. *Nursing Education Perspectives, 36*(5), 317–323. https://doi.org/10.5480/15-1671

Letksy, M. P. (2008). *Macrocognition in teams: Theories and methodologies.* Ashgate.

Lloyd, R. (2008). Milestones in the quality measurement journey. In E. Ransom, M. Joshi, D. Nash, & S. Ransom (Eds.), *The healthcare quality book* (2nd ed., pp. 87–108). Health Administration Press.

Lockman, J. L., Ambardekar, A., & Deutsch, E. S. (2015). Optimizing education with in situ simulation. In J. C. Palaganas, J. C. Maxworthy, C. A. Epps, & M. E. Mancini (Eds.), *Defining excellence in simulation programs* (pp. 90–97). Wolters Kluwer.

Locsin, R. C. (2001). The culture of technology: Defining transformation in nursing, from "the lady with a lamp" to "robonurse"? *Holistic Nursing Practice, 16*(1), 1–4. https://doi.org/10.1097/00004650-200110000-00004

Lowens, T. L., & Gliva-McConvey, G. (2015). Standardized patients. In J. C. Palaganas, J. C. Maxworthy, C. A. Epps, & M. E. Mancini (Eds.), *Defining excellence in simulation programs* (pp. 199–212). Wolters Kluwer.

Mathieu, J. E., Heffner, T. S., Goodwin, G. F., Salas, E., & Cannon-Bowers, J. A. (2000). The influence of shared mental models on team process and performance. *Journal of Applied Psychology, 85*(2), 273–283. https://doi.org/10.1037/0021-9010.85.2.273

McGaghie, W. C., Issenberg, S. B., Cohen, E. R., Barsuk, J. H., & Wayne, D. B. (2011). Does simulation-based medical education with deliberate practice yield better results than traditional clinical education? A meta-analytic comparative review of the evidence. *Academic Medicine, 86,* 706–711. https://doi.org/10.1097/acm.0b013e318217e119

McGaghie, W. C., Issenberg, S. B., Petrusa, E. R, & Scalese, R. J., (2010). A critical review of simulation-based medical education research: 2003–2009. *Medical Educator, 44,* 50–63. https://doi.org/10.1111/j.1365-2923.2009.03547.x

McGaghie, W. C., Siddall, V. J., Mazmanian, P. E., & Myers, J. (2009). Lessons for continuing medical education from simulation research in undergraduate and graduate medical education: Effectiveness of continuing medical education: American college of chest physicians evidence-based educational guidelines. *Chest, 135*(3), 62S–68S. https://doi.org/10.1378/chest.08-2521

McLaughlin, S., Fitch, M. T., Goyal, D. G., Hayden, E., Kaugh, C. Y., Laack, T. A., Nowicki, T., Okuda, Y., Palm, K., Pozner, C. N., Vozenilek, J., Wang, E., & Gordon, J. A. (2008). Simulation in graduate medical education 2008: A review for emergency medicine. *Academic Emergency Medicine, 15,* 1117–1129. https://doi.org/10.1111/j.1553-2712.2008.00188.x

Merriam-Webster. (2020). www.merriam-webster.com

Michaelson, J. D., & Manning, L. (2008). Competency assessment in simulation-based procedural education. *American Journal of Surgery, 196*(4), 609–615. https://doi.org/10.1016/j.amjsurg.2007.09.050

Monachino, A. M., & Tuttle, S. A. (2015). Just-in-time training programs. In J. C. Palaganas, J. C. Maxworthy, C. A. Epps, & M. E. Mancini (Eds.), *Defining excellence in simulation programs* (pp. 127–134). Wolters Kluwer.

Morrison, J. B., & Deckers, C. (2015). Common theories in healthcare simulation. In J. C. Palaganas, J. C. Maxworthy, C. A. Epps, & M. E. Mancini (Eds.), *Defining excellence in simulation programs* (pp. 500–501). Wolters Kluwer.

Motola, I., Devine, L. A., Chung, H. S., Sullivan, J. E., & Issenberg, S. B. (2013). Simulation in healthcare education: a best evidence practical guide. AMEE Guide No. 82. *Medical Teacher, 35*(10), e1511–30. https://doi.org/10.3109/0142159x.2013.818632

Mudumbai, S. C., Gaba, D. M., Boulet, J. R., Howard, S. K., & Davies, M. F. (2012). External validation of simulation-based assessments with other performance measures of their-year anesthesiology residents. *Simulation in Healthcare, 7*(2), 73–80. https://doi.org/10.1097/sih.0b013e31823d018a

Murray, D., Boulet, J., Ziv, A., Woodhouse, J., Kras, J., & McAllister, J. (2002). An acute care skills evaluation for graduating medical students: A pilot study using clinical simulation. *Medical Education, 36*(9), 833–841. https://doi.org/10.1046/j.1365-2923.2002.01290.x

Owei, L., Neylan, C. J., Raghavendra, R., Caskey, R. C., Morris, J. B., Sensenig, R., Brooks, A. D., Dempsey, D. T., Williams, N. N., Atkins, J. H., Baranov, D. Y., & Dumon, K. R. (2017). In situ operating room-based simulation: A review. *Journal of Surgical Education, 74*(4), 579–588. https://doi.org/10.1016/j.jsurg.2017.01.001

Paige, J., Fairbanks, T., Rollin, J., & Gaba, D. (2018). Priorities related to improving healthcare safety through simulation. *Simulation in Healthcare, 13*(3S), S41–S50. https://doi.org/10.1097/SIH.0000000000000295

Parry, M., & Fey, M. K. (2019). Simulation in advanced practice nursing. *Clinical Simulation in Nursing, 26*, 1–2. https://doi.org/10.1016/j.ecns.2018.11.004

Palaganas, J. C., & Rock, L. K. (2015). Simulation-enhanced interprofessional education: A framework for development. In J. C. Palaganas, J. C. Maxworthy, C. A. Epps, & M. E. Mancini (Eds.), *Defining excellence in simulation programs* (pp. 108–119). Wolters Kluwer.

Person, R. (2013). *Balanced scorecards & operational dashboards with microsoft excel*. Amazon.com.

Reason, J. (2004). Beyond the organizational accident: The need for "error wisdom" on the frontline. *Quality and Safety in Health Care, 13*(Suppl. 2), ii28–ii33. https://doi.org/10.1136/qhc.13.suppl_2.ii28

Rudolph, J. W., Simon, R., Raemer, D. B., & Eppich, W. J. (2008). Debriefing as formative assessment: Closing performance gaps in medical education. *Academic Emergency Medicine, 15*, 1010–1016. https://doi.org/10.1111/j.1553-2712.2008.00248.x

Russ-Eft, D., & Preskill, H. (2001). *Evaluation in organizations*. Perseus Books Group.

Ruth-Sahd, L. A. (2003). Reflective practice: A critical analysis of data-based studies andimplications for nursing education. *Journal of Nursing Education, 42*(11):488–497. PMID: 14626387.

Sanko, J. S., Shekhter, I., Kyle, R. R., & Birnbach, D. J. (2015). Using embedded simulated persons. In J. C. Palaganas, J. C. Maxworthy, C. A. Epps, & M. E. Mancini (Eds.), *Defining excellence in simulation programs.* (pp. 213–226) Wolters Kluwer.

Schocken, D. M., & Gammon, W. L. (2015). Hybrid simulations. In J. C. Palaganas, J. C. Maxworthy, C. A. Epps, & M. E. Mancini (Eds.), *Defining excellence in simulation programs* (pp. 235–240). Wolters Kluwer.

Slone, F. L, & Lampotang, S. (2015a). History of modern-day mannequins. In J. C. Palaganas, J. C. Maxworthy, C. A. Epps, & M. E. Mancini (Eds.), *Defining excellence in simulation programs* (pp. 172–182). Wolters Kluwer.

Slone, F. L, & Lampotang, S. (2015b). Mannequins, terminology, selection, and usage. In J. C. Palaganas, J. C. Maxworthy, C. A. Epps, & M. E. Mancini (Eds.), *Defining excellence in simulation programs.* Wolters Kluwer (pp. 185–190).

Smith, P., & Ragan, J. (1999). *Instructional design*. John Wiley & Sons.

Society for Simulation in Healthcare. (n.d.). http://www.ssih.org

Society of Simulation in Healthcare. (2012). *Simulation terminology and concepts committee.* www.ssih.org.

Suliburk, J. W., Buck, Q. M., Pirko, C. J., Massarweh, N. N., Barshes, N. R., Singh, H., & Rosengart, T. K. (2019). Analysis of human performance deficiencies associated with surgical adverse events. *JAMA Netw Open, 2*(7), e198067. https://doi.org/10.1001/jamanetworkopen.2019.8067

Todd, M., Manz, J., Hawkins, K., Parsons, M., & Hercinger, M. (2008). The development of a quantitative evaluation tool for simulation in nursing education. *International Journal of Nursing Education Scholarship, 5*(1), 1–17. https://doi.org/10.2202/1548-923x.1705

Totten, A. M., McDonagh, M. S., & Wagner, J. H. (2020). *The evidence base for telehealth: Reassurance in the face of rapid expansion during the COVID-19 pandemic.* Agency for Healthcare Research and Quality.

Walker, S. E., & Weidner, T. G. (2010). The use of standardized patients in athletic training education. *Athletic Training Education Journal, 5*(2), 87–89. https://doi.org/10.4085/1947-380x-5.2.87

Willhaus, J., Burleson, G., Palaganas, J., & Jeffries, P. (2014). Authoring simulations for high-stakes student evaluation. *Clinical Simulation in Nursing, 10*(4), e177–e182. https://doi.org/10.1016/j.ecns.2013.11.006

Wilkes, M., & Bligh, J. (1999). Evaluating educational interventions. *British Medical Journal, 318*, 1269. https://doi.org/10.1136/bmj.318.7193.1269.

RECOMMENDED RESOURCES

Bristol, T., Walls, D. ,Weber, C., Murphy, H., Searles, S., & Sportsman, S. (2019). *Learning gets real: A hands-on simulation guide for teaching tomorrow's clinical practitioners.* Elsevier. https://evolve. elsevier.com/education/expertise/simulation-success/learning-gets-real-a-hands-on-simulations-guide-for-teaching-tomorrows-clinical-practitioners/
International Nursing Association for Clinical Simulation and Learning (INACSL). https://www.inacsl.org/
Society for Simulation in Healthcare. http://ssih.org/

EVALUATION OF POPULATIONS AND HEALTH POLICY

THIRTEEN

EVALUATION OF POPULATIONS AND POPULATION HEALTH

Joanne V. Hickey

The health of the people is really the foundation upon which all their happiness and all their powers as a state depend.
—Benjamin Disraeli

INTRODUCTION

The transformation of health care has brought about changes in the fundamental definitions of health and health care reflected in updated definitions of public health and population health and how health care delivery is provided. A greater appreciation of the prominence of the influence of the determinants of health on the health of individuals, populations, and communities has fueled changes in health policies, organizational structures and processes, and payment for health care. Health has been redefined with a focus on health, wellness, and prevention of illness rather than on just illness care alone. The focus on populations and community health has reframed how health professionals practice. Professional nurses recognize an expansion of their role from simply caring for individual patients in a clinic/hospital/nursing facility to caring for a panel of patients seen regularly in those settings to ongoing prevention of illness and promotion of wellness. Nurses understand that their patients have health problems similar to those of the populations from which they come. Doctor of nursing practice (DNP) graduates increasingly find themselves working to change health and health care for populations served through ongoing assessment and evaluation to determine the needs and way to correct their unmet needs. Some population health evaluations are large-scale evaluations conducted by state and national agencies such as state health departments and national organizations such as the Centers for Disease Control and Prevention (CDC). DNP graduates may be employed by such agencies and be members of various teams engaged in the evaluation. However, most DNP graduates will more likely be involved in evaluating population health initiatives for groups of patients with the same medical diagnoses or risk factors or those from the same ethnic groups in a clinical setting. For example, the medical diagnoses of a population in a practice could be atrial fibrillation, stroke, or rheumatoid arthritis. Many commonalities will be noted in the characteristics, symptoms, risks, and responses to the particular health problem. Evidence-based guidelines implemented by nurses are often available to guide care that is implemented by nurses. Regardless of the scope (e.g., CDC or smaller specialty practice) of the evaluation of a population, the principles for evaluation are similar. The purpose of this chapter is to help DNP nurses to understand populations and population health and how to evaluate their health outcomes.

EXPECTATIONS OF THE DOCTOR OF NURSING PRACTICE GRADUATE FOR POPULATION HEALTH

The American Association of Colleges of Nursing (AACN) recognized the importance of the health of populations in their document *The Essentials of Doctoral Education for Advanced Nursing Practice*. The focus of Essential VII is clinical prevention and population health for improving the nation's health (AACN, 2006, p. 16). Graduates are expected to possess broad knowledge in social sciences, statistics, and environmental sciences to be able to interpret these data as applicable to both the individual and population levels for the prevention and management of health problems with equity and best practices to support the health of the nation. These competencies require abilities in analysis, synthesis, and evaluation of scientific information to build and support the multiple strategies for a healthy nation. The new Essentials (AACN, 2021) continue to support population health and use a framework of a domain, descriptor, contextual statement, and competencies model. See the link provided in the reference list for definitions of these terms (AACN, 2021). Domain 3: Population Health has been revised in the new Essentials. In addition, the concept of social determinants of health is included in the new Essentials (AACN, 2021), under the heading of concepts.

TERMINOLOGY

A *population* is a group of people who have common characteristics such as age, geography, political boundaries, race/ethnicity, religion, environmental exposures, occupation, education, sexual preference, and so on. According to the AACN, a *population* is a discrete group that the nurse cares for across settings at local, regional, national, and global levels.

Population health has been defined as "the health outcomes of a group of individuals, including the distribution of such outcomes within the group" (Kindig & Stoddart, 2003, p. 380). These groups are often geographic populations such as nations or communities, but can also be other groups such as employees, ethnic groups, disabled persons, prisoners, patients, or organizations or any other defined group. The health outcomes of such groups or institutions are of relevance to policy-makers in both the public and private sectors as well as to evaluators for purposes of decision-making. According to the AACN (2021), *population health* describes collaborative activities among stakeholders for the improvement of a population's health status across the continuum. The purpose of these collaborative activities, including interventions and policies, is to strive toward health equity in which diversity, equity, inclusivity, and ethics are emphasized and valued. Accountability for outcomes is viewed as shared by all, since outcomes arise from the multiple factors that influence the health of a defined group. Population health includes *population management* achieved through systems thinking, including health promotion and illness prevention, to achieve population health goals (AACN, 2021; Storfjell et al., 2017).

Winslow, a founding father of public health, defined *public health* as "the science and art of preventing disease, prolonging life, and promoting health through the organized efforts and informed choices of society, organizations, public and private communities and individuals" (Winslow, 1920, pp. 183–191). Public health provides the critical functions through local and state health departments and national centers (e.g., CDC) that include the prevention of epidemics, control of environmental hazards, and the encouragement of healthy behaviors. A broader vision of the public health system offered by *The Future of the Public's Health in the 21st Century* calls for "building a new generation of intersectoral partnerships that draw on the perspectives and resources of diverse communities and actively engage them in health action" for the population (Institute of Medicine [IOM], 2002, p. 4).

Patient-centered care is defined as "providing care that is respectful of and responsive to individual patient preferences, needs, and values, and ensuring that patient values guide all clinical decisions" (IOM, 2001, p. 49). This definition implies a goal of advocacy for the patient. Patient-centered care is one of the six interrelated elements constituting high-quality health care that the IOM (2001) report identified. In addition, *patient-centered* means considering a patient's cultural traditions, personal preferences, values, family situation, social circumstances, and lifestyles. It supports active involvement of patients and their families in the design of new care models and in decision-making about individual options for treatment (IOM, 2001).

Community engagement is defined as "the process of working collaboratively with groups of people who are affiliated by geographic proximity, special interests or similar situations with respect to issues affecting their well-being" (CDC, 2011, p. xv). It is a fundamental value of public health based on the belief that the public has a right to participate. The public health community believes that by using the "collective intelligence" and working together, problems will be more accurately identified and more effective solutions will be developed. Through this process, individuals and communities have an opportunity to understand and to engage collaboratively in the processes of changes.

DETERMINANTS OF HEALTH

What are the conditions that contribute to disparities in health among individuals and populations? These conditions are commonly called the determinants of health. The *determinants of health* are the personal, social, economic, and environmental factors that impact the health status of individuals and populations. These determinants of health have been defined more formally as the "combined effects of individual and community physical and social environments and the policies and interventions used to promote health, prevent disease, and ensure access to quality healthcare" (U.S. Department of Health and Human Services [DHHS], 2002, p. 7; Wilkinson & Marmot, 2003; World Health Organization & Commission on Social Determinants of Health, 2008).

The *Healthy People* initiatives have been instrumental in addressing the determinants of health. The latest 2030 version, *Healthy People 2030* (*HP2030*), includes many changes. *HP2030* reflects a more focused, evidence-based, and statistically rigorous set of objectives. The following summarizes the major differences in *HP2030* from previous versions. The following data-related criteria were applied in the selection of objectives and data sources:

- Data are reliable, valid, and nationally representative with no major methodological issues (e.g., limited population coverage, inadequate sample size, unknown or low response rates, and inadequate studies of nonresponse bias).
- Data are timely with baseline data no older than 2015 and include a measure of variability and assurance of at least two additional data points throughout the decade.
- Data are publicly available with complete documentation, generally with federal government management or oversight.

In addition to the data-related criteria listed above, *HP2030* core objectives were selected based on the following criteria: national importance, evidence-based, and disparities and equity. There are three categories of objectives: core, developmental, and research. Currently, there are 355 core objectives that cut across a number of disease entities and problems with targets for achieving each objective (National Center for Health Statistics, 2020). More information about *HP2030* is available at the CDC *Healthy People 2030* (2020) website at https://www.cdc.gov/nchs/healthy_people/index.htm.

Since the term *determinants of health* was coined, the numbers and types or categories of determinants have changed over time. Originally, there were four general determinants (i.e., human biology, health system, environment, and lifestyle), which were included in the Lalonde Report (Glouberman & Miller, 2003), but changes have occurred in versions of *Healthy People* including the 2030 version with new categories and the numbers of determinants. The determinants of health depicted in the *HP2030* (Figure 13.1) include the following: (a) economic stability, (b) education access and quality, (c) health care access and quality, (d) neighborhood and built environment, and (e) social and community context. These five categories of determinants are described in the following section. A visit to the website for each one provides multiple objectives and supporting data including targets for the specific determinant of health.

Economic Stability

The goal of the economic stability determinant of health is *to help people earn steady incomes that allow them to meet their health needs.* HP2030 focuses on helping more people achieve economic stability. One of 10 people in the United States lives in poverty, and many others cannot afford basics such as healthy food, health care, and housing (Semega et al., 2019). By comparison, people employed on a regular basis are less apt to live in poverty and more likely to be healthy although some people have difficulty finding and keeping a job. Others have chronic conditions or disabilities with related limited physical or mental capabilities, which are also limitations. Still others who have steady employment may not earn an adequate

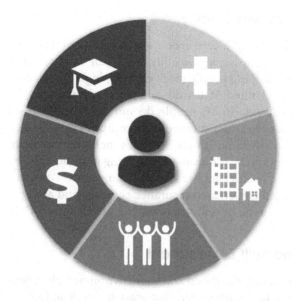

Figure 13.1 Determinants of health for *Healthy People 2030*.

Source: Healthy People 2030. (2020). USDHHS, Office of Disease Prevention and Health Promotion. Retrieved September 28, 2020, from https://health.gov/healthypeople/objectives-and-data/social-determinants-health

salary to support a healthy lifestyle. Activities designed to support economic stability include employment programs, career counseling, and high-quality child care opportunities designed to help more people find and keep jobs. In addition, policies to help people pay for food, housing, health care, and education can reduce poverty and improve health and well-being (DHHS, 2020a, https://health.gov/healthypeople/objectives-and-data/browse-objectives/economic-stability#cit1).

Education Access and Quality

The goal of the education access and quality determinant of health is *to increase educational opportunities and help children and adolescents do well in school*. It is recognized that people with higher levels of education are more likely to be healthier and live longer. Children and adolescents from low-income families, those with disabilities, and those who experience forms of social discrimination (e.g., bullying) are more apt to have academic difficulties. These children and adolescents are at a higher risk for not graduating from high school or attending college. This profile is one of children and adolescents less likely to secure safe, high-paying jobs, in the future. Children and adolescents with these characteristics are more likely to have health problems such as cardiovascular disease, diabetes mellitus, and depression. In addition, some schools, especially those in poverty areas, are poor performers, so attendees do not receive a quality education that makes them ill-prepared for jobs or higher education. Interventions to help children and adolescents do well in school and help families pay for higher education can have long-term health benefits (DHHS, 2020b).

Health Care Access and Quality

The goal of the health care access and quality determinant of health is *to increase access to comprehensive, high-quality health care services.* HP2030 focuses on improving health by helping people receive timely, high-quality health care services. Many people in the United States do not receive health care services that they need. Approximately one in 10 people do not have health insurance (Berchick et al., 2018). Without health insurance and a primary care provider, people may be unable to access and afford health care services including screening, preventive care, and health promotion. In addition, people living in rural and underserved areas may not have access to health care because of distance/travel or unavailable local providers. What is needed is increased insurance coverage and access to health care providers either via in-person or remote access (e.g., telehealth; DHHS, 2020c).

Neighborhood and Built Environment

The goal of the neighborhood and built environment determinant of health is *to create neighborhoods and environments that promote health and safety.* The neighborhoods in which people live have a major impact on their health and well-being (CDC, 2018). HP2030 focuses on improving health and safety in places where people live, work, learn, and play. Many people in the United States live in neighborhoods with high rates of violence, crime, unsafe air or water, and other health and safety risks. Racial/ ethnic minorities and people with low incomes are more likely to live in places with these risk factors. In addition, some people are exposed to situations at work that can harm their health such as secondhand smoke or loud noises. Interventions and policy changes at the local, state, and federal levels that can help reduce these health and safety risks and promote health are needed. For example, providing opportunities for people to walk and bike in their communities, by adding sidewalks and bike lanes, can increase safety and help improve health and quality of life (DHHS, 2020d).

Social and Community Context

The goal of the social and community context determinant of health is *to increase social and community support.* HP2030 focuses on helping people receive social support they need in places where they live, work, learn, and play. An individual's relationships and interactions with family, friends, coworkers, and community members can have a major impact on their health and well-being. Social environment may also include access to resources in the community (public safety, parks, and recreational facilities), social institutions (law enforcement, school systems, and governmental and social service agencies), and cultural supports and opportunities. Many people face challenges and dangers beyond their control such as unsafe neighborhoods, discrimination, or difficulty affording basic needs. This can have a negative impact on health and safety throughout their life. Positive relationships at home, at work, and in the community can help reduce these negative impacts. However, some people, such as children whose parents are incarcerated and adolescents who are bullied, often don't receive support from loved ones or others. Interventions to help people receive the social and community support they need are critical for improving health and well-being (DHHS, 2020e).

OTHER INFLUENCES ON HEALTH

Policies and Interventions

Governmental policies at the local, state, and federal levels may profoundly affect individual and population health. Individual- and population-level behavior change may occur with changes in government regulations. Cuts in programs, such as Medicaid, for dependent and low-income families due to changes in political structure at the state and federal levels may greatly alter the resources of struggling, working-class families.

Individual Behaviors or Lifestyles

Individual behaviors and lifestyle choices impact health outcomes. These factors include an individual's responses to internal stimuli and external conditions and often interact with an individual's biology. Lifestyle factors include risk behaviors such as alcohol, tobacco, and other kinds of substance abuse; unprotected sexual behaviors; sedentary lifestyle and lack of regular physical activity; poor diet; and poor safety practices, such as neglecting seat belt and child restraint use in motor vehicles. Persons who use tobacco, alcohol, or illegal drugs, including injection drugs and crack cocaine, are at an increased risk for infection and other health problems. Many population health interventions target such individual behaviors designed to reduce the rates of chronic disease and injury acquired from risky behaviors.

Biology and Genetics

Biological factors include the effects of an individual's genetic makeup, family history, and physical and mental health problems acquired over the course of the individual's lifetime. Genetic factors may affect certain population groups more than others. Older individuals are more likely to acquire cancers due to the physical effects of aging on cells. Examples of genetic and biological determinants of health in certain inherited conditions (e.g., sickle cell anemia, hemophilia, and cystic fibrosis); the *BRCA1* or *BRCA2* gene that increases the risk of breast and ovarian cancer; and a family history of certain forms of heart disease (DHHS, 2009).

RISK, RISK FACTORS, AND POPULATIONS AT RISK

Risk is simply the probability that something will occur. With respect to health, risk is the increased probability that a disease, an injury, a disability, or a death will occur to an individual or a population. *Risk factors* are those characteristics of an individual and/or a population that increase their risk for a disease, an illness, a disability, or a death. Frequently identified risk factors include age, gender, family history, ethnicity, immune state, and others. Two types of risks deserve mention. The first is an *attributable risk,* that is, a measure of the increased prevalence in a population attributable to a specific condition or disease. The attributable risk, or risk difference, is the absolute difference in incidence between an exposed and unexposed group. It quantifies the risk of disease in the exposed group attributable to the exposure by removing the risk that would have occurred due to other causes.

Expressed differently, the attributable risk calculates the number of cases of disease among the exposed that could be eliminated if the exposure was eliminated. This is a useful measure of the public health impact of an exposure, assuming there is a cause–effect relationship (Rothman & Lash, 2020).

Relative risk is a second important measure of risk that estimates the magnitude of an association between exposure and disease, based on the incidence of disease in the exposed group relative to the unexposed group. A relative risk of 1.0 indicates that there is no association between the exposure and outcome; a relative risk greater than 1.0 indicates a positive association or an increased risk; and a relative risk less than 1.0 indicates an inverse association, or a decreased risk considered a protective effect (Rothman & Lash, 2020). Unlike the attributable risk, the relative risk does not provide any information about the absolute risk of the event occurring, but rather the higher or lower likelihood of the event in the exposure versus the nonexposure group (Tenny & Hoffman, 2020).

The term *populations at risk* refers to all individuals and populations who have a similar types of risk, such as health care workers (HCWs) with continuing exposure to patients with COVID-19, older adults (65 years and older), and immune-compromised individuals. A population at risk can be identified only in probabilistic terms. Populations can also be identified in terms of current need rather than risk. A *population in need* can be identified by a population's health status, disabilities, medical conditions, or other determinants of health (e.g., housing and education). Based on scientific evidence, it is known that these conditions can lead to other problems if not addressed properly. A population in need can also be identified by their risks for certain conditions such as obesity and heart disease or smoking and lung cancer. All of these concepts are considerations in the evaluation of populations.

ASSESSING THE DISTRIBUTION OF DISEASE IN A POPULATION

The novel COVID-19 pandemic is like no other pandemic in history. To begin with, coronavirus (COVID-19) is a new virus that has spread throughout the world at an unprecedented rate. Because it is a new virus, nothing was known about it until the pandemic struck. Since then, a steep learning curve has typified what is known about the pathogen, signs and symptoms, course of the disease, treatment, recovery, and prevention. What has been reported as the state of the science one day has often been corrected the next day as new knowledge is developed. A discussion of COVID-19 is being used to describe the distribution of diseases in a population.

COVID-19 symptoms can range from mild (or no symptoms) to severe illness. COVID-19 is primarily spread from person to person from respiratory droplets when an infected person coughs, sneezes, or talks. Another transmission mode is touching a contaminated surface and then touching the mouth, nose, or eyes. The list of signs and symptoms is long and general and includes fever, chills, shortness of breath, fatigue, muscle or body aches, headache, new loss of taste or smell, sore throat, nausea or vomiting, congested or runny nose, and diarrhea. Signs of severe illness and need for emergency care include trouble breathing, persistent pain/pressure in the chest, new onset of confusion, inability to wake up or stay awake, and bluish lips or face. Symptoms may appear 2 to 14 days after exposure to the virus. Mortality rates have been high especially in high-risk groups as discussed in the following.

How will a DNP nurse apply the previous discussion of risk and determinants of health to implement the CDC COVID-19 guidelines, which have been rapidly evolving and updated as new information emerges (CDC, 2020b)? Some of the questions to consider are the following:

- What is the incidence of COVID-19 in your community (county or region served by the health care setting), and how does it compare with the state and national average?
- What is the incidence of COVID-19 in your facility and specific settings, and how do those rates compare with other entities?
- Are patients with suspected or confirmed COVID-19 encountered in your setting (inpatient and outpatient)? If yes, how many are treated in your health care setting daily/weekly?
- Currently, does your health care setting have a cluster of persons with confirmed COVID-19 that might be a result of ongoing transmission of COVID-19?

A review of basic concepts and methods pertaining to these measures of morbidity may be helpful here. *Distribution of disease* refers to the occurrence of a disease, an injury, a disability, or a death according to the extent of the problem in the population during a given time period. The common questions are as follows: What is the disease or other health problem? How much is occurring? To whom? When? For example, if one is counting new events in a nursing facility, such as new cases diagnosed by positive COVID-19 testing, the new infections are called *incidence*. Newly diagnosed active cases of COVID-19 during a time period are also called incidence. A count of all of the residences demonstrating a positive COVID-19 test at one time, regardless of when they were infected, is called *prevalence*.

It is also important to relate cases, whether new or existing, to the population from which they were counted. This process involves relating the cases (the numerator) to the whole (the denominator) to calculate a proportion, percentage, or rate. *Rates* are the basic measures of disease, injury, disability, or death in a defined population over a specified period of time. *Rates* allow comparisons between populations, between geographic areas, and over periods of time. *Incidence* rates are calculated by the number of events occurring in a population during a specific time period divided by the number of persons in the population at risk for those events, and multiplied by a base number (100, 1,000, 10,000, or 100,000) that will result in a whole number answer. For example, one might calculate the incidence rate of COVID-19 in a month in one country as follows:

$$\frac{\text{No. of new cases of COVID in April, 2020}}{\text{No. of residents in the country in April, 2020}} \times 100,000$$

$$= \text{Incidence of COVID per 100,000 population}$$

Prevalence rates are calculated by the number of existing events in a population during a time period or at one time divided by the number of persons in the population at risk for those events and multiplied by a base number (100, 1,000, 10,000, or 100,000) that will result in a whole number.

$$\frac{\text{No. of persons with COVID hospitalized today}}{\text{Total no. of patients in the hospital today}} \times 100$$

$$= \% \text{ of hospitalized COVID patients today}$$

The incidence rates of new COVID-19 cases can be compared with a state or national distribution of the disease. The state or national distribution of COVID-19 is sometimes called a *standard population*, that is, one that encompasses the population being studied. The process of comparison is similar to comparing one's weight with a standard weight chart for one's height and age. State or national COVID-19 incidence rates serve as a standard for comparing the local or regional rates. Therefore, the assessment of the distribution of COVID-19 could include the comparison of incidence rates of COVID-19 in the local population during a week or month with those of the state or nation during the same time period, as well as incidence over time, incidence in certain high-risk groups, and incidence in the health care facility or clinic.

It is equally important to assess the characteristics of the populations who have COVID-19 by a positive test and those who are ill with COVID-19. What are their demographic characteristics such as ages, genders, race, or ethnicity? Where do they live (urban, rural, or suburban areas)? What is the geography and climate of their locale? What are their living conditions (single-family dwellings, multiple-family households, or congregate living facilities)? What do members of the population do for a living and where do they work? Do they have comorbidities, such as heart disease or diabetes mellitus, which may exacerbate COVID-19?

The CDC, state and local municipalities, and other organizations collect COVID-19 data, and those data are available for review by the general public. The presence of COVID-19-positive persons without illness and persons with COVID-19 with clinical symptoms who are residents in health care facilities such as nursing facilities may be monitored by laboratory data and patient records.

ASSESSING RISK FACTORS AND POPULATIONS AT RISK

Understanding the mechanisms (i.e., risk factors) whereby a disease or health problem exists in a population provides a roadmap for developing interventions. With respect to an infectious disease, an examination of such factors as the nature and virulence of the pathogen, mode of transmission, natural history of the disease, susceptibility of the potential host, and environmental factors that may increase the probability of transmission is important to understand in terms of disease control and prevention.

As discussed earlier in this chapter, risk, risk assessment, and prevention are major foci of the CDC guidelines. DNPs are frequently responsible for the care of populations afflicted by an infectious disease, for example, COVID-19 allegedly spread by droplet transmission. To prevent spread, the principles inherent in these guidelines may be used by the DNP nurse in caring for patient populations, by the hospital/clinic administrator responsible for the health of the staff, and by ancillary personnel who have contact with ill patients.

Since COVID-19 has had such a huge impact on health care globally, information about COVID-19 will be used as examples for the following discussion. The information on COVID-19 in this chapter comes exclusively from posted CDC COVID-19 guidelines found on the CDC (2020b) website at https://www.cdc.gov/coronavirus/2019-ncov/index.html. This site should be visited often because it is updated frequently as new information is learned about COVD-19.

The CDC guidelines identify risks associated with the transmission of COVID-19, risk factors in certain groups that increase the risk of transmitting COVID-19, populations at risk for acquiring COVID-19 infection, and populations at risk for acquiring COVID-19. These are discussed in the following sections.

Risk Associated With Transmission of COVID-19

COVID-19 is transmitted in airborne particles (i.e., droplets) released when a person with laryngeal, oral, or nasal COVID-19 organisms coughs, sneezes, or talks. The particles are small enough that air currents may keep them airborne for prolonged periods, allowing the droplets to travel. COVID-19 can also be transmitted by contact with surfaces (e.g., desktops, cell phones, and table tops) that might be contaminated with COVID-19 droplets.

Risk Factors That Increase the Risk of Transmitting COVID-19

The more airborne particles released when a person coughs, the more the risk of transmission. Perhaps the greatest risk for transmitting COVID-19 is not following the CDC recommendations for prevention that include wearing a mask and social distancing. Wear a mask in public settings when around people not living in your household and particularly where other social distancing measures are difficult to maintain, such as grocery stores, pharmacies, and gas stations. Masks may slow the spread of the virus and help people who may have the virus, and do not know it, from transmitting it to others. COVID-19 can be spread by people who do not have symptoms and do not know that they are infected. That's why it's important for everyone to practice social distancing (i.e., maintaining a distance of at least 6 feet from another person) and wearing a mask in public settings. Masks provide an extra layer to help prevent the respiratory droplets from traveling in the air and onto other people. In addition, guidelines for avoiding groups and contact with people not in your household should be followed. Finally, if you are sick, stay home and avoid all contact with other people.

Populations at Risk for Acquiring COVID-19

The characteristics of persons exposed to COVID-19 that may increase their risk for infection and severe illness are related to age and preexisting health conditions. Among adults, the risk for severe illness from COVID-19 increases with age, with older adults at a highest risk. Severe illness means that the person with COVID-19 may require hospitalization, intensive care, or ventilator support, or they may even die. Risk increases with advanced age, and the greatest risk for COVID-19 and serious illness is in the 85 or older age-group. Eight of 10 COVID-19 deaths reported in the United States have been 65 years old or older. Increased risk of severe illness is also associated with several underlying medical conditions that include cancer, chronic kidney disease, chronic obstructive pulmonary disease, immunocompromised states, obesity, heart disease, sickle cell disease, and type 2 diabetes mellitus. By understanding the risk factors that put a particular population at an increased risk, decisions can be made about what recommendations should be made about precautions in order to avoid COVID-19 and related illness.

Populations at Risk for Acquiring Symptomatic COVID-19

Not every person infected about COVID-19 will progress to having active disease. What is noteworthy about COVID-19 has been the rapidly developing information about testing and criteria for who should be tested. Two types of tests are available for COVID-19: a *viral test* that indicates if a person has a current infection and an *antibody test* that indicates past infection. Much discussion has been reported about the sensitivity and specificity of each test, and the discussion continues.

The CDC guidelines for testing for *suspected current infection* include the following: people who have symptoms of COVID-19; people who have had close contact (within 6 feet of an infected person for at least 15 minutes) with someone with confirmed COVID-19; and people who have been asked or referred for testing by their health care provider or local/state health department. Testing for *past infection* is conducted by examining blood for antibodies that suggest a past infection with the COVID-19 virus. Antibodies are disease-specific proteins that help fight infections and can provide protection against a future infection. An antibody test may not show if a person has a current COVID-19 infection because it can take 1 to 3 weeks after infection for the body to make antibodies. Not everyone needs to be tested although clear determination of who should be tested is still being discussed. If a person is tested, they should self-quarantine/isolate at home pending test results and follow the advice of their health care provider or a public health professional.

The results of COVID-19 testing must be placed in perspective. The more people tested in the general population, the more positives will be found. Many of these people may be asymptomatic although they can still infect others and therefore need to quarantine for a recommended period of time. In some instances of active disease, it may be advised to engage in contact tracing as a key to slow the spread of COVID-19 and protect others within a community. Further, more testing equals more positives. What is the impact on reports of incidence and prevalence for a population and local, state, and national statistics? Comparison of prevalence statistics between countries may be distorted if the other country does not have comparable numbers of testing. Therefore, caution is advised in comparing reported statistics.

Summary

DNP nurses frequently encounter infectious diseases in their practices and patient populations. Inadequate infection control practices in the health care facility increase the risk for nosocomial infections, which constitute a major population health hazard to patients, their families, and health care professionals. Readers are encouraged to access the CDC COVID-19 guidelines for more information about recognizing the risks and preventing the transmission of COVID-19 (2020b) at https://www.cdc.gov/coronavirus/2019-ncov/index.html.

ANALYZING A HEALTH PROBLEM IN A POPULATION

A population of patients may experience multiple health problems. Some are overt health problems such as diabetes mellitus, asthma, or COVID-19. Others are risk factors for future health problems such as smoking, poverty, or environmental hazards. Still others may be categorized as a lack of resources, which is the case for populations who are uninsured, homeless, or live in areas remote from health care facilities. Further, some health problems are categorized as a population-in-need with unmet needs such as a need for help with an elderly parent, a need to have someone with whom to talk, or a need to have a place to go during a hurricane.

In order to analyze a problem, such as a high incidence of new COVID-19 infections, one begins with a measure of the extent of a problem in a specific group or population during a specific time period. An example could be finding that 30% of nursing facility residences were symptomatic with COVID-19 during the past 2 weeks. Although health status problems are the easiest to quantify in a population, it is also possible to have measures of the extent of risk factors and lack of resources. For example, it may have observed that 80% of staff working with nursing facility residences do not wear face masks or engage in social distancing.

Knowing what is causing the problem is extremely helpful. Therefore, the next step in analyzing a health problem is to organize the evidence on determinants of the problem in the population. Some of this evidence may be available from first-hand experience with the population; other evidence is available from published research and guidelines.

The Health Problem Analysis Model (Exhibit 13.1) is useful to analyze complex problems in a population. The model is an adaptation of a worksheet published by the CDC and Public Health Practice Program Office in 1991 and reprinted in Turnock (2009, p. 74). It has similarities to a driver diagram discussed in Chapter 9. An examination of the components of the model helps to clarify the organization of the information collected. Turnock (2009, p. 74) defined a *determinant* as a "scientifically established factor that relates directly to the level of the health problem. A health problem may have any number of determinants identified for it." For example, inhalation of COVID-19 in aerosolized droplets is a determinant of infection with COVID-19. A *direct contributing factor* is a "scientifically established factor that directly affects the level of the determinant." For example, near proximity to a person with COVID-19 is a direct contributing factor.

An *indirect contributing factor* is a "community-specific factor that affects the level of a direct contributing factor. There may be many indirect factors contributing to a direct factor, and indirect factors may vary considerably from one community to another" (CDC, cited by Turnock, 2009, p. 73). An example of an indirect contributing factor is crowded living conditions or a crowded waiting room, which may increase the risk for exposure to the COVID-19. Exhibit 13.2 provides an analysis of a *specific problem*: 30% of nursing facility residents were symptomatic with COVID-19 during the past 2 weeks. Note that both the direct and indirect contributing factors provide opportunities for early intervention to prevent or ameliorate the problem.

EVALUATING POPULATION HEALTH OUTCOMES

Assessing and analyzing health problems in a population are not easy tasks. They are undertaken to provide a sound foundation to bring about change in the problem and, ultimately, to intervene to improve the health status of the population. Multiple manuals, books, and websites are available to assist in planning, implementing, and evaluating new and existing programs to improve the health status of the populations. See Box 13.1 for a few examples of websites.

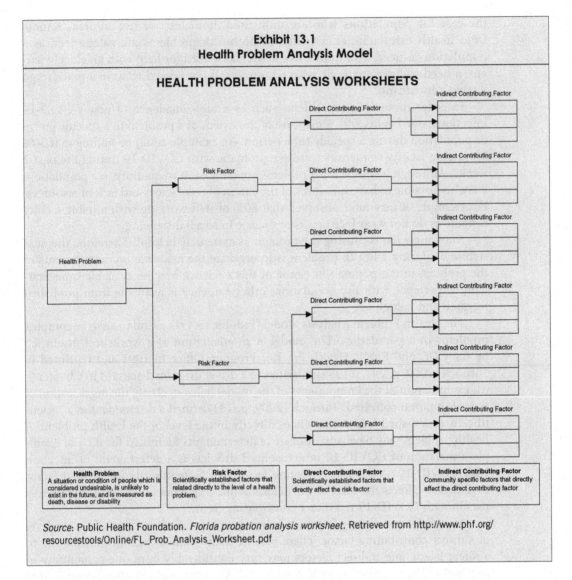

Exhibit 13.1
Health Problem Analysis Model

HEALTH PROBLEM ANALYSIS WORKSHEETS

Health Problem	Risk Factor	Direct Contributing Factor	Indirect Contributing Factor
A situation or condition of people which is considered undesirable, is unlikely to exist in the future, and is measured as death, disease or disability	Scientifically established factors that related directly to the level of a health problem.	Scientifically established factors that directly affect the risk factor	Community specific factors that directly affect the direct contributing factor

Source: Public Health Foundation. *Florida probation analysis worksheet*. Retrieved from http://www.phf.org/resourcestools/Online/FL_Prob_Analysis_Worksheet.pdf

Evaluating outcomes from a population-focused intervention is facilitated if the problem has been adequately assessed and analyzed. Evaluation includes the measurement of performance and identifying standards or criteria by which performance is to be judged. Knowing the answers to the following questions will provide guidance for the change that is desired:

- What is the extent of the problem and how is it distributed in the population?
- How does the extent compare with the extent and distribution of the problem in a standard population?
- Is the problem increasing or decreasing with time?
- What population is affected by the problem and what are their demographic characteristics?

If it is determined that the problem is greater than expected in some segments of the population, appropriate interventions may be targeted to that population.

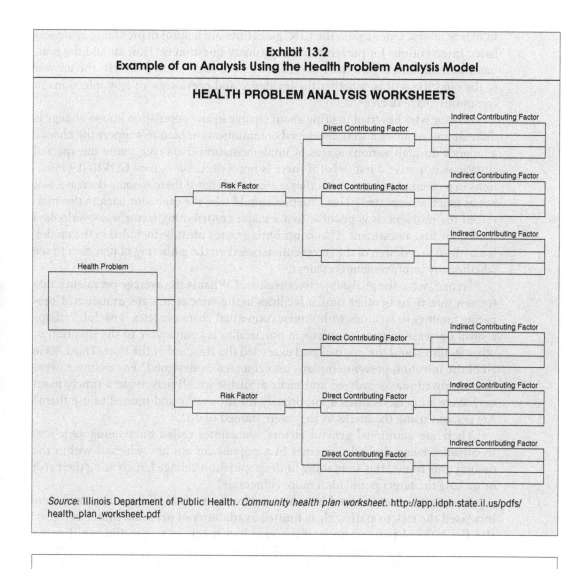

Exhibit 13.2
Example of an Analysis Using the Health Problem Analysis Model

HEALTH PROBLEM ANALYSIS WORKSHEETS

Source: Illinois Department of Public Health. *Community health plan worksheet.* http://app.idph.state.il.us/pdfs/
health_plan_worksheet.pdf

BOX 13.1   Population Health Websites

www.cdc.gov
www.inequality.org/
www.ahrq.gov
www.populationhealthalliance.org
www.who.org
www.thecommunityguide.org/index.html

Along with the stated problem statement, there are always assumptions made
that must be clearly understood. For example, assuming that the analysis of the
problem in Exhibit 13.2 is realistic and based on accurate information concerning
COVID-19, the evaluator can develop interventions to improve infection control
practices. Such interventions could be to improve the availability, use training, and

fit of face masks. Once again, the CDC guidelines are helpful in providing evidence-based interventions for prevention. The primary question is "How should the evaluator determine whether the interventions were successful?" Clearly, the answer to the question will be whether the incidence and prevalence of new infections in community have decreased.

Anyone who has tried to bring about change in any population knows change is difficult and requires a well-developed communication plan to support the change as it goes through various stages of implementation. However, many unexpected situations can arise. First, what if there is not a decrease in new COVID-19 infections in a given population? Another scenario is what if there is some decrease, but not as much as expected? This situation should take the evaluator back to the analysis of the problem. It is possible that a major contributing factor was overlooked during the first assessment. That contributing factor must be included in the model. It may lead to redesign of the intervention based on the gathering of new data to see whether any improvement is evident.

Second, were the goals/objectives realistic? What is the average prevalence rate for new infections in other similar facilities in the same area, state, or nation? Comparing findings to facilities with similar contextual characteristics is useful. Perhaps a small decrease in new infections in one facility is comparable to the situation in other facilities, and the original goal exceeded the standard at the time. Third, were all of the infection prevention plans implemented as designed? For example, were new approved masks ordered and made available for all persons in a timely manner? Were all persons fitted appropriately for the masks and trained to use them? Are persons using the masks as they were trained to do?

There are additional general factors, sometimes called intervening variables, to consider when desired outcomes in a population are not achieved within the desired time frame. Has something in the population changed, increasing their risk or making the target population more vulnerable?

The environment should be examined for contextual changes that may have increased the risk to staff such as limited availability of personal protective gear. Has the ratio of patients to staff increased so much as to preclude staff using adequate infection control practices? The new information learned from the evaluation can then influence the further analysis of the problem and further planning.

In summary, the process of improving the health of populations is not unlike that of improving the health of an individual patient. The process begins with an understanding of basic social, behavioral, biological, and physical environmental concepts influencing individuals and populations. It then proceeds to assess and diagnose health problems in both individuals and populations. Part of the diagnosis is to quantify a problem by comparing its characteristics to a standard or criterion. The next step is to analyze the problem by applying scientific evidence and direct observation of the conditions surrounding the problem to highlight the factors contributing to the problem. This step provides direction for the intervention to prevent the progression of the problem. The final step is to determine the outcome that is desired with respect to the problem and plans and interventions to achieve that goal. If the goal is not reached, the problem is further assessed and analyzed and the planning circuit continued. If the goal is achieved, the individual patient or the population experiences a higher level of health.

PROCESS OF EVALUATION OF A POPULATION

How is a DNP nurse going to evaluate a population? Chapter 8 provides a basic framework for the evaluation of a program or project. The steps of the evaluation include the following: (a) *purpose and scope*; (b) *design and methodology*; (c) *data collection, acquisition, and management*; (d) *data analysis and interpretation*; (e) *project management*; and (f) *dissemination*. Although these steps are listed as separate entities, there is a back-and-forth approach to these steps as the work progresses. One step is never considered completed because of the dynamic nature of the evaluation process and the entity being evaluated. Table 13.1 provides a list of activities and questions/focus to consider in planning an evaluation of a population.

TABLE 13.1   Activities and Questions/Focus to Consider in Evaluating Populations

Activities	Questions and Focus
1. Purpose and Scope	
• Determine the purpose(s) of the population evaluation. • Determine the scope (boundaries) and focus of the evaluation. • Learn all you can about the population. • Describe the population; refine as new information becomes available. • Focus the evaluation. • Negotiate your role. • Establish time line for the evaluation.	• What are the purposes of the evaluation? • What is the scope of the evaluation? • Who is requesting it and how will the report be used? • Investigate the historical background of the population (demographics, determinants of health, etc.). • How would you succinctly describe the population? • Based on the purpose and characteristics of the population, how will you narrow the focus of the evaluation? • How will you participate in the evaluation? To whom are you responsible? Will you be given access to the people and information that you need to conduct the evaluation?
2. Design and Methodology	
• Determine the design based on purpose. • Determine the best methods to conduct the evaluation based on purpose, available resources, culture, etc. • Prepare the plan for evaluating the population. • Decide what to measure as related to the purpose. • Determine any associated costs with the evaluation.	• Do you have an overall plan? • What will you measure and observe? • Do you have a written plan? • What will the evaluation cost? • Are you clear about your role and responsibilities?
3. Data Collection, Acquisition, and Management	
• Construct or purchase instruments for measurement and data collection. • Set deadlines for data collection.	• How will you collect the data? • What resources are available for data collection (e.g., people, technology)?

(continued)

TABLE 13.1 Activities and Questions/Focus to Consider in Evaluating Populations (*continued*)

Activities	Questions and Focus
• Determine where data will be found. • Plan how the data will be acquired and captured and when will be collected. • Verify that your data collection plan is implemented as designed (fidelity).	• Do you have a written time line for data collection (e.g., Gantt chart)? • Address inter-rater reliability if others are collecting data.
4. Data Analysis and Interpretation	
• Determine who and how data will be analyzed. • Involve the team in reviewing the data and its interpretation. • Determine recommendations based on data analysis and interpretations.	• Who is responsible for data analysis? • Is there a plan for data analysis? • Is the analysis free of bias? • Who is responsible for data interpretation? • How is the interpretation verified?
5. Project Management	
• Assume to be responsible and accountable for leadership and all activities for implementation of the evaluation. • Determine evaluator personnel and their responsibilities. • Provide needed resources as negotiated. • Develop policies and procedures for evaluation implementation. • Provide a plan for data storage and security. • Manage the agreed upon time line using a Gantt chart or other means.	• Has an overall plan of all activities and time line for the evaluation been developed? • Has it been communicated to all involved in the evaluation? • Have team assignments been made and clarified with team members including responsibilities and expectations? • Have data been collected and stored for accuracy and security? • Is the time line being followed?
6. Dissemination	
• Determine the format for reporting your findings. • Meet with appropriate stakeholders to verify factual information. • Present the report (e.g., written and/or oral report) to designated audiences. • Return any documents or other resources used for the evaluation to owner. • Come to closure.	• How will you verify with the team leader or team members that your facts are correct? • How will you disseminate a report of the evaluation and your findings (informal, formal, memo, email, written, oral, etc.) and to whom? • How will you come to closure with the project?

In the following section, the six steps discussed in the preceding will be implemented with a focus on the evaluation of a population. The information provided is applicable regardless of whether the DNP nurse is an internal or external evaluator to the organization or the scope of the evaluation is focused on a smaller or large population. The reader is referred to Chapter 8 for further discussion of planning and implementing an evaluation.

Purpose and Scope

In order to conduct a useful evaluation of a population, the DNP nurse (i.e., evaluator) must clearly understand the purpose and scope of the evaluation in order to set the specific focus and boundaries (i.e., scope) for a doable evaluation. This information comes from a joint discussion with the person or persons requesting the evaluation (e.g., director, chief nurse or executive officer, board, committee, or another initiator) and evaluator. The purpose or purposes of the evaluation are varied and may include the outcomes of an intervention such as strategies of COVID-19 spread in a designated community; examination of the population's compliance with evidence-based practice guidelines; or unmet needs of a population. Another way to focus an evaluation is from the perspective of problems. What are the specific health problems within the population being addressed? The problem approach also helps to identify desired evaluation outcomes and helps to set the evaluation criteria to be used to evaluate the performance. Because information from an evaluation will most likely be used for decision-making, it is helpful to know who is going to receive the information and how the information will be used (e.g., continued funding of a service). All of this information helps to shape the evaluation process.

The DNP nurse may or may not have knowledge about the population and should take the time to conduct a comprehensive assessment of the population. Even if the evaluator thinks they know the population, take a fresh unbiased look at the population from the eyes of an evaluator. Examples of areas to consider are listed in Table 13.1. This information can be gathered through discussions, observations, and review of databases, literature, and written materials. When necessary information has been collected, the evaluator will be able to describe the population in detail.

Once the DNP nurse has collected information and formulated a description of the population, the evaluator can begin to clarify the rationale and objectives for the evaluation and narrow the scope. This should lead to a brief written outline of purpose, rationale, objectives, and scope, which should be shared with those requesting the evaluation to verify and clarify a common focus of the evaluation. This is also a time to negotiate the evaluator role. Be clear about the expectations, responsibilities, deliverables, time line, and the person to whom the evaluation is reported. Verify access to both information and people for the conduct of the work, and determine what the representative of the population has been told about the evaluation as well as who provided that information. In addition, identify the contact person who will act as a facilitator if issues occur in the conduct of the evaluation. Discuss what format the final report should take and who should receive it. Finally, the conditions under which the work will be conducted should be addressed. If the evaluator is an outside consultant, conditions of work and compensation are addressed through a contract. If the evaluator is internal to the organization, how will this work be calculated into their current workload? Is there anyone available to help or provide support for data gathering or other phases? These and other questions need to be addressed prospectively to avoid misunderstandings later.

Design and Methodology

In selecting an appropriate design and evaluation method, the evaluator should further refine and double-check the population characteristics and the goals/objectives of the evaluation. This may seem redundant, but as the evaluator continues to work and plan, there may be new information and subtle changes in direction that influence the approach including what data need to be collected in order to get to the heart of the evaluation. The evaluator should also clarify the outcomes on which to focus (e.g., processes, outcomes) and include the details in a written format for clarity of communications. A clear understanding of how the resultant information will be used is important to maintain congruency between purposes and collected information.

The next step in the evaluation is to develop a detailed, step-by-step written plan of activities, data to be collected, methods of collection, time line for collection, and sources of data. To map the evaluation process in a concise and an efficient format, a written plan should be created or a logic model framework used to guide the evaluation. The evaluator should decide what to measure and observe including demographics, contextual characteristics, and so forth. The variables selected must be operationally defined to determine how they can best be measured. For example, to investigate population compliance with preventive measures, it must be clear what behaviors are of interest for evaluating compliance. How the concept is operationalized will drive options for measurement. For example, wearing a mask by population members may include wearing an approved mask that covers the mouth and nose. The evaluator must decide what method or methods of measurement are available to measure performance and which will best meet the objectives of the evaluation.

Data Collection, Acquisition, and Management

In this phase, a protocol to evaluate performance based on accepted standards and criteria, and to set time lines for data collection, acquisition, and management is needed. Depending upon the evaluation's purposes and objectives, the evaluator may create an investigator-developed data collection instruments, purchase validated instruments, or use a combination of both. Follow a realistic time line for data collection. If others are assisting with data collection, the evaluator will need to orient them to the instrument and data collection process and verify acceptable inter-rater reliability.

Data acquisition has to do with gaining possession of the desired data. This means that the evaluator needs to know what data are required, location/source of the data, the process for extracting the data, and appropriate storage of data. See Table 8.1 in Chapter 8 for location and sources of data. Chapter 8 also addresses data extraction, storage, and management.

Data Analysis and Interpretation

Data analysis is conducted once data are collected and organized in a usable format. Quantitative data may be entered into a spreadsheet of statistical analysis programs such as the Statistical Package for Social Sciences (SPSS) if not been previously entered. Qualitative data may be analyzed using content analysis or other qualitative data analysis methods. Data analyzed should be related clearly to the evaluation objectives. As the evaluator analyzes these data, an eye is kept on opportunities for quality improvement of population components around the areas evaluated. Are there any national standards or benchmarks that may be useful to frame the data interpretation? The evaluator should think about recommendations that may assist the decision-makers who will receive the final report.

Project Management

The section on project management presented in Chapter 8 is generic and applies to all evaluations. The reader is directed to the project management section in Chapter 8 for further information.

Dissemination

Once data analysis is completed and findings are formulated, the evaluator may wish to meet with stakeholders to discuss and follow up on the findings. This meeting is directed at transparency and provides the opportunity to correct any factual information that was reported incorrectly.

The final step in the evaluation process is dissemination of the findings of the evaluation in both written and oral reports. Content on dissemination of findings has been provided in Chapter 8 in the section on dissemination.

SUMMARY

DNP-prepared nurses are expected to understand populations at the micro-level and macro-level and the critical importance of population health to support a healthy nation. DNP nurses are also expected to have the competencies to assess and evaluate populations, both small and large, to determine compliance with science-based standards and identify opportunities for change in areas in which problems exist. In this chapter, the examples related to the evaluation process have been the COVID-19 pandemic that has challenged local/state/national medical professionals to learn rapidly about this unknown pathogen while also advising public health authorities and the populace about the prevention of spread of this virulent pathogen. As new knowledge is acquired almost on a daily basis, DNP nurses and members of health care professional teams partner with public health professionals to utilize and update information in their clinical practice and community to protect the populace from infection. The COVID-19 pandemic has created immense challenges that are being addressed through partnerships with health professionals and communities. DNP nurses are members of these teams focused on population health for a healthy nation and have significant contributions to this work.

REFERENCES

American Association of Colleges of Nursing. (2006). *The essentials of doctoral education for advanced nursing practice.* www.aacn.nche.edu

American Association of Colleges of Nursing. (2021). *The essentials: Core competencies for professional nursing education.* Author. https://aacnnursing.org/Portals/42/Downloads/Essentials/Essentials-Draft-Document.pdf

Berchick, E. R., Hood, E., & Barnett, J. C. (2018). *Health insurance coverage in the United States: 2017* [PDF file]. https://www.census.gov/content/dam/Census/library/publications/2018/demo/p60-264.pdf

Centers for Disease Control and Prevention. (2011). *Principles of community engagement* (2nd ed.). http://www.atsdr.cdc.gov/communityengagement/pdf/PCE_Report_508_FINAL.pdf

Centers for Disease Control and Prevention. (2018). *Social determinants of health: Know what affects health.* https://www.cdc.gov/socialdeterminants/index.htm

Centers for Disease Control and Prevention. (2020a). *Healthy people 2030*. Retrieved September 28, 2020, from https://www.cdc.gov/nchs/healthy_people/index.htm

Centers for Disease Control and Prevention. (2020b). *Coronavirus disease 2019 (COVID-19)*. https://www.cdc.gov/coronavirus/2019-ncov/faq.html

Glouberman, S., & Miller, J. (2003). Evolution of the determinants of health, health policy, and health information systems in Canada. *American Journal of Public Health, 93*, 388–392. https://doi.org/10.2105/ajph.93.3.388

Healthy People 2030. (2020). https://www.cdc.gov/nchs/healthy_people/index.htm

Institute of Medicine. (2001). *Crossing the quality chasm: A new health system for the 21st century*. National Academies Press.

Institute of Medicine. (2002). *The future of the public's health in the 21st century*. National Academies Press.

Kindig, D., & Stoddart, G. (2003). What is population health? *American Journal of Public Health, 93*(3), 380–383. https://doi.org/10.2105/ajph.93.3.380

National Center for Health Statistics. (2020, August). *NCHS fact sheet: Healthy People 2030*. https://www.cdc.gov/nchs/about/factsheets/factsheet-hp2030.htm

Rothman, K. J., & Lash, T. L. (2020). *Modern epidemiology* (4th ed.). Lippincott Williams & Wilkins.

Semega, J., Kollar, M., Creamer, J., & Mohanty, A. (2019). *Income and poverty in the United States* [PDF file]. https://www.census.gov/content/dam/Census/library/publications/2019/demo/p60-266.pdf

Storfjell, J. L., Winslow, B. W., & Saunders, J. S. D. (2017). *Catalysts for change: Harnessing the power of nurses to build population health in the 21st century*. https://www.rwjf.org/en/library/research/2017/09/catalysts-for-change--harnessing-the-power-of-nurses-to-build-population-health.html

Tenny, S., & Hoffman, M. R. (2020, July). *Relative risk StatPearls*. https://www.ncbi.nlm.nih.gov/books/NBK430824/

Turnock, B. J. (2009). *Public health: What it is and how it works* (4th ed.). Jones and Bartlett Publishers.

U.S. Department of Health and Human Services. (2002). *Healthy People 2010* (2nd ed.). U.S. Government Printing Office.

U.S. Department of Health and Human Services. (2009). *Healthy People 2020*. http://www.healthypeople.gov/2020/about/DOHAbout.aspx

U.S. Department of Health and Human Services. (2020a). *Determinants of health*. https://health.gov/healthypeople/objectives-and-data/browse-objectives/economic-stability#cit1

U.S. Department of Health and Human Services. (2020b). *Education access and quality*. https://health.gov/healthypeople/objectives-and-data/browse-objectives/education-access-and-quality

U.S. Department of Health and Human Services. (2020c). *Health care access and quality*. https://health.gov/healthypeople/objectives-and-data/browse-objectives/health-care-access-and-quality#cit1

U.S. Department of Health and Human Services. (2020d). *Neighborhoods and environments*. https://health.gov/healthypeople/objectives-and-data/browse-objectives/neighborhood-and-built-environment

U.S. Department of Health and Human Services. (2020e). *Social and community context*. https://health.gov/healthypeople/objectives-and-data/browse-objectives/social-and-community-context

Wilkinson, R., & Marmot, M. (2003). *The solid facts: Social determinants of health*. Center for Urban Health, World Health Organization. http://www.euro.who.int/__data/assets/pdf_file/0005/98438/e81384.pdf

Winslow, C. E. A. (1920). The untilled field of public health. *Modern Medicine, 2*, 183–191. https://doi.org/ 10.1126/science.51.1306.23

World Health Organization, & Commission on Social Determinants of Health. (2008). *Closing the gap in a generation: Health equity through action on the social determinants of health*. Final Report of the Commission on Social Determinants of Health. World Health Organization.

FOURTEEN

EVALUATION OF HEALTH POLICY: FROM PROBLEM TO PRACTICE

Joyce L. Batcheller, Peggy L. Landrum,
Nancy Manning Crider, and Patricia S. Yoder-Wise

> *"(Nurses) must engage in the policymaking process to ensure that the changes they believe in are realized ... [and] ... envision themselves as leaders in the process" [and seek out new partners to share their goals].*
> —*The Future of Nursing: Leading Change, Advancing Health,*
> Institute of Medicine 2011, p. 246

INTRODUCTION

Evaluating policy is a complex process, beginning with the inception of an idea or a concern all the way through the implementation and reevaluation. Policy evaluation, by its very nature, is a rather drawn-out process. For example, seldom do policies reflect actual practice. In a large part, this is due to the more rapid advancement of knowledge as opposed to what many view as a sluggish policy process. To be effective, however, policy must be built on science and ethics. Because the process of developing the policy is typically a political one, not every policy reflects the best scientific thinking, nor the best tests of ethics. The intent is always to develop the most effective policy the political process can tolerate. This chapter discusses two key elements of evaluating policy—the policy itself and the process of creating the policy.

People, including nurses, evaluate policy all of the time. As an example, nurses say they hate some policies because they always have to do a work-around to provide needed care. Or nurses say they think another policy truly promotes equitable health care because of how patients are admitted to a hospital in emergent situations. That casual level of evaluation, however, is insufficient if policy needs to be examined for its effectiveness or if the process of creating policy at the organizational, community, or governmental levels needs to be evaluated to determine whether the process inhibits or facilitates policy development.

As noted in the introduction, both elements of policy evaluation (the policy itself and the policy process) are equally important. Without a clear policy, a statement of what is expected, being engaged in the policy process would be ineffective.

Similarly, without a clear perspective of the process, nurses can expend a great deal of energy on a policy statement without success.

Policy often is the result of the intersection of practice, research, and education. When something doesn't work well for patients or colleagues, we become concerned about the current approach. We look to research to determine what the latest findings are, and we then educate ourselves and others about the discrepancy between what is and what should be. In some cases, that gap is wide because no policy currently exists; in other cases, the gap is narrow because only a small adjustment to an existing policy needs to be made.

In addition to ranking at the top of the annual Gallup poll (2020) about trusted professions, nurses also were cited in a study conducted in 2019, which was sponsored by the Commonwealth Fund, the *New York Times*, and Harvard University's T.H. Chan School of Public Health (2019). The polling group was asked what group they trusted most to fix the existing health care insurance issue. Overwhelmingly, nurses were seen as the *only* group to be trusted to fix the crisis. Consistently, nurses were listed as the first (most preferred) in the various subcategories. Nurses were almost twice as likely to be seen as preferred to the second group—physicians. Again, in 2020, NursesEverywhere commissioned a study by the Harris poll to investigate the public's view of nurses and several key issues that were dramatically highlighted during the COVID-19 pandemic. This poll of more than 2,000 adults found the following: People believed they should be able to receive the same level of care postpandemic as they received during the pandemic; 91% said that hospitals should be required to meet minimum safe staffing standards (90% said the same for nursing facilities); and 75% believed nurses should be able to treat patients via telehealth (NursesEverywhere, 2020). In short, the public expects that we will also fix the policy issues about their care.

WHAT IS POLICY?

Nurses typically are concerned with three types of policy: public policy, health policy, and employment policy. The first is broad-reaching and is often enacted for reasons other than direct health benefits. An example of public policy might be policies regulating utilities. Such policies aren't addressed because they do not affect health directly, but public utilities definitely provide better living conditions that support better health. The second type of health policy includes policies with which we are most familiar because people's health is directly affected by them. An example might be policies related to immunizations for individuals and populations. These policies are based on science related to health and are designed to provide better conditions for a healthy life. The third type of policy relates to fair treatment in employment settings. An example of those might be the protections against discrimination. These policies also contribute to health, in this case the psychological or physical health of employees. Each of these policy types affects nurses and patients although some are more direct and have a greater impact than others.

Policy can be defined as "a consciously chosen course of action: a law, regulation, rule, procedure, administrative action, incentive or voluntary practice of governments and other institutions" (Milstead & Short, 2019, p. 3). This definition is presented in descending order in relation to the weight of the policy. Laws, for example, if broken have specified consequences and in health care might lead to loss of licensure. On the other end of the spectrum of policies is the incentive or voluntary practice where norms and peer pressure push for compliance, but other than social sanctions, the violation of those has few dramatic repercussions.

NURSES' ROLES IN HEALTH POLICY

Nurses have a professional responsibility to be involved in policy-making, especially at the state and federal levels. Frontline caregivers are advocates for patients and families they care for every day. They have ideas on how to prevent readmissions, decrease costs, and improve quality and access to care. While many organizations create workplaces conducive to engaging staff, such as having shared governance structures and processes, that is not enough. The Institute of Medicine's (IOM) *Future of Nursing: Leading Change, Advancing Health* report (2011) cites the importance of nurses being involved in the policy-making process to ensure that changes they believe in are actually realized. Nurses are leaders at all levels and need to develop the skills to lead policy changes. This may be done at an organizational, a local, a state, or a national level.

Several nurses have served in major policy roles. Perhaps most prominently, three nurse members of the 111th Congress (Eddie Bernice Johnson [D-TX], Lois Capps [D-CA], and Carolyn McCarthy [D-NY]) were instrumental in sponsoring and supporting health care legislation related to acquired immunodeficiency syndrome (AIDS) research and gun control. More recently, Representative Lauren Underwood (D-IL) has been influential on many pieces of health-related legislation, both as a nurse and as an individual with a chronic health condition. Other examples include State Senator Paula Hollinger of Maryland, who successfully sponsored one of the nation's first stem cell research bills, and the appointment of Rear Admiral (RADM) Sylvia Trent Adams as Acting Surgeon General of the United States and Lieutenant General Dorothy Hogg as the first nurse to fill the Surgeon General role in the United States Air Force. Additionally, Dr. Mary Wakefield has had an illustrious career at the federal level where she ultimately served as U.S. Deputy Secretary of Health and Human Services. No matter where these nurses served, they were involved in positions that developed policy and had accountability for policy—either implementing it as it was or advocating for changing the policy. Unfortunately, nurses have not made many inroads over the past two decades into politics and policy work (Rasheed et al., 2020).

Although several other nurses have been engaged in running for office, supporting candidates, advocating for legislation, and working on policy, the real educational emphasis of this role is vested in the graduates of doctor of nursing practice (DNP) programs. The American Association of Colleges of Nursing (AACN) has advocated for involvement in policy since its adoption of the *Essentials of Doctoral Education for Advanced Nursing Practice* (AACN, 2006). DNP graduates are expected to design and implement policies that promote access to health care that is safe, timely, effective, and equitable (IOM, 2011). In the new *The Essentials: Core Competencies for Professional Nursing Education* (AACN, 2021), health policy is identified as a featured concept that is evident in many of the domains. It defines *health policy as* involving goal directed decision-making about health that is the result of an authorized public decision-making process (Keller & Ridenour, 2021).

It represents an important aspect of advocacy for patients and for the profession by speaking with a united voice on policy issues that affect nursing practice and health outcomes. Nurses can have a profound influence on health policy by becoming engaged in the policy process on multiple levels; they must be prepared to interpret, evaluate, and lead policy change (AACN, 2021, p. 15). The terms "health policy" and "policy" are found abundantly across domains and competencies in the new 2021 Essentials.

The intent of DNP programs related to policy is to prepare graduates to proactively participate in the development, implementation, and evaluation of health policy at all levels, ranging from institution to local, state, regional, federal, and international levels (IOM, 2011). An example of the impact of federal legislation on health care can be found in Box 14.1, the 2010 Patient Protection and Affordable Care Act (ACA; 2010). This legislation remains highly relevant to nurses because it often is the source of support for many vulnerable patients with whom we interact on a regular basis. Further, because laws, as an example, seldom provide sufficient information to be practical, nurses, including DNP-prepared nurses, have the opportunity and obligation to participate in the development of rules and regulations that allow for the practical implementation of the law.

One set of laws and resultant rules and regulations that DNP graduates frequently engage with are those governing the practice of nursing. The current approach to regulating advanced practice relies heavily on the expectations of the various specialties. Add to that perspective the variations among states regarding what authority nurses in advanced practice roles have, we can easily see why we must monitor what is happening with the Nurse Practice Act in each state. During the early phases of the COVID-19 pandemic in 2020, for example, governors quickly created emergency orders to expand what this group—and others—could

---

BOX 14.1   Patient Protection and Affordable Care Act of 2010

Advanced practice nurses were actively involved with the passage of the landmark Patient Protection and Affordable Care Act of 2010 (ACA) legislation and spent countless hours preparing policy briefs and providing testimony to key stakeholders and decision-makers. The passage of the ACA in 2010 provided access to health care coverage to millions of U.S. citizens who had previously been ineligible due to the high cost of insurance, limited benefit packages, and pre-existing conditions. In addition to access to care, the ACA also addressed quality of care, cost of care, and the health care workforce (ANA, 2010; National Conference of State Legislatures [NCSL], 2011).

While the ACA mandated an essential benefit package and access to care, much of the implementation was left to the states. Among the major decisions left to the states was the decision to expand Medicaid programs to low-income populations with monetary assistance from the federal government or retain state control and defer the financial incentive. Other decisions related to the creation of high-risk pools and state-run health benefit exchanges (NCSL, 2011).

Since its passage in 2010, there have been many attempts to repeal the ACA. With each challenge DNP-prepared nurses have worked individually and in collaboration with multiple professional organizations and key stakeholders to protect vulnerable populations and educate the public and decision-makers how advanced practice registered nurses (APRNs) including nurse practitioners, clinical nurse specialists, certified nurse midwives, and certified registered nurse anesthetists are prepared to help provide affordable care for all (ANA, 2010). In 2016, the American Nurses Association (ANA) developed *Principles for Health System Transformation 2016* (ANA, 2016).

do in order to mount a more effective response. These emergency orders change the landscape of nursing practice.

EVALUATION AND OUTCOME FOCUS OF HEALTH POLICY

Nurses have the expertise and experience to make a difference in health policy. This begins with nurses being prepared to use the nursing process, the systematic guide to client-centered care. Irrespective of the specific nursing process model used, the process always starts with assessment and ends with evaluation. It typically includes the following five sequential steps: assessment, diagnosis, planning, implementation, and evaluation (American Nurses Association [ANA], 2020).

By following this process, nurses are well positioned to identify needed changes and strategies for closing gaps they may find in patient populations and in their communities. The last step is an essential part of the nursing process—evaluating and analyzing the effectiveness of care. Nurses are outcome-focused, build relationships with key stakeholders, and communicate what changes may be needed. Undergirding all of what nurses do is how to think critically about the effectiveness of the plan of care to be able to make changes as needed. This kind of knowledge and experience in health care positions nurses to lead health policy changes effectively.

In addition, nurses are well positioned to build relationships especially with new partners from the community. Their communication skills and ability to assess both verbal and nonverbal communication are invaluable. For example, many nurses have enhanced their communication skills through the use of standardized communication tools such as the Situation–Background–Assessment–Recommendations (SBAR) tool. This tool is commonly used by nurses to frame a conversation, especially in critical situations, which requires a clinician's immediate attention and action. Many leaders find this framework to be useful in just about any conversation, including those related to policy (Institute for Healthcare Improvement, 2017). Being able to communicate clearly is an essential attribute of someone engaged in policy. Policies are often complex, and often the process is, too. The "glue" that holds the work together and allows for advancement of a policy is the ability to communicate clearly.

SPECIFIC POLICY ANALYSIS

One of the more common frameworks for analyzing a policy is that of the Centers for Disease Control and Prevention (CDC, 2018). Specifically, Domains 1 and 2 apply to the policy itself (see Figure 14.1). Domain 1 relates to identifying the problem or issue. This may be a proactive step, as in considering a new policy, to address an issue for which no policy exists. At the microlevel of policy analysis, we saw this happening regularly during the COVID-19 pandemic when little was known about the disease, how it was spread, how to treat it, or what care was to be provided. Nurse leaders in health care organizations found their days overtaken by creating policies and rewriting them, sometimes within a matter of hours due to emerging information. The problem or issue identification may also be retrospective, for example, when a policy exists and is not achieving the desired results. An example of this might be seen in the changes to rules and regulations associated with the ACA. Policies were put in place to implement the law, and as they were tested, some were determined to be

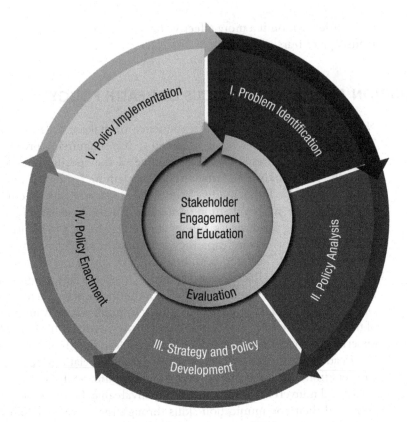

Figure 14.1 Centers for Disease Control and Prevention policy process (2018).

Source: Centers for Disease Control and Prevention. (2018). *The CDC policy process model.* Retrieved April 11, 2020, from https://www.cdc.gov/policy/polaris/training/policy-cdc-policy-process.html

ineffective. The response to the existing policies was to modify, create a new one, or provide new avenues for implementing the intent of the policy. Another example is when volte-face (a policy reversal) occurs. This is most commonly seen by legislators who took a position for or against a position and then, typically over time and after intervening variables, reversed their position to the opposite view. This reversal may precipitate a whole new view of what the policy should now be.

Domain 2 involves identifying and describing policy options. This step is based on how best to address the issue identified in Domain 1. This process requires several activities with which nurses are actively engaged. For example, DNP graduates commonly addressed an issue in their educational program in which they are interested and developed an extensive review of the literature. Although this review may relate to only one element or one discipline or one phase of the identified problem, that information is useful to a legislative staff as they create positions for the legislators. Additionally, much of that work or our own practice experiences relate to identifying best practices. DNP graduates can become the local resource for various issues. For example, a policy being developed might look appropriate to a legislator who represents a district with both large urban and rural populations. Knowing how a particular viewpoint might affect care differently in those two populations is invaluable information in forming the policy and the legislator's position.

As nurses engage in the direct work of the policy itself, they need to consider some key steps in the process. One of the steps most critical to what the policy should be or whether nurses should support a particular policy is the filter of a nursing ethical perspective (Yoder-Wise, 2019). Specifically, Provision 9 of the ANA Code of Ethics states that the nursing profession should maintain the profession's integrity, describe professional values, and integrate into health policy and nursing practice and the principles of social justice (ANA, 2015). If we are unable to see how a particular policy meets those expectations, why would we support it? At this point, nurses need to recall that a lot of policy is developed in an incremental manner. In other words, it might not meet our expectations of fully articulating nursing values, yet the wording more closely approximates those values than a prior stance. The enactment of the ACA, as an example, is a platform on which to advance additional policy changes to address elements that haven't worked in the past. The development of a policy statement relies heavily on exquisite and precise communication to be as clear as possible about what the desired action is—unless, of course, the intent of the policy is to obfuscate the full potential. Then, the policy may be written in ambiguous terms and clarified through the far less rigorous work of creating rules and regulations or procedures.

A specific strategy commonly used in creating a policy statement is the Overton window (Overton, 2013). Simply stated, this "window" represents the point where the majority of a group of voters (e.g., legislators) will support something. The ideas or policy statements range from radical to very radical (worst/best; most costly/least costly; most freedom/least freedom). Somewhere midway in the range of possibilities is the idea that likely can become policy. If that idea can't be proposed, the idea is to move to something that is popular or sensible or at least acceptable. Getting to an ideal policy is a major challenge, so voters often look for what would seem to be popular or sensible. They aren't usually happy with an acceptable policy, but they definitely don't want a radical idea (from the individual's or party's perspective) adopted. Additionally, because none of us is only one thing (e.g., nurse), we are influenced by our other views on life (e.g., gender, religion, age, or social status). Thus, something that might seem an absolutely reasonable policy may be equally opposed by another nurse who understands our view, but is driven by a value different from nursing. This is why a policy process is so critical.

SYSTEM MODELS FOR POLICY ANALYSIS

Policy models are built to provide information to policy-makers who are trying to develop policies intended to solve real-world problems, usually for a future situation. Models provide information that can help policy-makers select knowledgeable choices among policy options. A system model is developed to provide the policy-maker(s) and other stakeholders with information about the way the system works presently and to explore the possible consequences of implementing different policies under different future circumstances, which is usually impossible to test in a real situation (Milstead & Short, 2019). Three models are presented here to assist readers in valuing the complexity of the process.

The Centers for Disease Control and Prevention Model

The CDC developed a policy process to enable common language and understanding (https://www.cdc.gov/policy/polaris/training/policy-cdc-policy-process.html).

It includes five specific domains: problem identification, policy analysis, policy development, policy enactment, and policy implementation (see Figure 14.1). Stakeholder engagement and education and evaluation are two main themes that are interwoven within the five domains.

Domain Descriptors. Problem identification focuses on clarifying a problem or an issue using data to correctly frame the problem or issue. Policy analysis includes a literature review and environmental scan to explore potential options that may be needed to determine the most effective, efficient, and feasible options. Once this is completed, a strategy needs to be developed to ensure the policy will be adopted. This includes identification of federal guidelines and regulations or standards that are needed. Identification of key stakeholders both for and against a proposal is needed. Different strategies to influence their perspectives need to be developed. The enactment phase is where ongoing monitoring of the policy occurs. Last, the policy implementation phase includes the steps needed to enact the policy, monitor uptake, and ensure full implementation (CDC, 2012; see Exhibit 14.1). Although each of the domains can take time and resources, the key work from the standpoint

---

Exhibit 14.1

CDC Domain Descriptions

From: *Overview of CDC's policy process.* (2012).

https://www.cdc.gov/policy/analysis/process/docs/CDCPolicyProcess.pdf

Domain 1: Problem Identification

- Collect, summarize, and interpret information relevant to a problem or an issue (e.g., nature of the problem and causes of the problem).
- Define the characteristics (e.g., frequency, severity, scope, and economic and budgetary impacts) of the problem or issue.
- Describe the characteristics of who the problem or issue affects (e.g., age, race/ethnicity, gender, socioeconomic status, education level).
- Determine whether there are gaps in the data or if there are areas in need of more information.
- Frame the problem or issue in a way that is factual and easy for the audience to understand.

Domain 2: Policy Analysis

- Research and identify policy options by conducting an environmental scan and engaging stakeholders.
- Describe (a) the health impact of the policy (morbidity and mortality), (b) the costs to implement the policy and how the costs compare with the benefits (economic and budgetary impacts), and (c) the political and operational factors associated with adoption and implementation (feasibility).
- Assess and prioritize policy options.

Domain 3: Strategy and Policy Development

- Follow internal or external procedures for getting policy enacted or passed.
- Define strategy for engaging stakeholders and policy actors.

Domain 4: Policy Enactment

- Enact laws, regulations, procedures, administrative actions, incentives, or voluntary practice.

(continued)

Exhibit 14.1
CDC Domain Descriptions (continued)

Domain 5: Policy Implementation

- Translate policy into practice and define standards for implementation.
- Implement regulations, guidelines, recommendations, directives, and organizational policies.
- Identify indicators and metrics to evaluate the implementation and impact of the policy.
- Coordinate resources and train personnel to implement policy.
- Assess implementation and ensure compliance with policy.
- Support postimplementation sustainability of policy.

Overarching domains: The following two activities should be considered throughout each of the five domains.

1. Stakeholder Engagement and Education

- Identify key stakeholders, including supporters and opponents.
- Assess relevant characteristics (i.e., knowledge, attitudes, and needs).
- Implement communication strategies and deliver relevant messages and material.
- Solicit input and gather feedback.

2. Evaluation

- Formally evaluate the appropriate steps of the policy cycle, including the impact and outcomes of the policy.
- Define evaluation needs, purpose, and intended users.
- Conduct an evaluation of prioritized questions (e.g., assess if the problem was defined in a way that prioritized action; how stakeholders were engaged, if the policy is being implemented as intended, and what the impact of the policy is).
- Disseminate evaluation results and facilitate use.

(https://www.cdc.gov/policy/analysis/process/docs/CDCPolicyProcess.pdf)

---

of evaluation of policy (as opposed to the process) is policy analysis. Typically, experts are engaged in policy analysis from their area of expertise, while major related professional associations are engaged in the broader analysis. If the policy is addressing a new issue (no current legislation addresses the issue), questions arise such as "Why do we think a policy is the answer to this issue? Does a related policy already exist? How many people would be supported by this policy? How many would be inconvenienced? Is the cost worthy of the anticipated outcome? What related evidence exists to support a particular position?"

Overarching Domains of the CDC Policy Model. Two domains should be integrated, as needed, throughout all of the domains that include (a) stakeholder engagement and education and (b) evaluation. Stakeholder engagement and education includes identification of and connection with key stakeholders, decision-makers, partners who may be affected by the policy, and the general public. Understanding what kinds of questions and potential barriers exist allows nurses to proactively address those issues. Evaluation occurs throughout the policy cycle because it is important to ensure the process, needs, purpose, and intent of the policy are clear to gain support and facilitate implementation(see Exhibit 14.1). An example of a specific policy is illustrated in Box 14.2, Preventing Readmissions for Heart Failure Patients.

BOX 14.2 Preventing Readmissions for Heart Failure Patients

Heart failure (HF) is a highly prevalent condition that affects approximately 6.5 million individuals in the United States every year. It was a contributing cause of 1 in 8 deaths in 2017 and costs the nation an estimated $30.7 billion in 2012. This number includes the cost of health care services, medications to treat, and missed number of days of work (CDC, 2019). Additionally, the prognosis for HF is poor, with more than half of the HF patients dying within 5 years of diagnosis (https://www. cdc.gov/heartdisease/heart_failure.htm).

The Centers for Medicare & Medicaid Services (CMS) developed the 30-day readmission measures to encourage hospitals and health systems to evaluate the entire continuum of care and more carefully transition patients to outpatient or other postdischarge care. The Hospital Readmission Reduction Program (HRRP) was implemented in 2012 and included an Inpatient Prospective Payment System (IPPS) for hospitals that would be penalized for excess readmissions in 30 days postdischarge (Bailey et al., 2019).

Excess readmissions are measured by a ratio, calculated by dividing a hospital's number of "predicted" 30-day readmissions for heart attack, acute myocardial infarction (AMI), HF, pneumonia, chronic obstructive pulmonary disease (COPD), total hip/knee arthroplasty (THA/TKA), and coronary artery bypass graft surgery (CABG) by the number that would be "expected," based on an average hospital with similar patients (Kilgore et al., 2017).

Policy Analysis

The business case for focusing on preventing readmissions within 30 days of discharge for HF patients is very strong. The economic burden of HF is related to a high readmission rate with almost 25% of patients being readmitted within 30 days and approximately 50% of those readmissions occurring within 2 weeks of discharge. Hospitalization and inpatient care are identified as the cost drivers of HF and accounted for 48% to 90% of the overall spending in multiple studies (Freeman et al., 2018).

This policy served as a call to action to align the care HF patients received in their community throughout the continuum with a special emphasis on preventing a readmission. The appropriateness of the transition process contributed to readmissions among Medicare beneficiaries within 30 days of discharge in approximately 20% of the cases.

Care transitions refer to the movement of patients from one health care provider or setting to another. For people living with serious and complex illnesses, transitions in setting of care (from hospital to home or nursing home, for example) are prone to errors. For example, one in five patients discharged from the hospital to home experience an adverse event within 3 weeks of discharge, when an adverse event is defined as an injury resulting from medical management rather than the underlying disease (Kilgore et al., 2017). The most common adverse events are medication related, which often can be avoided or mitigated. Since this policy was implemented, other studies found that the average cost of a HF readmission compared to the initial admission was about 30% higher for Medicaid, over 5% higher for Medicare, 11% higher for uninsured patients, and nearly 32% higher for private patients (Bailey et al., 2019).

Unfortunately, the policy does not address (a) the impact on the quality of life for the HF patients and (b) barriers they may be facing. For example, differences in access to care may exist in various communities, and being able to afford the care that is needed may be a challenge for some patients. Patients who are underinsured or uninsured often will delay seeking care or may not fill needed prescriptions if it means their families will not be able to eat. Access to care may be more challenging for patients who live in rural areas and whose job is the main source of income for their families. Additionally, demographic variables such as race, ethnicity, preferred language, and socioeconomic variables are not included when Medicare does the analysis of readmissions rates and costs.

Studies found that people with low incomes and who are representative of racial and ethnic minorities experience worse health because of inequitable social conditions. One study estimated

(continued)

SIDEBAR 14.2 **Preventing Readmissions for Heart Failure Patients (*continued*)**

---

that eliminating racial/ethnic health disparities would reduce health care costs by $230 billion and indirect costs of excess disease and mortality by more than $1 trillion over four years (Braveman et al., 2019). Inequities in health care—such as lack of health insurance, unaffordable medical expenses, and structural racism in health care—create disparities in care and make the system more costly and less effective. Health care providers and health care systems must play a major role in advancing health equity to prevent needless suffering, premature deaths, and avoidable costs.

Policy Enhancements Needed

Payments for telehealth visits should be included so that HF patients can be managed from home and thus avoid missing work. During the COVID 19 pandemic, telehealth emerged as a strategy of choice in an effort to reduce the exposure of people to settings, such as emergency departments and clinics, where contamination was more likely. While the technology was established quickly and many people took advantage of this approach, the financial mechanism for provider payment lagged. This care management can be provided by advanced practice registered nurses (APRNs) as well as registered nurses (RNs) who are working to their full extent by licensure law. The effectiveness of this strategy in terms of decreasing costs and the number of hospital visits each year and preventing readmissions would need to be studied. Nurse-managed HF clinics can provide care management on an outpatient basis for patients who have more advanced HF. The nurses can provide patients and families with knowledge and support, manage symptoms through close monitoring of weight and other essential metrics, adjust medications, and refer patients as needed if symptoms worsen. Employers of large groups of workers could offer onsite telehealth services and provide some kind of incentive to employees who utilize the telehealth services and complete the follow-up care that is needed.

When HF patients are classified as having more advanced stages of the disease, another important addition to this policy could be a requirement that palliative/supportive care be discussed with patients and their families. *Palliative care*, also increasingly known as *supportive care*, may be one of the most misunderstood terms in health care. Many people believe it's the same as hospice care and it means the end of life. Palliative care, however, is different from hospice care, and when put in place, palliative care can potentially bring hope, control, and a chance at a better quality of life for seriously ill patients and their caregivers (Family Caregiver Alliance, 2016). Supportive care is a collaborative, interdisciplinary team approach that may be comprised of the following kinds of professionals: RNs, physicians, social workers, chaplains, dieticians, pharmacists, and licensed mental health professionals. Some teams also include music therapists, massage therapists, and other holistic care providers. Most insurance companies provide coverage for palliative/supportive care. While this may seem to be a sensitive issue, the individuals who provide this kind of care have completed special training, so discussions about advance directives and power of attorney can be done in a very caring manner. The idea of Advanced Directives and Medical Power of Attorney experienced a surge in importance when the COVID-19 pandemic occurred in the United States in 2020. As a result, people had the opportunity to become aware of the spectrum of care for people with advanced stages of illness, including HF.

Culture of Health Implications

The Robert Wood Johnson Foundation has advocated to build a culture of health for several years. It specifically focused on scalable solutions that can begin in a targeted, local community. Its action framework includes ten underlying principles (see Figure 14.2). The framework consists of four action areas and a fifth area on outcomes. The overall goal is for all individuals to reach their full health potential by eliminating health disparities. It challenges us to think of incentives that can be used to promote individual health and engage investors and leaders within organizations, communities, or policy changes that are needed to promote health and well-being. One example is to have incentives to provide workplace wellness programs and invest in employee health. A second is to include investors to finance health and well-being and for individuals to be incentivized to make behavior changes that will improve overall health. These principles need to redirect our thinking from a disease or a setting to the wholeness of care.

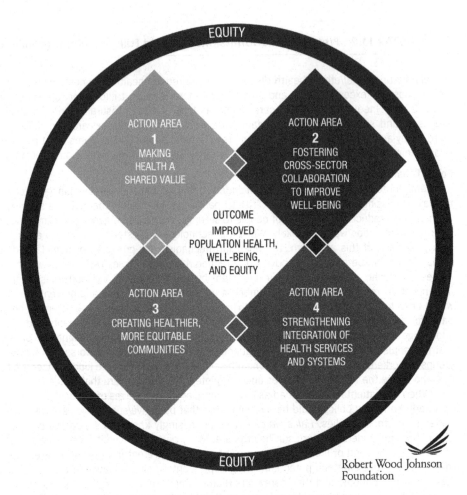

Figure 14.2 The Culture of Health Action Framework (2018).

Source: Robert Wood Johnson Foundation. (2020). Culture of health action framework. https://www.evidenceforaction.org/what-culture-health

THE FRAMEWORK FOR PLANNED POLICY CHANGE

The Framework for Planned Policy Change (Yoder-Wise, 2019) builds on several policy development models, but primarily on the Policy Circle Model (Hardee et al., 2004). The Framework for Planned Policy Change is applicable to any setting in which policy is developed, from clinical settings to governmental institutions. Each of the nine steps comprising the framework is important to address to increase the odds of success in promoting adoption of a policy. However, the steps are not always sequential. Also, some steps may need attention more than once; flexibility is important in the policy arena as in other areas.

The steps of the framework provide a guide for moving through the development of a policy. Once an individual or a group of individuals identify a need for change, the possibility for policy development or modification is established. Key stakeholders must be identified at an early stage to promote meaningful

TABLE 14.1   The Framework for Planned Policy Change

Steps/Components	Action
1. Precipitator	Identify events that cause experience of distress
2. Critical point	Understand magnitude, intensity, duration, or urgency that moves precipitator to greater prominence
3. Assessing	Determine further action and engage stakeholders
4. Planning	Consider multiple factors to choose the most appropriate approach to resolving the issue or restrategizing to take additional steps
5. Detailing	Identify and create consensus around tactics of promoting the policy
6. Monitoring	Determine status of policy and of stakeholder's continued support
7. Adopting/celebrating	Recognize accomplishments by supporters to encourage continued enthusiasm and energy by supporters
8. Implementing, monitoring, and refocusing	Ensure the policy is enacted as intended and determine any necessary adjustments
9. Evaluating	Review success of the policy, effectiveness of the process, and further actions

Source: Adapted from Yoder-Wise, P. S. (2019). A framework for planned policy change. Nursing Forum, 55(1), 45–53. https://doi.org/10.1111/nuf.12381

collaboration. As the precipitating event or situation reaches a critical point, it is crucial to assess assorted relevant variables in order to recommend and begin planning for further action. Including both broad and specific perspectives in planning will expand the scope of involvement and thus influence. Details matter and must be considered (e.g., cost, engagement, relevance, connections). As the appropriate policy action is determined and taken, monitoring the progress will help determine what further modifications may be needed. Finally, recognizing and celebrating policy adoption energizes the team, including stakeholders. Evaluating outcomes reveals impact, unintended consequences, and possible future actions. Table 14.1 summarizes these steps.

EVIDENCE-INFORMED HEALTH POLICY MODEL

In the clinical setting, evidence-based practice (EBP) models provide a mechanism for incorporating research findings into clinical nursing care. Actual evidence is used to create models of care that address clinical problems, thus improving both effectiveness and safety of patient care. The PICOT question format provides a structure for designing a solid clinical question that can be researched and answered, serving as a guide to find evidence (Melnyk & Fineout-Overholt, 2018). The PICOT acronym represents the elements of the guiding question: What is the Patient population; what is the Intervention; how does the intervention Compare to the status quo; what is the Outcome of interest; and what is the Time frame if applicable (Loversidge, 2016).

Evidence is also a significant factor when addressing health policy problems (Loversidge, 2016). Health policy development is a complex affair, whether at the level of a heath care organization or in a governmental legislative setting, and it can affect many aspects of consumer health, including safety and quality care. The complicated nonlinear process by which policy is developed means that informing policy with evidence can be quite a challenge (Morgan, 2010). However, evidence used in support of the policy can, at the very least, help to raise questions/doubts and, at best, can be compelling enough to persuade stakeholders. Ultimately, when evidence is used to inform policy-making, it is most effective in influencing and guiding discussion (Campbell et al., 2009).

In the Evidence-Informed Health Policy Model, Loversidge (2016) showed how an EBP model can be adapted to use evidence to influence the development of a forthcoming policy or critically review an existing one. When addressing a policy issue rather than a clinically based patient care problem, the traditional PICOT question must be adapted. When applied to policy, the elements of the guiding question are modified as follows: a consumer population replaces "patient"; a policy development or revision serves as the "intervention"; an existing condition, or status quo, provides the point of "comparison"; and the expected effect of the policy change represents the "outcome." Table 14.2 summarizes this model.

EVALUATING THE PROCESS OF NURSING MODELS

Evaluating the process of policy-making, that is, how each component or step evolves and is enacted, provides the areas of interest. The approach to evaluating the policy process presented here is based on both the Framework for Planned

TABLE 14.2 The Evidence-Informed Health Policy Model

Step	Rationale
0. Cultivate spirit of inquiry	Encourages receptiveness to policy initiatives
1. Ask policy question—PICOT format	Facilitates presentation of issue in a succinct relevant way
2. Collect relevant best evidence	Informs policy dialogue
3. Critically appraise evidence	Legitimizes basis for policy development and ultimate adoption
4. Integrate evidence, issue expertise, and stakeholder values and ethics	Allows most diverse and inclusive justification for policy
5. Contribute to health policy development and implementation process	Capitalizes on professional expertise to advocate for policy
6. Frame policy change for dissemination to affected population	Engage in promoting awareness of policy/influencing
7. Evaluate effectiveness of policy change and disseminate findings	Assess impact and determine effectiveness of policy and identify needed revisions

Source: Adapted from Steps of Evidence-Informed Health Policy Model: Loversidge, J. M. (2016). An evidence-informed health policy model: Adapting evidence-based practice for nursing education and regulation. *Journal of Nursing Regulation, 7*(2), 27–33. https://doi.org/10.1016/S2155-8256(16)31075-4.

Policy Change (Yoder-Wise, 2019) and the Evidence-Informed Health Policy Model (Loversidge, 2016). Both models address critical elements of the policy process that can be considered when evaluating the overall progression, from identified deficit or need to outcomes and "what comes next." The components of this approach are relevant in any setting, from small organizations to health policies that affect entire nations. The following six areas of policy process evaluation will help to determine both successes and challenges, thus informing future work in the same and/or related policy arenas.

Articulated Need

Was the need to originate, modify, or end a policy clearly articulated? Typically, a problem or an opportunity prompts the beginnings of a policy development or change process. Yoder-Wise (2019) referred to this as a precipitator, something that triggers action. Something prompted someone or a group of people to take action to change the status quo. Precipitators can escalate into critical points, in which case they are more likely to gain traction with stakeholders. However, if the need to change was not convincing to a broad range of stakeholders, then the policy likely was compromised from its inception. Likewise, if the proposed action, or policy, is not consistent with professional values, gaining traction would be improbable.

Was the appropriate decision made regarding the action to take? In some cases, a theoretically appropriate policy is already in place, but regulatory guidelines have not been established, or funding for implementation is inadequate. In these cases, perhaps a focus on garnering resources to support the existing policy components is more suitable than creating yet another policy.

Was the need for a change, as well as the recommended change itself, presented in a clear and logical way, and specifically was the benefit to the consumer obvious (Loversidge, 2016)? A PICOT format ensures that key components of the policy problem are concisely stated: who is affected, action requested by the policy, current state of affairs, and expected outcome following enactment. Combining these elements in one statement helps to identify the basic meaning of the policy as well as what effect is expected. Perhaps the most significant is that the benefit to the consumer can clearly be shown (Loversidge, 2016).

Assessed Evidence and Support

Was the evidence gathered to support the need for a change both relevant and thorough, and was it critically appraised? Data may be considered internal, such as the organization or the political component (e.g., city, state, and nation) in which the policy would apply. External sources of data may be other organizations, or different political components (e.g., other cities, states, and nations). Data may also come from a number of sources, including the literature and issue experts. If evidence intended to support the need for change is of poor quality or is irrelevant, the policy dialogue suffers and the risk of ineffective decision-making is high (Loversidge, 2016).

Was the evidence clear enough to be convincing to key stakeholders, those individuals who align around a strong belief in the need for change? Before individuals can commit to bringing about change, they first must be clear about the current state, or the status quo. Otherwise, it is impossible to identify and understand what is needed and to move forward with purpose (Yoder-Wise, 2019).

Were the appropriate stakeholders engaged? At least a portion of stakeholders must have influence in the system. If stakeholders are to sustain support for a project, their values must align with the ethical underpinnings of the policy development team (Loversidge, 2016; Yoder-Wise, 2019).

Was the political climate of the organization or legislative body assessed? The perspectives of organizational or legislative decision-makers will determine how policy issues are framed. A particular policy may be expected to result in both cost-effectiveness and improved access to health care, but one may be emphasized more than the other in order to better appeal to those in charge (Yoder-Wise, 2019).

Were both unintended and unavoidable consequences considered? Unintended consequences may occur even with very thorough planning. The sooner they are recognized, the more quickly they can be addressed and the lower the political cost. Unavoidable consequences are those that accompany the expected outcomes of the policy but cannot be changed (Yoder-Wise, 2019). The policy team, including stakeholders, should have identified whatever unavoidable consequences will be created and be prepared to address them, including rationale for acceptability.

Prepared Policy Statement

Was a clear decision made to move ahead? What was considered in the decision? To ensure effective work, the policy team would have decided on several issues before moving forward. The issues of concern may be addressed by either informal or more formal action. Attempts may be made to change the culture toward informally adopting specific behaviors, or based on the evidence gathered, a formal policy may be deemed appropriate. Discussions of realistic desired outcomes will assist in decision-making to move forward, maintain the status quo, or restrategize to improve the likelihood of success (Yoder-Wise, 2019).

Were individuals with differing views involved in making key decisions about the policy? Both "sides" of an issue must be represented in the preparation stage of policy development. Individuals in positions of power will hold varying views of what is most relevant about this policy, as will stakeholders. Diverse views are very useful for framing the policy to better appeal to various factions. A single policy may effectively serve the goals of different groups, both stakeholders and authority groups, but both factions must be convinced. Having considered multiple views will help the policy team as they determine realistic outcomes as well as the most effective framing for the policy (Yoder-Wise, 2019).

During preparation, were stakeholders presented with multiple perspectives? As the actual policy is being formed, consideration of broad perspectives is important. Typically, the developers have a specific irritant (precipitator) that has rallied a group of people. Thus, the specific situation is already primary. A diverse group of stakeholders increases the network of connections, which means greater exposure to the ultimate decision-makers. Some stakeholders will care about one outcome, while others will only be convinced to invest because of a different outcome.

Did the preparation include identification of specific tactics to be used moving forward, including very intentional wording of the policy? A sponsor will be needed. In the governmental arena, the sponsor would be a legislator; for organizational policy, someone with authority or with issue expertise should be sought to sponsor the policy (Loversidge, 2016). Choosing a sponsor is critical and should be based on specific and detailed considerations (Yoder-Wise, 2019). Determining realistic estimates of the cost of preparing and implementing the policy will improve the tactics for framing the policy to stakeholders, who need to be as informed as possible.

Nurses are almost always stakeholders in health-related policies, whether in legislative or in health care organizational settings. They may be instrumental in initiating an exploration of possibilities for change, or they may be content experts, or they may be advocates for personnel and/or patients—or they may be in all three roles. Nurses are often very effective at demonstrating clearly that a change is needed. Regardless of role, it is critical that nurses provide their expertise to the policy process, including evaluation (Loversidge, 2016).

Monitored Progress

Were the status and progress of the policy monitored throughout the process? Monitoring allows the developers of the policy to understand who is talking to whom about the pros and cons of the policy, either in legislative circles or in the organization. Consequently, modifications can be made if necessary and the policy can be reframed appropriately for those who would be affected by the policy. Stakeholders can be updated on the new or modified policy and as any additional information becomes available. Even if no modifications are necessary, stakeholders need ongoing support so that interest and energy does not wane. As issue experts, nurses are often well positioned to provide this support, in both the form of information and actual stories that bring life to the issues (Loversidge, 2016; Yoder-Wise, 2019).

Were outcomes clearly stated so that the policy team knew exactly what to monitor? This is the point at which additional and/or unintentional consequences may have been identified and addressed, with both stakeholders and decision-makers. If extreme opposition to the policy has arisen, a decision may be made to terminate the policy process.

Determined Outcomes

Once the policy is adopted, was the implementation process monitored? A policy can be adopted, but not implemented if the appropriate regulations and procedures are not also in place. It could be partially implemented, without achieving the expected outcomes that were the drivers for developing the policy from the beginning of the project. Possibilities for action toward further implementation of the policy and/or to refocus the policy can be explored by the policy team with input from stakeholders.

Were the successes, challenges, and unintended consequences identified and explored? Most policies are not developed in isolation but rather are part of a larger vision. Likely, related policy action will be taken in the future. What would the team do differently? What additional stakeholders and perspectives would be helpful? Even if this policy was not adopted, understanding as much detail as possible about the process of moving the policy forward can inform future related work on the same or related issues. Clear articulation of successes, both within the team and to the stakeholders at large, both will serve as an affirmation and will be energizing for future work (Yoder-Wise, 2019).

Were the outcomes of policy implementation evaluated and was that information disseminated? The policy team, stakeholders, and consumers care about the differences the policy will make for whatever conditions it addresses. The important point of comparison is the analysis of the changes brought about by the new policy as compared to the activities and outcomes of the prior policy. Do the outcomes of this policy implementation result in improvement (Loversidge, 2016)? Understanding the impact of the policy informs future endeavors. Dissemination of information about the policy and the outcomes is essential. Consumers must be informed about implications of the policy in order to fully realize its benefits (Loversidge, 2016).

Created Future Cycle

Was a plan created for continuing the work that has begun? In most instances, a policy "win" is one aspect of a broader vision. Is additional work needed to ensure that procedures and/or regulations are established to support the intended outcomes of the policy? If procedures are either not in place or ignored, or if the policy is not adequately funded, then it likely will not be implemented without additional efforts. Additionally, policy updates or modifications may be necessary to address unintended consequences, and additional policies may be needed to develop related new goals.

Were additional stakeholders identified for the next phase of work? The project may benefit from greater diversity in perspective and skills. Perhaps additional content experts are needed, or more individuals who wield influence, or those skilled in public relations or fund-raising. Additions to the team can help to maintain enthusiasm and morale and should be carefully considered to expand the sphere of influence.

SUMMARY

Nurses perform the work of nursing in many venues. Few nurses work in formal policy positions at the organizational, local, state, or federal level. However, every nurse can be engaged in shaping policy and in the process of evaluating existing and proposed policies and problems that need policy attention. They can also participate in the process of evaluating the process of creating, maintaining, and changing policy. Unless nurses are engaged with policy and the process associated with it, we are limiting our potential to effect quality care.

REFERENCES

American Association of Colleges of Nursing. (2006). *The essentials of doctoral education for advanced nursing practice.* https://www.aacnnursing.org/Portals/42/DNP/DNPEssentials.pdf

American Association of Colleges of Nursing. (2021). *The essentials: Core competencies for professional nursing education.* Author. https://www.aacnnursing.org/Portals/42/AcademicNursing/pdf/Essentials-2021.pdf

American Nurses Association. (2010). *ANA issue brief, health system reform: Nursing's goal of high quality, affordable care for all.* https://www.nursingworld.org/~4ae32b/globalassets/docs/ana/health-system-reform---final--haney---6-10-10.pdf

American Nurses Association. (2015). *Code of ethics for nurses with interpretive statements.* Author. https://www.nursingworld.org/coe-view-only

American Nurses Association. (2016). *ANA's principles for health system transformation 2016.* https://www.nursingworld.org/~4afd6b/globalassets/practiceandpolicy/health-policy/principles-healthsystemtransformation.pdf

American Nurses Association. (2020). *The nursing process.* Retrieved April 5, 2020, from https://www.nursingworld.org/practice-policy/workforce/what-is-nursing/the-nursing-process/

Bailey, M. K., Weiss, A. J., Barrett, M. L., & Jiang, H. J. (2019, February). *Characteristics of 30-day all-cause hospital readmissions (2010-2016).* Retrieved April 11, 2020, from https://www.hcup-us.ahrq./reports/statbriefs/statbriefs/sb248-Hospital-Readmissions-2010-2016isp

Braveman, P., Gottlieb, L., Francis, D., Arkin, E., & Acker, J. (2019). *What can the healthcare sector do to advance health equity?* University of California San Francisco and Robert Wood Johnson Foundation. https://www.rwjf.org/en/library/research/2019/11/what-can-the-health-care-sector-do-to-advance-health-equity.html

Campbell, D. M., Redman, S., Jorm, L., Cooke, M., Zwi, A. B., & Rychetnik, L. (2009). Increasing the use of evidence in health policy: Practice and views of policy makers. *Australia and New Zealand Health Policy, 6,* 21. https://doi.org/10.1186/1743-8462-6-21

Centers for Disease Control and Prevention. (2012). *Policy analysis.* Retrieved April 11, 2020, from https://www.cdc.gov/policy/analysis/process/docs/CDCPolicyProcess.pdf

Centers for Disease Control and Prevention. (2018). *The CDC policy process model.* Retrieved April 11, 2020, from https://www.cdc.gov/policy/polaris/training/policy-cdc-policy-process.html

Centers for Disease Control and Prevention. (2019). *Facts about heart failure in the United States.* https://www.cdc.gov/heartdisease/heart_failure.htm#:~:text=About%206.5%20million%20adults%20in,in%208%20deaths%20in%202017.&text=Heart%20failure%20costs%20the%20nation,and%20missed%20days%20of%20work

Commonwealth Fund, New York Times, & Harvard School of Public Health (2019, October). *Americans' values and beliefs about national health insurance reform.* https://www.nytimes.com/2019/10/30/upshot/Survey-health-3-way-tie.html

Family Caregiver Alliance. (2016). *Understanding palliative/supportive care: What every caregiver should know.* Retrieved April 11, 2020, from https://www.caregiver.org/understanding-palliativesupportive-care-what-every-caregiver-should-know

Freeman, J. V., Tabada, G. H., Reynolds, K., Sung, S. H., Liu, T. I., Gupta, N., & Go, A. S. (2018). Contemporary procedural complications, hospitalizations, and emergency visits after catheter ablation for atrial fibrillation. *The American Journal of Cardiology, 121*(5), 602–608. https://doi.org/10.1016/j.amjcard.2017.11.034

Gallup. (2020). *Most trusted professions.* Retrieved August 30, 2020, from https://news.gallup.com/poll/274673/nurses-continue-rate-highest-honesty-ethics.aspx

Hardee, K., Feranil, I., Boerwinkle, J., & Clark, B. (2004, June). *The policy circle: A framework for analyzing the components of family planning, reproductive health, maternal health, and HIV/AIDS policies.* Policy Working Paper Series No. 11.

Institute for Healthcare Improvement. (2017). *SBAR: Situation-Background-Assessment-Recommendation.* Retrieved April, 11, 2020, from www.IHI.org

Institute of Medicine. (2011). *Future of nursing: Leading change, advancing health.* National Academies Press.

Keller, T., & Ridenour, N. (2021). Ethics. In J. Giddens (Ed.), *Concepts for nursing practice.* Elsevier.

Kilgore, M., Patel, H. K., Kielhorn, A., Maya, J. F., & Sharma, P. (2017). *Economic burden of hospitalizations of medicare beneficiaries with heart failure.* Retrieved April 11, 2020 from https://www.ncbi.nlm.nih.gov/pmc/articles/PMC5436769/

Loversidge, J. M. (2016). An evidence-informed health policy model: Adapting evidence-based practice for nursing education and regulation. *Journal of Nursing Regulation, 7*(2), 27–33. https://doi.org/10.1016/S2155-8256(16)31075-4

Melnyk, B. M., & Fineout-Overholt, E. (2018). *Evidence-based practice in nursing & healthcare: A guide to best practice* (4th ed.). Wolters Kluwer.

Milstead, J. A., & Short, N. M. (2019). *Health policy and politics: A nurse's guide.* Jones & Bartlett Learning.

Morgan, G. (2010). Evidence-based health policy: A preliminary systematic view. *Health Education Journal, 69*(1), 43–47. https://doi.org/10.1177/0017896910363328

National Conference of State Legislatures. (2011). *The Affordable Care Act: A brief summary.* https://www.ncsl.org/research/health/the-affordable-care-act-brief-summary.aspx

NursesEverywhere. (2020). Retrieved August 30, 2020, from https://www.nurseseverywhere.com/

Overton, J. P. (2013). *The Overton window. Mackinac Center for Public Policy*. Retrieved August 30, 2020, from https://www.mackinac.org/OvertonWindow

Patient Protection, & Affordable Care Act. (2010). *Public Law 111–148*. 111th Congress. An Act. Entitled the Patient Protection and Affordable Care Act. Retrieved March 23, 2010, from https://www.govinfo.gov/content/pkg/PLAW-111publ148/pdf/PLAW-111publ148.pdf

Rasheed, S. P., Younas, A., & Mehdi, F. (2020). Challenges, extent of involvement, and the impact of nurses' involvement in politics and policy making in last two decades: an integrative review. *Journal of Nursing Scholarship*, 52(4), 446–455. https://doi.org/10.1111/jnu.12567

Robert Wood Johnson Foundation. (2020). *Culture of health action framework*. Retrieved September 8, 2020, from https://www.evidenceforaction.org/what-culture-health

Yoder-Wise, P. S. (2019). A framework for planned policy change. *Nursing Forum*, 55(1), 45–53. https://doi.org/10.1111/nuf.12381

FIFTEEN

DRIVERS OF CHANGE, IMPACT, AND CHALLENGES FOR EVALUATION OF HEALTH CARE

Joanne V. Hickey and Eileen R. Giardino

Evaluation is as natural as a chef tasting vegetable soup or a basketball player watching to see if a hook shot goes through the hoop. Of course, evaluation gets more complicated when we seek to evaluate the impact of efforts of a team rather than a solitary individual, when success is harder to define than getting the ball through the hoop, when scarce resources are used to support a program.
—Emil J. Posavac (2016, p. xv)

INTRODUCTION

Evaluation includes two distinct and interrelated components, a description of performance and standards or criteria established to judge that performance (Rossi et al., 2019). The primary purpose of evaluation is to inform and support decision-making based on relevant data that are collected, organized, and analyzed according to the high standards of evaluation. The Posavac quote that frames this chapter states that health care is fundamentally a "team sport" that exists in a resource-constrained environment (Posavac, 2016). This concept is also applicable to evaluation in that evaluation requires cooperation and collaboration of several individuals working together around a common goal.

Evaluation models, unlike models in other areas, often lack the precision found in other models in that they provide general principles rather than clear and specific direction of process. Rather, evaluation requires the evaluator to apply those principles of evaluation to fit the goals and objectives of the specific evaluation project in a given setting. The evaluator must also customize the details of the evaluation, identify the performance of interest, and either find suitable standards for measuring performance or design criteria to measure performance. Health care has been described as the most complex of all organizations and systems. When the dynamic nature of health care is coupled with the magnitude of health care complexity, the challenges of evaluation are intensified. In the final analysis of evaluation in health care, the question is—does the evaluation capture any differences in outcomes of quality of care for patients/populations as compared with current performance?

The purpose of this final chapter is to briefly discuss current major drivers of change and their impact on health care and practice, and to address the challenges that these changes bring to evaluation of quality in health care. As Doctor of Nursing Practice (DNP) nurses are employed at all levels within health care systems, they need to be aware of all of the changes in which they work in order to identify opportunities for innovative changes and be empowered to function effectively. DNP nurses need to be leaders in implementing innovation, evaluating the effects of the innovations in the clinical arena, and lead nurses in understanding trends as they unfold.

Although there are many drivers of change within the health care system, the authors have chosen to address eight drivers as they relate to evaluation, recognizing that there is overlap and interrelatedness among these entities. This chapter discusses the following eight drivers of change: COVID-19 pandemic; health policy and other policy changes; organizations and systems; population health; informatics and health care technologies; interprofessional partnerships; personalized health and precision medicine; and workforce competency.

COVID-19 PANDEMIC

The major driver of the COVID-19 pandemic is the need to control and eradicate this pandemic infection. The COVID-19 pandemic has been and continues to be a devastating crisis unlike any other experienced by the global community. It has created an unprecedented impact on all aspects of life including health care, education, national and global economies, and individual everyday normal activities as we have known them to be. COVID-19 is a mega driver of change that is so powerful that it has impacted every level and institution of society. It has interacted with current drivers of change in specific areas such as health care organizations and workforce and revised the previous drivers, made them irrelevant, or created new drivers for change.

Along with all of the negative effects of COVID-19, there have also been positives that resulted from the pandemic such as increased innovation, collaboration, rapid change and nimbleness, and a willingness to try new approaches without the long-term processes usually required for organizational change. People have been forced to think differently, take risks, and become more innovative than ever. Disruptive innovation has occurred at an accelerated pace with new products and processes replacing available daily. The willingness to try new things without a prolonged testing period or required for 100% evidence of success has been replaced by "just-in-time" solutions that seem reasonable to achieve needed outcomes, including a willingness to abort and try another solution if something does not work. The reduced resistance to change has freed usual caution and fueled innovative solutions. Unprecedented collaborations have crossed boundaries among competitors, systems, communities, and nations to share knowledge and resources to address common problems. A new level of comfort has been accepted as new knowledge is made available on a daily basis. What was the state of the science and evidence-based practice yesterday is replaced today by new knowledge for practice. Traditional knowledge is likely to be replaced as we live in the moment and accept the tentative nature of life in the COVID-19 era.

Given these variables, challenges for evaluation of this ultra-macrosystem level of population and organizational health are significant as well as evaluation in microsystems of practice. The focus on evaluation addresses the question of what performance indicators are useful and, more importantly, what is evaluated related to quality outcomes. For example, if you wish to compare the impact of COVID-19 in a certain country's health care system, the number of positive COVID-19 tests may not be the best indicator of prevalence because the more people tested in a population, the more positives will be found, many of whom may be asymptomatic. Another example is evaluating outcomes based on deaths. It does not tell you anything about the age groups affected or deaths per 1,000 or other comparative denominator. Therefore, evaluation at this macro level may not have reliable indicators of quality for comparison.

HEALTH POLICY AND OTHER POLICIES

Inadequate policies related to health are drivers of change and have a significant impact on health care delivery and outcomes as well as effectively addressing equity and disparity of care. Policy makers at the organizational, local, state, national, and international levels have had to respond quickly to urgent needs for policy changes to address unprecedented situations and move forward effectively because some policies may have been barriers to progress in this COVID-19 era. The usual long-term processes for developing and approving policies have given way to expedited and innovative approval methods. The red tape for Food and Drug Administration (FDA) approval of new drugs is one example of expedited review at the national level. Organizations have also had to revise their policies, for example, on personal protective equipment for frontline providers and admission policies for COVID-19 patients to specialized, quickly adapted units.

Other health-related policy revisions have occurred in licensure and scope of practice. Many states have prescribed numbers of direct practice hours for students in basic nursing programs to be eligible for licensure examination. With COVID-19 and the closing of clinical practicum sites for students, policies had to be modified with subsequent acceptance of virtual clinical experiences and simulation as a substitute for hands-on patient care experiences. Scope of practice policies have also undergone changes to allow nurse practitioners to assume greater responsibilities as a means to supplement shortages of health care providers. Finally, Medicare reimbursement policies to pay for telehealth visits at a time of quarantine and social distancing have been revised to include payment for such services. Attempts for payment for telehealth in the past failed, but the COVID-19 environment necessitated policy change so that people could receive needed health care.

ORGANIZATIONS AND SYSTEMS

The drivers for change in organizations have been unacceptable outcomes for a number of health-related quality measures and the absolute need to improve these outcomes to acceptable levels of performance. At a time when organizations have been engaged in improving outcomes and transformational change, the COVID-19 impact on organizations and systems has been profound. Executive management teams are faced with concerns regarding losses in all areas of their enterprise, their personnel, their clinical capabilities, their supply chain activities, as well as their finances. The near-term consequences of this public health crisis require action planning not only to help leadership teams care for their communities and employees but also concurrently to address the newfound nature of their business and the way in which they deliver services. Leadership teams and national organizations have an incredible opportunity to collaborate and align in the creation of the future state of health care globally (A. Scanlon-McGinity, personal communication, October 8, 2020).

POPULATION HEALTH

Perhaps the major driver for change in population health is disparity and equitable care for all. Both equity and disparity are at the root of poor health outcomes. Concern for equity and disparity is reflected in the long-standing triad of the access–cost–quality model and the Institute of Healthcare Improvement (IHI) framework. Both are designed to optimize health care system performance. The IHI model includes improving the patient experience of care (i.e., quality and satisfaction), improving the health of populations, and reducing the per capita cost of health care (IHI, 2020). With a national renewed focus on population health and refocusing health care from illness care to health care (includes wellness and preventive care), organizations have had to re-envision their vision, goals, and strategies. The refocusing of health care and population health has recognized an underutilized link of community engagement partnerships for equitable, cost-effective care. The link to the community, where people live and work, has created innovative partnerships to create environments that promote safety, health, and wellness, as noted in *Healthy People 2030* (U.S. Department of Health and Human Services, 2020). Community partnerships have included adding new stakeholders to the health care team (e.g., community health workers, firefighters) and incorporating informatics and health care technologies such as telehealth and wearable and smart home technologies to provide health care and monitor persons with chronic conditions in their homes. With community involvement including the voices of all constituents, a focus on providing health care for all of the diverse subgroups within a population can be addressed including equity and disparity.

INFORMATICS AND HEALTH CARE TECHNOLOGIES

Informatics and health care technologies are drivers for change in the 21st century. Informatics has combined information and communication technology with health care to improve all aspects of patient care. Data-based electronic systems are helping to decrease medical errors and the time from test or procedure to the clinicians who make diagnostic decisions based on those tests. The safe transfer of important knowledge reduces errors, increases communication among and between health care providers, and improves efficiency in the health care systems. All of these processes have led to improved patient-centered outcomes and improved safety of care provided.

The digital revolution has driven change in all areas of health care as the shift from mechanical and analogue electronic technology to digital electronics strengthened technology. Digital technology enables health care professionals to collect and analyze big data, improve safety and outcomes of care, and implement processes that save time, costs, and energy.

The COVID-19 pandemic was a catalyst for record changes in technological health care systems. An unprecedented rise in patient cases caused an immediate need to increase the efficiency of electronic health record (EHR) systems to store a higher volume of patient admission details, treatment decisions, and diagnostic actions and to mitigate supply shortages. There has been an unprecedented 20% to 55% increase in the use of telehealth services and health care visits in primary and acute care settings within a 5-month period from the time mitigation processes started. The COVID-19 crisis was a driver for health care organizations and providers to use a technology that many did not want to use prior to the pandemic. The COVID-19 crisis also accelerated the use of remote patient monitoring systems, mobile devices, and wearables, to name a few. The acceleration of the use of monitoring technology to assess patient status from a distance due to the pandemic fostered new expectations such that once people are aware of the use and effectiveness of new technology, they expect more of the same technology in the future. It would be impossible to go back in time and take away the technology that has become a norm in peoples' lives.

INTERPROFESSIONAL PARTNERSHIPS

The major driver for the proliferation of interprofessional partnerships in health care delivery is the need to improve outcomes of care in patients with complex chronic and acute health care conditions. The concept of interprofessional collaboration is not new. The Institute of Medicine (IOM) called for team-based patient care as a way to improve safety and patient outcomes in 2001 (IOM, 2001). *The Future of Nursing: Leading Change, Advancing Health* (IOM, 2011) described the significant role that team-based care would play in the delivery of health care. As the delivery of care continues to become more complex across a variety of settings, the need for multispecialty (e.g., cardiology, radiology, infectious disease) and interdisciplinary providers to coordinate care and improve outcomes is crucial (IOM, 2011).

The focus on quality health care in the 21st century centers on providing safe, effective, patient-centered care that is timely, efficient, and equitable (IOM, 2001). Interprofessional collaboration enables the timely diagnosis and treatment of acute and chronic conditions in ways that cannot be achieved when working in a silo. Interprofessional partnerships are a way to achieve the IOM characteristics of safe, timely, efficient, and effective care and can improve the patient experience, prevent medication errors, and achieve better patient outcomes.

An interprofessional partnership was the driver of an organizational change when the COVID-19 pandemic created complex demands on hospitals and care providers. The need for surge planning that occurred in locations outside of epicenters in northern Italy and New York City was replicated across the world. Interprofessional collaboration between hospital operations personnel and inpatient care providers prepared for a COVID-19 patient surge by developing innovative ways to integrate adult and pediatric care and maximize bed capacity. The expertise of many disciplines enabled hospitals to provide efficient, effective, and high-quality patient care during a time when traditional approaches to patient management were insufficient to address the overwhelming numbers of acutely ill patients with life-threatening conditions. Interprofessional collaboration helped to identify and implement innovative approaches to care in multisystem organizations. The immediate and overwhelming patient and institutional needs created by the COVID-19 pandemic were drivers for innovative changes in the health care system. The urgent need to develop new ways to provide care under the auspices of interprofessional collaboration across continents was the driver of a successful change that addressed patient care needs with effective quality outcomes (Natale et al., 2020).

PERSONALIZED MEDICINE

The major driver for personalized medicine is the advances in science and medicine that recognize that genetics, genomics, and other individual characteristics result in different responses to treatment and drugs, thus suggesting the need to individualize care. *Personalized medicine*, also referred to as *precision medicine*, is a medical model that separates people into different groups so that medical decisions, practices, interventions, and/or products are tailored to the individual patient based on their predicted response or risk of disease (Academy of Medical Sciences, 2015). According to the Precision Medicine Initiative, *precision medicine* is "an emerging approach for disease treatment and prevention that takes into account individual variability in genes, environment, and lifestyle for each person" (National Institutes of Health, n.d.). Precision medicine allows physicians and researchers to predict more accurately which treatment and prevention strategies for a particular disease will work in which groups of people. The precision medicine approach, in contrast to a one-size-fits-all approach, is one in which disease treatment and prevention strategies are developed for the average person, with less consideration for the differences between individuals (National Institutes of Health, n.d.).

Usage of the term "personalized medicine" has increased in recent years because of rapid scientific discoveries and the growth of new diagnostic and informatics approaches that provide understanding of the molecular basis of disease, particularly genomics. Taking the concept down to a personal level, *personalized health care* is about providing the right treatment for the right group of patients at the right time (Snyderman, 2012).

Science has made incredible advances in diagnosing and treating diseases even with the profound complexity of human biology. Every person is unique in many ways, but so are diseases in how they present and affect the individual. The digital revolution in health care has provided new ways to both collect high-quality data from each individual and link it to data from large patient data pools for analysis with artificial intelligence (AI)-based algorithms. AI has provided a paradigm shift toward precision medicine (Mesko, 2017). AI and machine learning algorithms enable a deeper understanding of how to treat an individual. Through analysis and drawing inferences from the vast amounts of data from patients and organizations, it is evident as to what distinguishes each individual from another (Ray, 2018). When applied to an individual patient, AI translates that information into a personalized approach to health care. Real-world evidence, molecular information generated from next-generation sequencing, data from wearable devices, mobile apps, and novel clinical trials are transforming the future of care (Roche Laboratories, n.d.).

It is clear that there are many underpinnings for precision medicine. AI applications to health care provide ultra-speed, accuracy, and an ability to manage and analyze large and complex datasets to answer complex clinical questions and uncover new knowledge. Interdisciplinary teams of scientists including physicians, geneticists, molecular biologists, nurses, and others come together to pool their knowledge and expertise to answer the daunting questions in health care for precision medicine and individualized care. Precision medicine is already changing outcomes. It is helping patients to live longer and better lives by ensuring each person receives the right treatment at the right time.

WORKFORCE COMPETENCY

The major driver for work competency is the unwavering expectation for consistent, high-quality, and safe care delivered by competent health providers who serve patients in all areas of practice. Traditional methods of learning and teaching such as classroom lectures and pedagogy have been the backbone of all levels of education. Since major concerns about health care quality and safety have been linked to workforce competency, competency-based training has gained popularity in recent years across many disciplines including education, medicine, public health, and global health (American Society for Training and Development, 2019). Competency-based education aims to move away from traditional learning assessment approaches such as counting hours spent learning to capturing the "knowledge, skills, and attitudes [or abilities] required for an acceptable level of practice" (Sawleshwarkar & Negin, 2017). Online learning that uses educational technologies and platforms has opened the doors to education for learners regardless of their physical location. The COVID-19 pandemic has further accelerated the use of learning technology as a means of supporting educational endeavors when traditional methods of education abruptly closed down. Even the reluctant persons who were against online education were forced to participate in this technology, and some even embraced it. But what about competency—how would that be measured?

Perhaps the newest educational strategy is simulation. Chapter 12, *Evaluation of Simulation to Support Ongoing Competency of the Health Care Workforce*, addressed simulation as a method of developing and assessing competency in health professionals. Technological advances in AI, robotic, and medical technology have been adapted to the teaching–learning processes. Manikins are life-like and can be programmed to simulate all kinds of clinical conditions and situations. The uses of simulation in health care include academic programs from basic to graduate level, residency training, onboarding of new employees, and ongoing updating and competency assurance of the workforce.

Continuing education of health professionals is critical to maintaining competency through professional conferences and online education. The expectation of physically attending professional conferences has changed when many innovative ways of conducting conferences virtually quickly developed in response to social distancing brought on by COVID-19. Resistance to conduct virtual conferences pre-COVID-19 would have been considered as heresy, but with constraints high and options few, virtual conferences have been accepted by many. Although online continuing education units (CEUs) have been available from a number of sources for many years, the number and technological quality of such offerings have increased. As CEUs represent completion of educational activities and are required for licensure and certification renewal, more nurses are engaged in online offerings as a means of earning required CEUs.

The previous content has addressed methods related to competency development and assessment. What about requiring new competencies for the 21st century such as those related to global health? COVID-19 has underscored that nurses are members of a global community. *Global health*, as defined by Koplan et al., is "an area for study, research, and practice that places a priority on improving health, and achieving equity in health for all people worldwide" (Koplan et al., 2009, p. 1994). Global health addresses the root causes of disease through an interdisciplinary and population-based effort, as well as an individual care perspective. Global health competencies are being developed based on what has been learned from the pandemic. The implementation of global health competencies must respond to the needs of specific agencies or particular groups of learners to be effective (Schleiff et al., 2020).

Maintaining a competent workforce is a challenging endeavor, but the link to the national and global imperatives for quality and safety is unmistakable. Communication and education technology continue to develop and support both workforce competency and the quality–safety mandate.

IMPACT ON DNP NURSES

The Future of Nursing: Leading Change, Advancing Health report described what the profession could do to address the demand for safe, effective, and high-quality health care services (IOM, 2011). While nursing is committed to patient-centered care, achieving quality outcomes, and improving patient safety, the DNP nurse is prepared to address macrosystem issues. The driving forces of the DNP-prepared nurse are to think creatively, strive for innovation in delivering health care, and evaluate every area of practice to improve delivery of care and achieve better patient, population, and organizational outcomes.

The challenge for the DNP nurse is to be a leader in the health care arena and a catalyst for change. A leader has the ability to think creatively and implement innovative ideas to an organization to strengthen practice. Nurses have a unique connection to the bedside that positions them to identify new and innovative ways to provide safe and effective patient-centered care. As such, nursing's leadership role in quality and safety comes with the expectation that nurses safeguard quality and safety by evaluating outcomes of care, determining to what extent current outcomes meet best quality outcome measures, and recommending ways to improve the effectiveness of health care and health care quality.

The Future of Nursing: Leading Change, Advancing Health (IOM, 2011) articulated a vision for a health care system in which nurses realize their full potential as contributors to the health care system. Ten years later, there is still room for the nursing profession to realize its full potential within the rapidly changing health care environment. However, no longer should we say "nurses have *great potential to lead* innovative strategies to improve the healthcare system" (IOM, 2011, p. 4).

Nurses *are* leading. No longer should we say that "nurses *should be* full partners, with physicians and other health professionals, in redesigning healthcare in the United States" (IOM, 2011, p. 4). DNP nurses *are* full partners who are prepared to be an active force in transforming and improving the health care system.

Health care organizations are an ever-changing environment that must respond to unexpected outside forces. The COVID-19 pandemic brought sudden and devastating circumstances to health care institutions that challenged all personnel to change how things were done. While nurses had to quickly adapt to a new normal of chaos, what did not change was the commitment to provide safe, effective, and patient-centered care. Nursing leadership was responsible for preparing for the surge of intensive care patients, adapting standards of care, supporting staff through difficult times, evaluating outcomes of care, and providing innovative ways to care for challenging patients. While all nurses stepped up to all of the challenges imposed by the COVID crisis, the focus of the DNP nurse is on all aspects of patient care from evaluating outcomes of care of the COVID-19 population to adapting standards of care to the patient with drastically different physical and psychological needs. Being able to be nimble and quickly change one's approach in a rapidly changing environment is a symbol of nursing leadership.

It is clear that DNP nurses by virtue of education and clinical competencies bring critical skills to the profession that enable them to navigate through the complex health care system. The evaluation skills that DNPs bring to the organizational setting enable them to assess systems of care and improve patient outcomes.

CHALLENGES OF EVALUATION OF QUALITY IN HEALTH CARE

The challenges of evaluation of the many facets of quality in health care are daunting. The many reasons for these challenges fall into the following overlapping areas: the complexity and dynamic nature of health care; the maze of measurements and methods; and the limited number of standards and criteria for judging outcomes.

First, changes in health status of individuals, populations, and organizations often occur because of complex interactions that cannot always be attributed to a linear cause–effect relationship to a particular variable. The particular variable may be one intervention or treatment provided by one provider or group. It is near impossible to determine what variable or combination of variables resulted in a desired outcome given the complexity of health care. Attempts by researchers to untangle the effect of each variable on an outcome have resulted in more confusion. For example, attempts to determine what nursing actions result in better patient outcomes have fallen short because many other providers other than the nurse impact patient care and because we practice in teams. In addition, findings of an evaluation at one point in time are only a one-time snapshot of quality because of the dynamic nature of health care. Longitudinal evaluations are more representative of the quality of an entity. All of these reasons suggest a need for better models and methods of capturing quality on health care.

Second, clearly identified measures to evaluate performance are needed. Currently, there is an overwhelming maze of measures available, and more are being developed. Various organizations have suggested characteristics of practical measures and typologies to organize measures into useful categories, with some success. In order to be practical and useful, a measure must be (a) sensitive to the performance of interest within the given context; (b) grounded in clinical evidence and science; (c) valid, reliable, and understandable; and (d) have available data sources for collection and analysis. A closer look at the maze of measures finds that most measures are process measures rather than outcome measures. Porter (2010) asserted that the majority of measures currently collected are process measures; while they may reflect current quality standards, they do not necessarily correlate with patient health or organizational outcomes. This assessment has not changed in the last decade. From a practical perspective, outcome measures can be more difficult to develop and collect than process measures. Developing health care quality measures, especially meaningful outcome measures, is a challenging work in progress.

Third, the limited number of standards and criteria for judging achievement of desired outcomes speaks to practicality and usefulness of both process and outcome measures. Standards and criteria for judging the achievement of outcomes come in many forms. Guidelines from various organizations, white papers, core competencies reports, and other authoritative publications attempt to base their criteria on evidence-based information that includes evaluation components of various investigations, including research. In tandem, the identification of useful and practical measures, as previously described, drives the development of standards and criteria for evaluation of quality in health care.

What is evident from this brief discussion of challenges of evaluation is that the entire enterprise of evaluation of quality in health care is a work in progress that is continually developing. Health care is recognized as the most complex areas for evaluation as compared to other areas such as education. The development and application of evaluation methods to health care are critically needed to evaluate the quality of health care as a means to guide providers and organizational leaders in the pursuit of high-quality and meaningful outcomes for individuals, populations, and organizations.

SUMMARY

This chapter has briefly touched upon drivers of change and the impact they have on the quality of health care. The approach to this chapter has been from the unique vantage point of how a mega driver of change has impacted other drivers' change in discrete areas of health care, the impact of those interactions on health care, and their influence on how DNP nurses practice. The challenges that a complex and dynamic rich environment brings to evaluation of quality of health care have been briefly summarized.

We conclude with the salutation, "may you live in interesting times." This saying is an English expression translated from a Chinese curse. While sounding like a blessing, the original expression was used to convey that life is better in "uninteresting times" of peace and tranquility rather than in "interesting" times, which are usually times of trouble (Wikipedia, n.d.). However, the "interesting times" in which we live bring unprecedented opportunities for change, innovation, leadership, and progress in achieving a higher quality of care that is measured through comprehensive science-based evaluations that support the bold decision-making needed to achieve desired outcomes. Will we ever go back to the "normalcy" of how we lived and provided health care in 2019? It is not likely. The steep learning curve through which we all have lived has made us wiser and better prepared for an unknown future.

REFERENCES

Academy of Medical Sciences. (2015, May). *Stratified, personalised or P4 medicine: A new direction for placing the patient at the centre of healthcare and health education* (Technical report). Author. https://acmedsci.ac.uk/viewFile/564091e072d41.pdf

American Society for Training and Development. (2019). *ASTD Competency Model*. Author.

Institute of Healthcare Improvement. (2020). *The IHI Triple Aim.* http://www.ihi.org/Engage/Initiatives/TripleAim/Pages/default.aspx

Institute of Medicine. (2001). *Crossing the quality chasm: A new health system for the 21st century.* National Academies Press.

Institute of Medicine. (2011). *The future of nursing: Leading change, advancing health.* National Academies Press.

Koplan, J. P., Bond, T. C., Merson, M. H., Reddy, K. S., Rodriguez, M. H., Sewankambo, N. K., & Wasserheit, J. N. (2009). Towards a common definition of global health. *Lancet, 373*(9679), 1993–1995. https://doi.org/10.1016/S0140-6736(09)60332-9

Mesko, B. (2017). The role of artificial intelligence in precision medicine. *Expert Review of Precision Medicine and Drug Development, 2*(5), 239–241. https://doi.org/10.1080/23808993.2017.1380516

Natale, J. E., Boehmer, J., Blumberg, D. A., Dimitriades, C., Hirose, S., Kair, L. R., Kirk, J. D., Mateev, S. N., McKnight, H., Plant, J., Tzimenatos, L. S., Wiedeman, J. T., Witkowski, J., Underwood, M. A., Tzimenatos, L. S., Wiedeman, J. T., Witkowski, J., Underwood, M. A., & Lakshminrusimha, S. (2020). Interprofessional/interdisciplinary teamwork during the early COVID-19 pandemic: Experience from a children's hospital within an academic health center. *Journal of Interprofessional Care, 34*(5), 682–686. https://doi.org/10.1080/13561820.2020.1791809

National Institutes of Health. (n.d.). What is the difference between precision medicine and personalized medicine? What about pharmacogenomics? *MedlinePlus.* Retrieved October 12, 2020, from https://medlineplus.gov/genetics/understanding/precisionmedicine/precisionvspersonalized/

Porter, M. E. (2010). What is value in health care? *New England Journal of Medicine, 363,* 2477–2481. https://doi.org/10.1056/NEJMp1011024

Posavac, E. J. (2016). *Program evaluation: Methods and case studies.* Routledge.

Ray, A. (2018). *Compassionate artificial intelligence.* Compassionate AI Lab. Retrieved October 12, 2020, from https://books.google.com/books?hl=en&lr=&id=wZt7DwAAQBAJ&oi=fnd&pg=PA14&dq=Ray,+A.+Artificial+intelligence+and+Blockchain+for+precision+Medicine&ots=fiSWfLeA5t&sig=1_kZMTJUy3IolY00s8Gzo0g7qtA#v=onepage&q=Ray%2C%20A.%20Artificial%20intelligence%20and%20Blockchain%20for%20precision%20Medicine&f=false

Roche Laboratories. (n.d.). *Personalized healthcare.* https://www.roche.com/about/priorities/personalised_healthcare.htm

Rossi, P. H., Lipsey, M. W., & Henry, G. T. (2019). *Evaluation: A systematic approach* (8th ed.). Sage.

Sawleshwarkar, S., & Negin, J. (2017). A review of global health competencies for postgraduate public health education. *Front Public Health, 5,* 46. https://doi.org/10.3389/fpubh.2017.00046

Schleiff, M., Hansoti, B., Akridge, A., Dolive, C., Hausner, D., Kalbarczyk, A., Pariyo, G., Quinn, T. C., Rudy, S., & Bennett, S. (2020). Implementation of global health competencies: A scoping review on target audiences, levels, and pedagogy and assessment strategies. *PLoS ONE, 15*(10), e0239917. https://doi.org/10.1371/journal.pone.0239917

Snyderman, R. (2012). Personalized health care: From theory to practice. *Biotechnology Journal, 7*(8), 973–979. https://doi.org/10.1002/biot.201100297

U.S. Department of Health and Human Services. (2020). *Healthy People 2030.* https://health.gov/healthypeople

Wikipedia. (n.d.). *May you live in interesting times.* Retrieved October 14, 2020, from https://en.wikipedia.org/wiki/May_you_live_in_interesting_times

INDEX

Printed in the United States
by Baker & Taylor Publisher Services

Printed in the United States
by Baker & Taylor Publisher Services